Basic Science in Obstetrics and Gynaecology

For Churchill Livingstone

Publisher: Peter Richardson
Editorial Co-ordination: Editorial Resources Unit
   Copy Editor: Rich Cutler
   Indexer: June Morrison
Production Controller: Neil A. Dickson
Design: Design Resources Unit
Sales Promotion Executive: Louise Johnstone

Basic Science in Obstetrics and Gynaecology
A Textbook for MRCOG Part I

Edited by

Michael de Swiet MD FRCP
Consultant Physician, Queen Charlotte's and Chelsea Hospital, London

Geoffrey Chamberlain RD MD FRCS FRCOG FACOG(Hon)
Professor of Obstetrics and Gynaecology, St George's Hospital Medical School, London

SECOND EDITION

CHURCHILL LIVINGSTONE
EDINBURGH LONDON MADRID MELBOURNE NEW YORK AND TOKYO 1992

CHURCHILL LIVINGSTONE
Medical Division of Pearson Professional Ltd

Distributed in the United States of America by Churchill
Livingstone Inc., 650 Avenue of the Americas, New York,
N.Y. 10011, and by associated companies, branches and
representatives throughout the world.

First edition 1986
Second edition 1992
    Reprinted 1994
    Reprinted 1995

ISBN 0-443-04229-2

British Library Cataloguing in Publication Data
A catalogue record for this book is available from the
British Library.

Library of Congress Cataloging in Publication Data
Basic science in obstetrics and gynaecology: a textbook for
    MRCOG, Part I/edited by Michael de Swiet, Geoffrey
V. P. Chamberlain. — 2nd ed.
        p. cm.
    Includes index.
    ISBN 0-443-04229-2
    1. Medical sciences.   2. Obstetrics.
3. Gynecology.   I. De Swiet, Michael.   II. Chamberlain,
Geoffrey, 1930—   .
    [DNLM: 1. Gynecology.   2. Obstetrics.
WQ 100 B311]
RG526.B37   1992
618.2 - dc20
DNLM/DLC
for Library of Congress   91-23088

The
publisher's
policy is to use
**paper manufactured
from sustainable forests**

Produced by Longman Singapore Publishers (Pte) Ltd
Printed in Singapore

Preface

We have been very gratified at the success of the first edition of *Basic Science in Obstetrics and Gynaecology*. In the preface to that edition we stated that 'little, if any, further reading will be required'. Unfortunately that has not been the case as the demands of MRCOG Part I have become more exacting. For this reason we have revised much of the text and asked new authors to contribute. These new contributions are particularly pertinent to areas where knowledge is expanding fast such as cell biology and molecular biology (Dr Bennett), biochemistry (Dr Knox) and immunology (Dr Manyonda).

We now believe that again most knowledge to pass the Part I MRCOG is in this book though the field of pathology is so large that readers may need to look further in this area.

We acknowledge with pleasure the effort and time that our previous and current contributors have put into revising their old and providing new material.

M. de S.
G.C.

Contributors

Graham Barker TD AKC MB FRCS MRCOG
Gynaecological Surgeon, St George's and
Bolingbroke Hospital, London
Drugs and drug therapy

Phillip Bennett BSc MD(Lond) MRCOG
The Action Research Laboratory for the
Molecular Biology of Fetal Development,
Institute of Obstetrics and Gynaecology, London
The cell, chromosomes and molecular genetics

Geoffrey Chamberlain RD MD FRCS FRCOG
FACOG (Hon)
Professor of Obstetrics and Gynaecology, St
George's Hospital Medical School, London
The fetus

T. M. Coltart PhD FRCS(Ed) FRCOG
Consultant Obstetrician and Gynaecologist,
Guy's Hospital, London and Queen Charlotte's
and Chelsea Hospital, London
Physiology

Sir John Dewhurst FRCOG FRCSE Hon DSc MD
FACOG FRCSI
Formerly Professor in Obstetrics and
Gynaecology, Institute of Obstetrics and
Gynaecology, Queen Charlotte's Maternity
Hospital, London
*The cell, chromosomes and molecular genetics,
Embryology, Endocrinology*

Robert Dinwiddie MB FRCP DCH
Consultant Paediatrician, The Hospitals for Sick
Children, London
The fetus

Ian Fergusson MA MB FRCS(Eng, Ed) FRCOG
Consultant Obstetrician and Gynaecologist, St

Thomas's Hospital, London
Embryology

H. Fox MD FRCPath FRCOG
Professor of Reproductive Pathology, University
of Manchester, Manchester
Embryology

S. L. Jeffcoate PhD FRCPath
Division of Endocrinology, National Institute
for Biological Standards and Control, South
Mimms, Hertfordshire
Endocrinology

Peter Knox MD DPhil
Senior Lecturer, St George's Hospital Medical
School, London
Biochemistry

E. Letsky MB BS FRCPath
Consultant Haematologist, Queen Charlotte's
and Chelsea Hospital, London
Physiology

T. L. T. Lewis CBE MB FRCS FRCOG
Emeritus Consultant Obstetrician and
Gynaecologist, Queen Charlotte's and Chelsea
Hospital, London
Anatomy

John de Louvois MSc PhD MRCPath
Honorary Senior Lecturer, RPMS Institute of
Obstetrics & Gynaecology, Queen Charlotte's
and Chelsea Hospital, London; Consultant
Clinical Scientist, Public Health Laboratory
Service, London
Microbiology

J. Malvern BSc FRCS(Ed) FRCOG
Consultant Obstetrician, Queen Charlotte's and
Chelsea Hospital, London
Anatomy, Physiology

Isaac T. Manyonda BSc MB MRCOG
Senior Registrar, Department of Obstetrics and
Gynaecology, St George's Hospital; formerly
MRC Clinical Research Fellow, Division of
Immunology, Department of Cellular and
Molecular Sciences, St George's Hospital
Medical School, London
Immunology

David Morris MD FRCS FRCOG
Consultant in Obstetrics and Gynaecology,
Guy's Hospital and Queen Charlotte's and
Chelsea Hospital, London
Anatomy

J. Osborn BSc PhD
Professor of Epidemiologic Methodology,
Istituto d'Igiene, University of Rome, La
Sapienza
Statistics

Peter Rubin MA DM FRCP
Professor of Therapeutics, University Hospital,
Queen's Medical Centre, Nottingham
Drugs and drug therapy

Michael de Swiet MD FRCP
Consultant Physician, Queen Charlotte's and
Chelsea Hospital, London
Physiology

D. G. Talbert BSc PhD MInstP
Senior Lecturer, RPMS Institute of Obstetrics
& Gynaecology, Queen Charlotte's and Chelsea
Hospital, London
Physics

Contents

1. The cell, chromosomes and molecular genetics

STRUCTURE AND FUNCTION OF THE NORMAL CELL

The human body consists of cells and intercellular matrix.

Cells

All cells possess certain basic structural features, regardless of their location, type and function (Figs 1.1 and 1.2). The major division is into nucleus and cytoplasm.

Nucleus

This is surrounded by a bilaminar nuclear membrane or envelope with occasional pores and contains the chromosomes, made from molecules of deoxyribonucleic acid (DNA), responsible for genetic coding and inheritance. Chromosomes are discussed later in this chapter. Within the nucleus, one or more mobile nucleoli are present; they contain ribonucleic acid (RNA), and are involved in cell protein synthesis. Nuclear RNA is a precursor of cytoplasmic ribosomal RNA (see later).

Cytoplasm

This comprises the remainder of the cell. It is enclosed within a trilaminar cell membrane which has a very complex biochemical structure, including many proteins and lipids; it is not rigid, but can alter its shape in response to various stimuli. The major function of the cell membrane is control and maintenance of the appropriate intracellular electrolyte and biochemical environment by energy-requiring active-transport mechanisms (e.g. sodium removal by the sodium pump). It also provides adhesion between adjacent cells, and bears the individual's major histocompatibility (transplant or HLA) antigens. In some cells (e.g. polymorphs) it determines motility and phagocytosis.

The cytoplasm contains many organelles:

Mitochondria are elongated, enzyme-rich bodies; each has a continuous external limiting membrane and an inner membrane folded into septa (cristae) which create partial subdivision of the matrix. Mitochondria oxidise proteins, carbohydrates and fats into energy, store it as adenosine triphosphate (ATP) and subsequently release it when required by the cell.

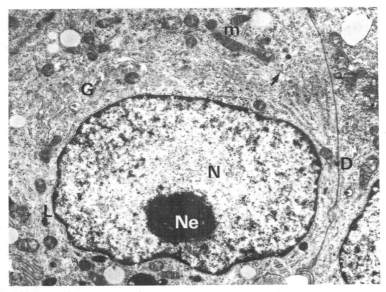

Fig. 1.1 Transmission electron micrograph showing normal cellular constituents, including nucleus (N), nucleolus (Ne), Golgi complex (G), mitochondria (m), desmosome (D), lysosomes (L) and polyribosomes (arrow). (From *The Breast in Pregnancy*, courtesy of Dr A. Ahmed.)

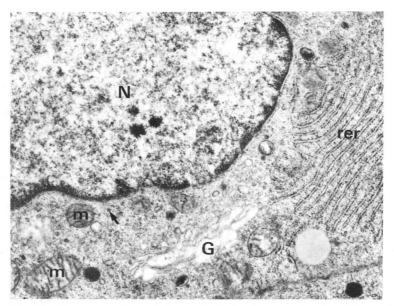

Fig. 1.2 Higher magnification of normal cell showing part of nucleus (N), rough endoplasmic reticulum (rer), a well-developed Golgi complex (G), mitochondria (m) and polyribosomes (arrow). (From *The Breast in Pregnancy*, courtesy of Dr A. Ahmed.)

Ribosomes are small granules containing RNA, the molecular structure of which is determined by nuclear DNA. They control synthesis of proteins required for intracellular metabolism. Aggregates of ribosomes are designated polysomes or polyribosomes.

The endoplasmic reticulum is a complex network of intercommunicating narrow tubules and vesicles (cisternae) mainly responsible for synthesising proteins subsequently secreted outside the cell. Two continuous types exist: rough endoplasmic reticulum, where ribosomes are attached to the outer surface, and smooth endoplasmic reticulum where ribosomes are absent.

The centrosome is a relatively clear area, usually near the cell centre, containing two centrioles.

Centrioles are hollow cylindrical bodies, 0.3–0.7 μm in length, which replicate before mitosis and orientate the mitotic spindle.

The Golgi complex is usually near the centrosome, and comprises numerous, small, irregular sacs, vacuoles and vesicles. It probably collects, modifies, packages and transports secretions from the rough endoplasmic reticulum to the cell membrane and, when necessary, adds carbohydrate residues.

Lysosomes are round or oval membrane-bound bodies containing proteolytic enzymes (acid hydrolases) for digesting unwanted endogenous and phagocytosed exogenous material.

Phagosomes are membrane-bound bodies containing material ingested by phagocytosis. To effect digestion, phagosomes combine with lysosomes to produce phagolysosomes. When indigestible material remains, residual or dense bodies are formed.

Microtubules, 200–270 Å (20–27 nm) in diameter, are found throughout the cytoplasm. They constitute the mitotic spindle filaments, and may also facilitate intracytoplasmic transport and maintain cell shape.

Microfilaments are 40–120 Å (4–12 nm) in diameter and of indefinite length. Some (tonofibrils) converge on intercellular junctions (desmosomes) to promote cell adhesion; functions of microfilaments elsewhere are unknown.

Specific structures are unique to, and characteristic of, specialised cells, e.g. myofilaments in muscle cells and melanosomes in melanocytes.

Several other structures may also be seen, including glycogen granules, lipofuscin granules, myelinoid bodies, siderosomes and lipid droplets.

Cell types

All cells are classified as one of two types — epithelial and connective tissue.

Epithelial cells cover or line body surfaces and internal cavities; in addition, most glands are epithelial, being derived embryologically from body surfaces. Epithelial cells therefore act as selective and protective barriers and synthesise most secretions.

Connective tissue cells are derived largely from embryonic mesoderm. Connective tissue exists in many types, and its composition varies in different parts of the body, depending on local requirements. Its main function is to provide structural support, generally as fibrous tissue and specifically as bone, cartilage, muscle and tendon. It is probably also responsible for body defences, since leucocytes and mononuclear phagocyte (reticuloendothelial) system cells are usually considered connective tissue in origin.

Intercellular matrix

This varies considerably in amount; very little is seen between epithelial cells, whereas connective tissue cells are often quite widely separated by matrix, the exact nature of which may provide the unique connective tissue structure (e.g. bone and cartilage). Interstitial extracellular fluid is located in the intercellular matrix.

Epithelial intercellular matrix is a narrow, mucopolysaccharide-rich layer traversed by intercellular junctions. Formerly designated cement substance, it is now thought, in some instances, to be an integral component of the cell membrane's external surface (glycocalyx).

Connective tissue intercellular matrix contains ground substance and fibres. The ground substance is a gel of variable consistency and viscosity, containing mucoproteins, glycoproteins and mucopolysaccharides; it is probably mainly secreted by fibroblasts. Of the fibres, collagen is the most important, being virtually ubiquitous and providing much structural rigidity. It is a trihelical structure derived from a soluble precursor (procollagen), secreted by fibroblasts and osteoblasts via an insoluble intermediate (tropocollagen). Four biochemical types, controlled by different structural genes, are described: types I (mature collagen in dermis, bone and tendon), II (unique to cartilage) and III (as 'reticulin' in early scar tissue, cardiovascular tissue and synovium) possess the triple helix and have a banded structure electronoptically; in contrast, type IV (in basement membranes) is probably not helical and appears amorphous ultrastructurally. Elastic fibres, comprising protein (elastin) and polysaccharide, provide resilience and are produced by smooth muscle cells and fibroblasts.

CELL DAMAGE INCLUDING IRRADIATION

Cell damage

Cell damage may result from various causes and may be manifest structurally in several ways. Early or mild injury produces either an excessive accumulation of normal metabolites (degeneration) or an accumulation of abnormal products (infiltration); these changes indicate functional derangement but are reversible if the initiating factors are removed. If severe or prolonged, irreversible cell death (necrosis) results.

Causes of cell damage include anoxia (usually due to impairment of blood supply), bacterial or viral infections, immunological injury, toxins, enzyme deficiencies, chemical poisons and physical agents (such as cold, heat, radiation and mechanical trauma).

Degenerations are usually given purely descriptive names, depending on cytoplasmic appearance: in cloudy swelling, it is swollen, hazy and granular; in hydropic degeneration, it contains vacuoles of clear fluid; in hyaline degeneration, it is uniformly pink staining and glassy; in mucoid degeneration, there are excess mucopolysaccharides. In all these types, sublethal damage and disruption have occurred within the various cellular components; thus the cell membrane is abnormally permeable, the endoplasmic reticulum and mitochondria are swollen and show loss of granules; polyribosomes are disaggregated and lysosomes are ruptured. In addition, there may be proliferation of intracytoplasmic organelles in an attempt to eradicate or neutralise the causative agent.

Infiltrations: of these, the accumulation of excess fat (fatty change) is the most important. This fat is considered exogenous, and is seen as numerous small intracytoplasmic lipid droplets. Inborn errors of metabolism, due to specific enzyme deficiencies, may cause infiltration by specific substances (e.g. glucocerebrosides in Gaucher's disease and various forms of glycogen in the glycogen storage diseases).

Necrosis indicates irreversible cell death. The cytoplasmic changes are often those of degeneration, but, in addition, coexisting, characteristic nuclear changes are seen. Initially, the nucleus shrinks and shows clumping and increased density of its chromatin (pyknosis). The nuclear membrane then ruptures, with chromatin fragmentation into small aggregates (karyorrhexis). Finally, nuclear material is digested and disappears (karyolysis). Once cell death has occurred, there is severe structural disorganisation and ultimate disappearance of cytoplasmic organelles, due to digestion by intracellular lytic enzymes (autolysis). Several types of necrosis are described, including coagulative necrosis, where outlines of dead cells are preserved, caseous necrosis, where cell outlines are absent, and colliquative necrosis, where necrotic tissue undergoes softening and liquefaction.

Radiation

Radiation is the emission, transmission and absorption of radiant energy, and may be particulate or electromagnetic (see Ch. 11).

Effects of ionising radiation

In the body, ionising radiation causes structural changes in atoms and molecules of cells in its path, with consequent functional and morphological abnormalities. It may be administered externally, or internally by injection, ingestion or implantation. Its effects are complex, resulting from both direct radiation damage and also the body's subsequent healing response.

Cellular effects are related largely to the character, duration and total amount of radiation given, but also are potentiated significantly by high local oxygen concentrations. Very mild irradiation produces no obvious effects whereas very heavy dosage causes immediate cell death. Intermediate levels delay mitosis; nuclear DNA synthesis may be inhibited, but it may continue, producing swollen cells with large distorted nuclei and disrupted cytoplasmic organelles. When mitosis finally occurs, abnormal chromosomes may be produced and ultimately cell degeneration and death may result; occasionally, there may be incomplete cell separation, producing multinucleated giant cells. Following irradiation, some cells lose their capacity to divide (reproductive death), whilst others, after a delay, show an increased mitotic rate. The exact mechanism of cellular damage following irradiation is unknown, but it is thought to be produced by formation of free radicals acting as strong oxidising or reducing agents.

Tissue effects vary, even when identical quantities of radiation are given. The greater the normal mitotic rate of the irradiated cells, the greater the sensitivity; thus, haemopoietic cells, germinal and gastrointestinal epithelium are the most radiosensitive whilst central nervous tissue, bones and muscles are radioresistant. Vascular changes are very important — initially, there may be dilatation or focal necrosis with rupture and haemorrhage; later there is often quite marked luminal narrowing by intimal and endothelial proliferation and hyalinisation. In most tissues, parenchymal epithelial cells are more radiosensitive than stromal connective tissue cells, and so, with intermediate radiation doses, there will be epithelial cell atrophy or destruction and replacement by dense connective tissue containing large pleomorphic fibroblasts.

Total body effects may be early or late, depending on dosage received. Early effects constitute the acute radiation syndrome (radiation sickness), with generalised depletion of mitotically active (radiosensitive) cells; if severe, death results within a few days. Late effects are carcinogenic or genetic.

Carcinogenic effects are reflected as an increased risk of subsequent chronic myeloid leukaemia, squamous cell carcinoma of skin and osteosarcoma.

Genetic effects: moderate gonadal irradiation will produce sterility; lesser doses may cause chromosomal aberrations resulting in mutations and a greater incidence of congenital abnormalities in offspring.

CHROMOSOMES

Our inheritance is determined by our genes which are carried on our chromosomes in the nuclei of all cells. Each adult cell contains 46 chromosomes which exist as 23 pairs, one member of each pair having been inherited from each parent. 22 pairs are homologous and are called autosomes. The 23rd pair are the sex chromosomes, X and Y in the male, X and X in the female.

The chromosomes in man may be examined directly in rapidly dividing tissue such as, for example, bone marrow; more often, however, they are examined following a tissue culture of peripheral blood lymphocytes or skin or other body tissues. Lymphocytes are cultured for 48–72 hours and a large number of dividing cells are obtained in the culture by using colchicine which inhibits the formation of the spindle and arrests cell division at metaphase (see below). Treatment with a hypotonic solution then allows the chromosomes to be spread more easily; they are fixed and stained either by conventional techniques or by other methods which reveal their characteristic banding patterns (Fig. 1.3). If skin or other tissue is cultured the process is more complex and prolonged and may take 2–4 weeks.

The chromosomes can only be detected in the nucleus of the cell at metaphase, i.e. shortly before cell division, when they condense to assume the characteristic shape in which we see them in a conventional karyotype (Fig. 1.3). Examination of the chromosomes then reveals them as roughly H-shaped structures joined at an area of constriction known as the centromere (Fig. 1.4). If the centromere is near the middle of the chromosome, it is said to be metacentric; if the centromere is near one end of the chromosome it is called acrocentric; and if it occupies a position midway between these

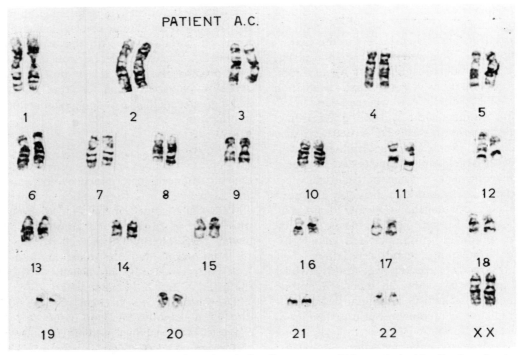

Fig. 1.3   A normal female 46,XX karyotype illustrating the banding patterns which permit the identification of each individual chromosome.

two it is submetacentric. Tiny pedunculated structures, known as satellites, are recognisable on some chromosomes and aid in identification; secondary constrictions are evident on other chromosomes. The chromosomes are numbered by convention with the largest being designated as 1 and the smallest as 22.

The chromosome pairs may be grouped into seven categories determined by their length and the position of the centromere: numbers 1–3 are large metacentric chromosomes; 4 and 5 are also large, but submetacentric; 6–12 and the X chromosomes are of medium size and submetacentric; 13–15 are medium sized and acrocentric; 16–18 are somewhat shorter than 13–15 and are submetacentric; 19 and 20 are short and metacentric; 21, 22 and Y are very short and acrocentric.

It is no longer necessary, however, to attempt to identify chromosomes solely by their size and centromere position, since with various staining techniques — the most commonly used being that of the Giemsa stain — a characteristic banding pattern (G banding) can be observed for each chromosome so permitting individual identification (Fig. 1.3).

An individual karyotype (or stylised chromosome arrangement as in Fig. 1.3) is by convention indicated by a figure for the total chromosome number — 46 — followed by the variety of sex chromosomes present, thus 46,XX (normal female) and 46,XY (normal male). When abnormalities exist they are similarly recorded as we will see later, for example, 45,X (monosomy X), 47,XXX (trisomy X), 45,X/46,XX (mosaicism), etc. For identification of structural faults the short arm of a chromosome is known as p, the long arm as q (Fig. 1.4). Accordingly a short arm with a portion missing (deletion) is written as 46X,del(Xp) and a deleted long arm as 46X,del(Xq). These abnormalities are considered in greater detail later.

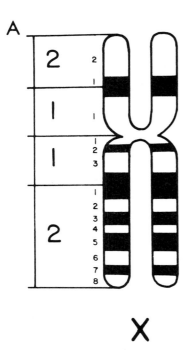

Fig. 1.4 Diagrammatic representation of an X chromosome at metaphase. Note that the short arm (referred to as p) and the long arm (referred to as q) are each divided into two main segments labelled 1 and 2 within which the individual bands are also labelled 1, 2, 3, etc.

Cell division

For further consideration it is necessary to distinguish two different cell types

1. Somatic cells
2. Germ cells

and two forms of cell division

1. Mitosis
2. Meiosis.

Somatic cells: mitosis

When somatic cells divide, which they do by mitosis, they normally reproduce faithfully the genetic constitution of the original cell. The process is as follows. Each cell has an ordered life cycle (Fig. 1.5). After a daughter cell is formed, it enters the G_1, or first gap, phase of its cycle and its chromosomes are disposed throughout the nucleus and cannot be separately distinguished although their number is diploid (46). The cell next enters its S period when DNA synthesis and reduplication is in progress; the chromosome number remains 46 but the quantity of DNA has been doubled. The cell then enters its next phase G_2,

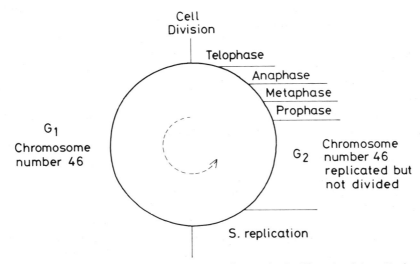

Fig. 1.5 Diagram illustrating the sequence of events in the life cycle of the cell.

or second gap, which lasts until active mitotic division begins. The G_1, S and G_2 stages of the cell life are known as interphase. During interphase the chromosomes remain dispersed throughout the nucleus and only two are identifiable; these are one X chromosome, by recognition of the Barr body (see below) which represents the inactivated X, and the Y body (if a Y chromosome is present), which is seen as a brightly fluorescent spot visible if the cell is treated with quinacrine.

The last stage of cell division is mitosis in somatic cells, or meiosis in germ cells undergoing gametogenesis. The stages of mitosis (Fig. 1.6) are:

1. Prophase: when the chromosomes condense and are thin and threadlike.

2. Metaphase: when the nuclear spindle appears the chromosomes align themselves singly at the equatorial plate of the spindle and the nuclear membrane disappears.

3. Anaphase: when the chromosomes separate at their centromeres and the daughter chromosomes migrate to opposite poles of the cell. The phase of replication of chromosome material has occurred during the S phase of the cell life cycle, the chromatids remaining attached by their centromeres until separation occurs at this stage.

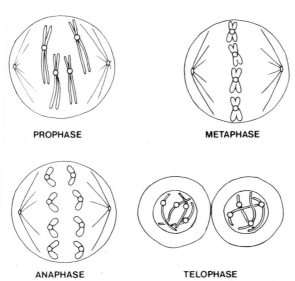

PROPHASE　　　　**METAPHASE**

ANAPHASE　　　　**TELOPHASE**

Fig. 1.6 Diagrammatic illustration of mitosis. Only four chromosomes are represented. For description see text.

4. Telophase: the chromosomes have reached the poles and begin once again to be dispersed into the nuclear material of the cell. At the same time the nuclear membranes close and cell division is accomplished.

Germ cells: meiosis

This is the process of reduction division by which the chromosome number of 46 is reduced to 23 during gametogenesis. It is a fundamental process of reproduction and is different in certain very important respects from mitosis.

There are two cell divisions in meiosis but only one replication. The first meiotic division is that in which the reduction in chromosome number occurs. Interphase is the same as in mitosis but the remaining phases are different. Prophase is very prolonged and is divided into several different parts. The first of these is leptotene in which the chromosomes appear as thread-like structures. Soon homologous chromosomes come to lie close together (zygotene): such a pair of homologous chromosomes is then termed a bivalent. At the next step, pachytene, each chromosome replicates itself so that each bivalent is now made up of four strands lying parallel to each other. The halves of each replicated chromosome, however, are still attached by the centromere. The chromosomes have shortened and it becomes evident that homologous chromosomes are fixed together at certain points called chiasmata; this step is called diplotene. There is further contraction of the chromosomes (diakinesis) and the chiasmata are seen to be moving towards the chromosome ends — terminalisation. Breaks occur in the chromosomes and genetic material crosses from one homologue to the other, part of one chromosome exchanging an identically sized fragment with the other. This crossing over or recombination occurs at one or more sites on each chromosome. There are areas, e.g. near to the centromere, where recombination occurs less frequently and other areas, known as *recombination hotspots*, where crossing over is more likely to occur. The nuclear membrane then disappears and prophase ends (Fig. 1.7a–e).

The first metaphase then begins with the chromosomes, in homologous pairs, lining up at the equatorial plate of the cell. One member of

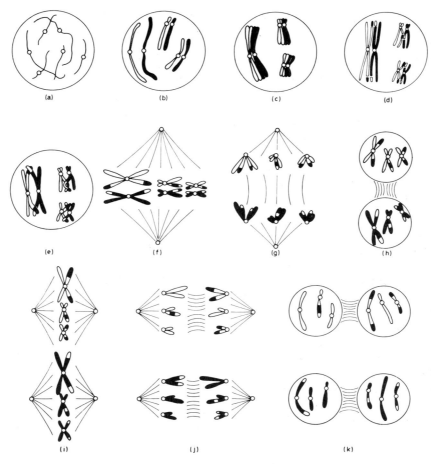

Fig. 1.7   The stages of meiosis. Normally the process of meiosis results in the chromosome number being reduced from 46 to 23. For simplicity in the examples shown, six chromosomes are reduced to three. Meiosis: **a** leptotene, six chromosomes; **b** zygotene; **c** pachytene; **d** diplotene; **e** diakinesis; **f** first metaphase; **g** first anaphase; **h** first telophase, three pairs of chromatids; **i** second metaphase; **j** second anaphase; **k** second telophase, three chromosomes in each of four cells. (By courtesy of the editors of *A Companion to Medical Studies* and Blackwell Scientific Publications.)

each pair then moves to opposite poles of the cell without any chromosome division having taken place (first anaphase) and the nuclear membrane closes (first telophase) around two cells with a haploid number of chromosomes — 23; these chromosomes have however replicated but remain attached at their centromeres (Fig. 1.7f–h).

The second meiotic division occurs in the same manner as mitosis with the result that four cells with 23 chromosomes have been created from the primary oocyte or spermatocye which began the meiotic process (Fig. 1.7i–k). The important process of crossing over ensures a redistribution of

genetic material between maternal and paternal chromosomes and ensures varied inheritance and species vigour.

Spermatogenesis: oogenesis

Important differences characterise spermatogenesis and oogenesis. In spermatogenesis (Fig. 1.8) four spermatids are produced from one primary spermatocyte. The spermatids then undergo a complex process of development to become mature sperms. The process of sperm formation is continually in progress throughout life. In oogenesis on the other

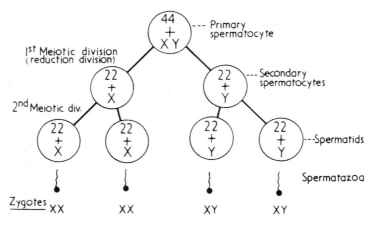

Fig. 1.8   Diagrammatic representation of spermatogenesis.

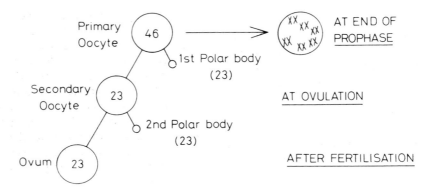

Fig. 1.9   Diagrammatic representation of oogenesis.

hand the first meiotic division results in an unequal distribution of cytoplasm between the two resulting cells, almost all the cytoplasm entering the secondary oocyte and only a tiny amount entering a small polar body (Fig. 1.9); the second meiotic division is the same. One ovum therefore is obtained from one primary oocyte; the two tiny polar bodies which are also produced appear to have no function other than the conservation of the cytoplasm of the ovum.

The process of oogenesis is different from spermatogenesis in a further important way. The early development of the primitive germ cells in the ovary during intrauterine life is mitotic and results in a great increase in the number of oocytes until these total about 7 million. The first division of

meiosis then occurs but is arrested during prophase at which stage the oocytes remain until they become involved in the process of ovulation during a menstrual cycle. An oocyte then either completes its development at the secondary oocyte stage, if it is the one that is to ovulate, or undergoes atresia if it is not in the favoured follicle. The completion of the process by division of the secondary oocyte and the casting off of the second polar body does not occur until after fertilisation.

It will be seen therefore that some primary oocytes remain in prophase for 12–50 years (Fig. 1.10). It will also be seen that the ovum has no maturation process like the sperm, since it is not finally formed from the secondary oocyte until after fertilisation has occurred.

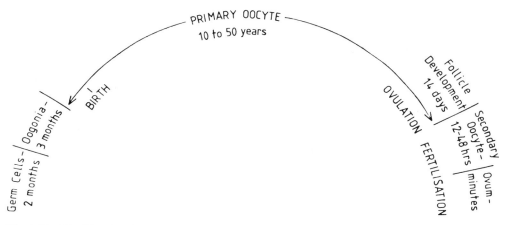

PRIMARY OOCYTE
10 to 50 years

Germ Cells - 2 months

Oogonia - 3 months

BIRTH

Follicle Development 14 days

Secondary Oocyte - 12-48 hrs

Ovum - minutes

OVULATION FERTILISATION

Fig. 1.10   The life cycle of human eggs.

Nuclear chromatin

When cells from a buccal smear of a female are suitably stained and examined, it is possible to discern at the periphery of some nuclei a darkly staining triangular body, known as the Barr body after its discoverer (Fig. 1.11). No such body will be seen in a buccal smear from a male. The presence of this body in females is explained by the Lyon hypothesis which postulates that in the female, at an early stage of embryogenesis, one of the two X chromosomes is inactivated; this inactivation is random and may be paternal or maternal. The inactivation is also permanent and the only function left to this chromosome is subsequent replication. During interphase this inactivated X appears as the Barr body and the individual is designated as chromatin positive.

The maximum number of Barr bodies in a nucleus is one less than the number of X chromosomes present. Thus, buccal smear examination will show the following results in various circumstances:

Normal female: 46,XX, chromatin positive, single bodies
Normal male: 46,XY, chromatin negative
Abnormalities: 47,XXX, chromatin positive, double bodies
48,XXXX, chromatin positive, triple bodies
48,XXYY, chromatin positive, single bodies
47,XXY, chromatin positive, single bodies
45,X, chromatin negative etc.

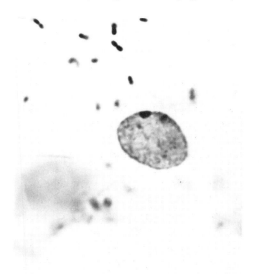

Fig. 1.11   The nucleus of a cell showing a characteristic triangular Barr body situated at the periphery of the nucleus at 12 o'clock.

Chromosome abnormalities

Aneuploidy

Aneuploidy is any deviation from the normal 46 chromosomes in a cell. It includes monosomy, trisomy and polyploidy.

Monosomy, the absence of one of a pair of chromosomes, is usually lethal to the embryo and therefore rare in live-born infants. The only exception is monosomy X or Turner's syndrome, which has an incidence in newborn females of approximately 1 in 2500. The features of Turner's syndrome include short stature, an apparently webbed neck and wide carrying angle of the arms, and frequently coarctation of the aorta. There is no gonadal differentiation, the gonads being represented by useless streaks of tissue. There is therefore no secondary sexual development at puberty and presentation is often with primary amenorrhoea. A much larger number of affected pregnancies abort. Monosomy X accounts for about 18% of chromosomal abnormalities seen in spontaneous abortion. Absence of the X chromosome leaving only the Y is incompatible with embryonic development and will always result in early abortion.

Trisomy is the presence of an extra chromosome. This can arise as a result of non-disjunction, when homologous chromosomes fail to separate at meiosis. This results in a germ cell containing 24 chromosomes. Trisomy of any chromosome can occur, but all except trisomies 21, 18 and 13 are lethal in utero. Trisomy 21 causes Down's syndrome. Trisomies 13 (Patau's syndrome) and 18 (Edward's syndrome) are associated with various malformations and severe mental retardation. Such infants usually die shortly after birth. Autosomal trisomies occur with increasing frequency as maternal age increases. The risk of Down's syndrome increases from 1 in 1500 live births at a maternal age of 23 years to 1 in 25 at the age of 45 years. Trisomy of sex chromosomes is compatible with normal development and since it causes no physical characteristics is often undetected.

Tetrasomy and pentasomy of sex chromosomes are compatible with normal development but affected individuals usually have some degree of mental retardation. It appears that the greater the number of X chromosomes, the greater the degree of mental impairment. Whatever the number of X chromosomes the presence of a normal Y chromosome always produces the male phenotype (see later).

Mosaicism, in which an individual has two cell populations each with a different genotype, may occur if non-disjunction occurs during early cleavage of the zygote. Similarly, anaphase lagging in which one chromosome fails to travel along the nuclear spindle to enter the nucleus and becomes lost may result in a normal/monosomy mosaicism.

Polyploid cells contain extra copies of all of the chromosomes. The commonest is triploidy – 69 chromosomes. Polyploidy nearly always causes spontaneous abortion although there are isolated reports of the live birth of affected infants. These are all severely malformed and die in the early postnatal period. Partial hydatidiform mole is a triploidy. The extra set of chromosomes are derived from the father. The triploid fetus usually dies *in utero*. Complete hydatidiform mole has the usual haploid chromosome number, 46, but all of these are paternally derived.

Structural chromosome abnormalites

Structural chromosome abnormalities occur when breaks occur in chromosomes. The nature of the chromosomal abnormality will depend upon the fate of the broken pieces.

Deletion occurs when the broken piece of a chromosome becomes lost (Fig. 1.12). Any part of either the long or the short arm of a chromosome may be lost. Identification of the missing portion can be made by examination of the G banding pattern. A chromosome with a deletion at both ends may circularise to form a ring chromosome. Ring formation always indicates that some chromosomal material has been lost, although identification of which portion is missing may be difficult.

Duplicated material may occur within a chromosome, may be attached to the chromosome elsewhere or may be attached to another chromosome. Because there is little or no loss of genetic material, duplications are more often compatible with life than other chromosomal abnormalities and are therefore found more frequently. Inversion occurs when a segment of a chromosome is reversed in its orientation. Paracentric inversion is confined to one single arm of a chromosome whilst pericentric inversion includes both arms either side of the centromere.

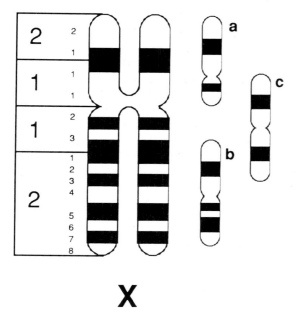

X

Fig. 1.12 Chromosome deletion and isochromosome formation. The large X chromosome at metaphase is seen on the left. **a, b** Deletion of the long arm at different points. **c** Isochromosome formation; it will be seen that only the two short arms of the X chromosome are represented here since division has been transverse instead of longitudinal and the isochromosome for the short arm of the X has been formed.

Isochromosome formation occurs during meiosis when the centromere divides transversely rather than longitudinally (Fig. 1.12). One of the resulting two chromosomes carries two long arms, the other carries two short arms. This abnormality has been often described in the X chomosome and may result in the Turner phenotype.

Translocations occur when chromosomes become broken during meiosis and the resulting fragment becomes joined to another chromosome. In a reciprocal translocation (Fig. 1.13), genetic material is exchanged between two chromosomes with no apparent loss. Provided that there is no loss of genetic material the translocation is balanced and results in normal development. Often there is loss of DNA at the break point which is too small to be detected by G banding. Usually this occurs in non-coding DNA and is inconsequential but rarely this may interrupt a gene

and cause a developmental abnormality. Translocation usually only occurs between one of two pairs of homologous chromosomes. There is therefore a 1 in 4 chance that any offspring will inherit both normal chromosomes, and have a normal phenotype. There is also a 1 in 4 chance of inheritance of both abnormal chromosomes, resulting again in a normal phenotype. There is, however, also a 1 in 4 chance of inheriting either additional genetic material and a 1 in 4 chance of inheriting reduced genetic material. Approximately 4% of individuals with Down's syndrome have additional chromosome 21 material attached to another chromosome, commonly 11. Breakage of the short arm of two acrocentric chromosomes near to the centromere may result in junction of the long arms and loss of the short arms. This is the Robertsonian translocation.

The terminology used to indicate precisely what variety of translocation has occurred is somewhat complex. The letter t is used to indicate that there has been a translocation and this is then followed in parentheses by the number of the chromosomes concerned with p or q relating to the involvement of long or short arms. Thus a translocation between the short arm of chromosome 4 and the short arm of chromosome 14 would be recorded as t(4p;14p). The chromosome having the lower number is recorded first, but if a sex chromosome is involved, this comes first. For example, a translocation between the Y chromosome and chromosome number 3 would be written t(Y;3).

SEXUAL DIFFERENTIATION

The sex-determining region of the Y chromosome

Sexual development depends upon the effect of the sex chromosomes on gonadal differentiation, the correct functioning of the differentiated testis and the response of the end organs to substances produced by the testis. A normal female has two X chromosomes and a normal male has one X and one Y. Both the X and the Y chromosomes carry genes other than those for sexual differentiation, although the Y chromosome is smaller than the X. There is a region at the top of the short arm of

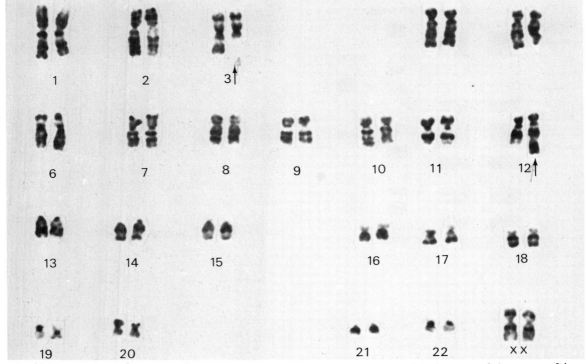

Fig. 1.13 Reciprocal translocation between chromosomes 3 and 12. A major portion of the long arm of chromosome 3 has broken off and has been exchanged with a small portion of the long arm of chromosome 12. This is a balanced translocation in an adult who was without abnormality.

the Y chromosome which is homologous to the same region of the X. Recombination occurs at meiosis between these two regions in the same way as between autosomes. This is therefore often known as the psuedoautosomal region of X and Y. There is also an homologous region in the mid part of the long arm of the X chromosome but it is not thought that recombination can occur here. In the normal situation, the presence of a Y chromosome causes differentiation of the undifferentiated gonads to testes. The Y chromosome carries a gene or genes which function as a testicular differentiating factor (TDF). For many years it was believed that this factor was a male-specific histocompatibility antigen known as H-Y. This theory was abandoned when it was demonstrated that certain species lack the H-Y antigen. Studies of individuals who were XX, but carried a small translocation from their father's Y chromosome onto X, showed that TDF must be on the long arm of the Y chromosome just below the X–Y

homology region. A gene in this region was found which was highly conserved and which coded for a protein whose structure suggested a DNA-binding transcription regulator. Since this protein contained zinc finger projections it was called ZFY. Again, several individuals were found who lacked ZFY but were undoubtable males. That area of the Y chromosome was searched again and another gene was found that coded for a protein which is expressed in the developing gonad. A mutation of this gene, 'sex determining region' of Y (SRY), has been found in a mouse which produced XY females. SRY is currently the best candidate for TDF but this is far from proved.

Mullerian inhibitor

The testes produce androgens which cause development of the Wolffian system and a Mullerian inhibitor. The Mullerian inhibitor is a protein. In the human it appears to have a local action, acting on the same side of the embryo in which it is produced. However, in cows, transplacental transfer of Mullerian inhibitor from a male to a female twin will result in masculinisation of the whole female, producing a freemartin. The Mullerian structures will develop unless inhibited so, if testes are present in the early embryo and function normally, the embryo will develop as male. If no testes are present, or if they fail to function, the embryo will develop as female. Female development does not require the presence of functioning ovaries. Turner's syndrome results from the inheritance of only one X chromosome and no Y chromosome (XO). Although there is no development of either testes or ovaries the embryo will develop as a female. The appearance of a child with Turner's syndrome is essentially female with minor dysmorphic features.

End organ insensitivity

Insensitivity of end organs to normally produced testicular androgens can also result in failure of masculinisation and a female phenotype, despite normal testes. Although the Wolffian tissues can respond to testosterone directly, differentiation of the external genitalia requires conversion of testosterone to dihydrotestosterone by the action of 5α-reductase. Deficiency in 5α-reductase, occasionally as a result of an autosomal recessive genetic abnormality, will result in partially or scarcely masculinised external genitalia and a female phenotype. Similarly, there are abnormalities of testosterone receptor function which may result in failure of masculinisation of the embryo.

MOLECULAR GENETICS AND RECOMBINANT DNA TECHNOLOGY

The study of the structure and function of the genome has undergone an explosion in the 1980s. The new recombinant DNA technology has allowed genes to be characterised at the DNA level, their nucleic acid sequence to be determined and the mutations causing disease to be identified. It is now clear that many single diseases, cystic fibrosis for example, may be caused by one of a number of different DNA mutations. It should be

noted that the word 'recombination' has two meanings in molecular biology. It can mean either the crossing over of genetic material from homologous chromosomes during meiosis, a recombination event, or it can mean the recombination of two DNA molecules in the test tube. For example, if a gene clone and plasmid are mixed together in an attempt to ligate the clone into the plasmid, plasmids which acquire the extra DNA are termed *recombinants* whilst those that do not are *non-recombinants*. Recombinant DNA technology will be considered here in principle to give the reader a basic understanding of the important techniques and concepts involved.

Gene structure and function

DNA is composed of a deoxyribose backbone, the 3 position (3') of each deoxyribose being linked to the 5 position (5') of the next by a phosphodiester bond. At the 2 position each deoxyribose is linked to one of four nucleic acids, the purines adenine or guanine or the pyrimadines thymine or cytosine. Each DNA molecule is made up of two such strands in a double helix with the nucleic acid bases on the inside. The bases pair by hydrogen bonding, adenine (A) with thymine (T) and cytosine (C) with guanine (G). DNA is replicated by separation of the two strands and synthesis by DNA polymerases of new complementary strands. With one notable exception, the reverse transcriptase produced by viruses, DNA polymerases always add new bases at the 3' end of the molecule. RNA has a structure similar to that of DNA but is always single stranded. The backbone consists of ribose, and uracil (U) is used in place of thymine (Fig. 1.14).

The central dogma of molecular genetics is that a gene, consisting of double-stranded DNA, is transcribed into single-stranded messenger RNA (mRNA), and this is translated into a protein (Fig. 1.15). In general, the concept of 'one gene, one protein' holds true, although there are examples of proteins coded for in parts, by genes on different chromosomes, and there are genes which code for RNA only, for example the transfer RNA (tRNA) genes. The amino acid sequence of the protein is coded in the DNA by triplets of nucleic acid bases. Each group of three bases, known as a codon, codes for a single amino acid. In most cases a single amino acid may be coded for by a variety of codons. The genetic code is therefore said to be degenerate. There are also three codons which code for the end of transcription, which are called stop codons (Fig. 1.16).

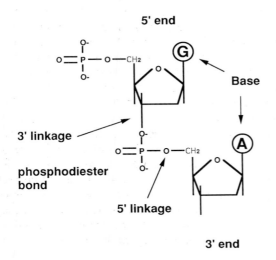

Fig. 1.14 The sugar phosphate backbone of DNA.

During transcription the RNA polymerase which constructs the complementary mRNA reads from the DNA strand complementary to the RNA molecule. This is known as the anti-sense strand whilst the opposite strand, which has the same base pair composition as the RNA molecule (with T in place of U) is the sense strand. Gene sequences are expressed as the sequence of the sense strand of DNA although it is in fact the anti-sense strand which is read.

In general, a gene consists of a 5′ untranslated region which may contain controlling elements to which modulating proteins may bind. The 5′ regions of genes are frequently characterised by elements such as the TATA and CAAT boxes and may be richer in GC pairs than elsewhere in the genome. There then follows the transcribed sequence. The coding portion of the gene is usually interrupted by one or more non-coding intervening sequences. The expressed coding parts of the gene are known as the *exons* whilst the intervening sequences are known as *introns*. Initially the mRNA molecule transcribes both introns and exons. The exons are perfectly spliced out before the mRNA exits the nucleus so that cytoplasmic

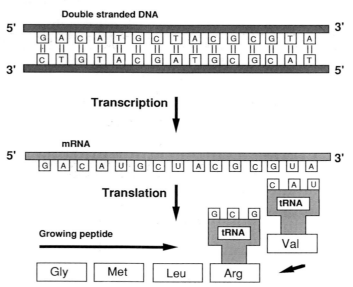

Fig. 1.15 Transcription and translation. Double-stranded DNA is transcribed forming a complementary single-strand mRNA. The mRNA is translated by tRNA to form the peptide chain.

mRNA consists only of coding regions and an untranslated region at the extreme 3′ end. A polyadenine (poly (A)) tail is added to most mRNA molecules at their 3′ end. The role of this poly(A) tail is not clearly established (it may act to control mRNA degradation) but its presence has proved to be useful in the laboratory manipulation of mRNA (Fig. 1.17).

Once in the cytoplasm the mRNA message is translated into protein by a ribosome. Ribosomes, consisting of a complex bundle of proteins and ribosomal RNA, attach to mRNA at the 5′ end. Protein synthesis begins at the amino terminal and amino acids are sequentially added at the freshly made carboxyl end. Amino acids are brought into the reaction by specific tRNA molecules. Each tRNA is a single-stranded molecule which folds in a way that allows complementary base pairing between parts of the same strand. The specific configuration allows the tRNA molecule to bind to its specific amino acid. There remains, unpaired, at one end of the molecule, three bases which are complementary to the codon coding for the amino acid. This *anticodon* binds to the codon of the mRNA and places the amino acid in the correct sequence of the protein. Usually several ribosomes translate a single mRNA molecule at any one time.

In lower organisms the majority of the DNA which constitutes the genome is coding. In higher

First Position	Second Position				Third Position
	U	C	A	G	
U	Phe Phe Leu Leu	Ser Ser Ser Ser	Tyr Tyr STOP STOP	Cys Cys STOP Trp	U C A G
C	Leu Leu Leu Leu	Pro Pro Pro Pro	His His Gln Gln	Arg Arg Arg Arg	U C A G
A	Ile Ile Ile Met	Thr Thr Thr Thr	Asn Asn Lys Lys	Ser Ser Arg Arg	U C A G
G	Val Val Val Val	Ala Ala Ala Ala	Asp Asp Glu Glu	Gly Gly Gly Gly	U C A G

Fig. 1.16 The genetic code.

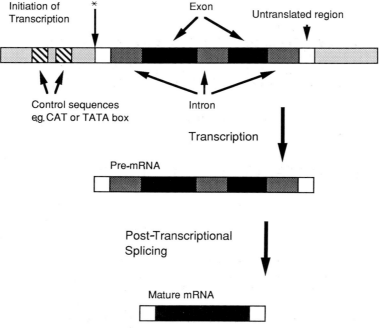

Fig. 1.17 Structure of a human gene and its RNA derivatives.

species the vast majority of the genome is non-coding. The amount of human DNA which actually functions as genes may be less than 10%. Much of the remainder consists of regions of DNA with repeating motifs. The function of this highly and moderately repetitive DNA is unknown although it may have a role in chromosome alignment at meiosis and mitosis.

Obtaining human DNA for study

Human DNA for research or clinical purposes can be obtained from a variety of sources. The most convenient is blood. Ethylenediaminetetraacetic acid (EDTA) inhibits the action of deoxyribonucleases (DNAses). Blood taken for DNA analysis should ideally be stored in EDTA anticoagulant tubes at $-20°C$. Leucocytes are separated from the anucleate erythrocytes and lysed. DNA is extracted by mixing the cellular lysate with phenol. Proteins and lipids dissolve in phenol whilst DNA and RNA remain in the aqueous phase. The RNA is then destroyed using specific ribonucleases (RNAses) and the DNA isolated by precipitation with alcohol. A similar procedure will extract DNA from most tissues including chorion villous biopsies. RNA can also be extracted using essentially similar principles but great care needs to be taken to avoid degradation by RNAses, which are found almost everywhere.

Restriction endonucleases

An enzyme which removes nucleic acids from either end of a DNA molecule is known as a DNA *exonuclease*. An enzyme which cuts within the molecule is an *endonuclease*. Most exonucleases show no specificity for particular bases or sequences of bases. The restriction endonucleases, however, will only cut at sites within specific sequences of DNA. Some recognise specific groups of four bases and therefore cut DNA into many small pieces (four cutters). Enzymes which recognise groups of six bases (six cutters) cut less frequently and yield larger fragments. Enzymes which recognise even larger groups cut rarely (rare cutters). Frequently, restriction sites are palindromic, for example the enzyme EcoRI recognises the 5'-3' sequence GAATTC. This

sequence has the palindromic complimentary sequence 3'-5' CTTAAG. The restriction enzymes used routinely usually cut the DNA within their recognition site. Those that cut on both strands at the same place produce a blunt-ended cut. Those that cut obliquely leave overhangs of single-stranded DNA. Since these overhangs are complementary and will tend to religate, in the presence of a DNA ligase, they are known as sticky ends.

One of the principle values of restriction enzymes in molecular biology is that they cut DNA molecules into consistent and predictable pieces. Digestion of total human DNA with a single restriction enzyme yields a series of fragments of varying size. The number of fragments is so large that after separation by electrophoresis the total DNA appears as a streak. On closer analysis it will be found that this streak is made up of a large number of individual DNA fragments each corresponding to the distance between two restriction sites.

Analysis of DNA by electrophoresis

Once DNA has been cut into fragments using a restriction enzyme the fragments may be separated using electrophoresis through a suitable medium, such as agarose. The rate of migration of DNA through an agarose gel is a function of its molecular size and the concentration of agarose. Once the DNA has been separated it can be visualised under ultraviolet light after staining with ethidium bromide. Ethidium bromide intercollates with DNA and RNA and once complexed will fluoresce in the visible range when illuminated by ultraviolet light. Southern blotting, developed in Edinburgh by Professor E.M. Southern, is a technique which allows specific regions to be identified from DNA that has been fragmented by a restriction enzyme. The DNA is separated using agarose gel electrophoresis. It is then treated with a denaturing agent, usually sodium hydroxide. This denatures the DNA and breaks the bonds between its two strands. In a large tray a thick piece of filter paper is laid over a raised support with its ends dipping in a high-salt solution. The gel is placed onto this filter paper wick on the raised support and a piece of nitrocellulose is placed upon the gel. On top of this is placed a stack of paper towels. Finally, all of the layers are kept compressed by a light weight. The high-salt solution rises up through the gel by capillary action taking with it the denatured DNA. The DNA is carried through to the nitrocellulose membrane to which it binds. Thus the filter becomes a replica of the original gel. Once transfer is complete the DNA may be irreversibly bound to the filter by baking or by treatment with ultraviolet light. More recently, improvements have been made to this technique. Nylon filters are available which are more robust and less flammable than nitrocellulose. The use of vacuum-mediated transfer can reduce the blotting time significantly.

Once a Southern blot has been made it can be hybridised to a radiolabelled DNA probe specific for the gene or region of DNA under study. A gene probe is usually a fragment of double-stranded DNA into which are incorporated radiolabelled nucleotides. The probe itself may be a clone from a cDNA library (see later), a piece of DNA from a non-coding part of the genome whose chromosomal location is known, a small oligonucleotide DNA molecule specifically synthesised *in vitro*, or an RNA molecule synthesised *in vitro*.

A similar process for blotting RNA molecules is known as *Northern blotting* and for proteins is known as *Western blotting*. At present no technique has been devised to be called Eastern blotting.

GENE-CLONING TECHNIQUES

Cloning vectors

Cloning a fragment of DNA means separating it from all other DNA and introducing it into a suitable vector so that it can be replicated in quantity. There are several types of cloning vectors. Plasmids are small circular DNA molecules found within bacteria. They replicate with and within the bacteria, can be passed from one bacterium to another and may carry with them genes for antibiotic resistance. Plasmids isolated from *Escherichia coli* have been modified to allow the insertion of foreign DNA. Replication of the plasmid within the bacteria also replicates the inserted DNA. These plasmids, with colourful names like

pUC19 or PBR328, contain an antibiotic resistance gene to allow selection of bacteria carrying the plasmid. They may also contain a method for distinguishing *recombinants*, those carring foreign DNA from *non-recombinants*. For example, pUC19 carries a gene for β-galactosidase which is interrupted if foreign DNA is cloned into it. If the host bacteria is grown on a plate containing the sugar, non-recombinant bacteria reduce the sugar, producing blue colonies. Recombinant colonies are white.

Plasmids can only accept foreign DNA up to about 10 kilo-base pairs (kbp) in size. Modified phage (bacterial viruses) can accept larger fragments, up to 20 kbp. Even larger fragments up to 50 kbp can be accommodated in cosmids. Cosmids are essentially phage from which virtually all of the genetic material has been removed leaving only the *cos-ends* needed to allow infection of the bacterium. Once inside the bacterium a cosmid cannot replicate as a phage but behaves more like a plasmid. Very large pieces of DNA in the region of 1000 kbp can be cloned into yeast artificial chromosomes.

There are essentially two strategies to gene cloning. The first relies on some knowledge of the protein to pick the relevant mRNA from a population of RNA molecules. For example, it was known that most of protein expression in pre-erythrocytes is globin so cloning the globin gene simply meant finding the commonest mRNA in that cell. Commonly, knowledge of fragments of amino acid sequence allows the design of small DNA molecules, known as *oligonucleotides*, which should detect the full-length sequence that originally coded for the protein. It is possible to induce bacterial expression of proteins coded for by genes cloned into phage *expression vectors*. The clone of interest may then be identified by screening with antibodies directed against the protein.

The second strategy, when a genetic mutation causes a disease but the nature of the relevant protein is not known, relies on tracking the mutated gene through affected families, identifying its chromosomal location and then moving in on the gene itself. This is so-called *reverse genetics*, *gene tracking* or *linkage analysis*. The protein itself is not characterised until the gene has been identified.

cDNA library construction and screening

One of the commonest ways of cloning a specific gene is to predict part of its nucleic acid sequence from knowledge of a fragment of the amino acid sequence and to use this to isolate its specific mRNA. RNA is readily degraded by robust RNAses present almost everywhere and is difficult to manipulate in the laboratory. Using *reverse transcriptase* it is possible to make a DNA copy of the mRNA. This double-stranded complimentary DNA (cDNA) can be cloned into a suitable vector, usually a phage, and conveniently propagated. Messenger RNA is extracted from a tissue known to express the protein of interest. A sephadex column with polythamine (poly(T) or oligo(dT)) molecules bound to it will trap mRNA by its poly(A) tail. A cDNA *library* made from this mRNA contains cDNA representations of all of the mRNA species expressed by the tissue. The

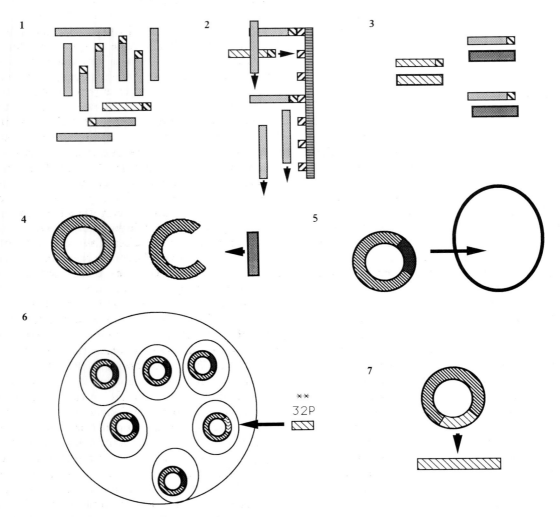

Fig. 1.18   cDNA library construction and screening. **1** Total RNA (▨▨▨) is extracted from a tissue known to express the gene of interest (▨▨▨). **2** mRNA is separated by chromatography using poly(T) which hybridises with the poly(A) tail (◩) of mRNA. **3** Reverse transcriptase produces a DNA copy of the RNA (cDNA). **4** A suitable vector is cut and the cDNA is ligated into it. **5** The vector is introduced into host bacteria. Antibiotic resistance selection ensures that only plasmid-carrying bacteria multiply. **6** A radiolabelled probe is used to identify the colony containing the cDNA of interest. **7** The specific colony is grown up, the vector isolated and the cDNA cut from it.

library is plated out on petri dishes. Phage, each containing a different cDNA, form plaques in the lawn of *Esch. coli*. Application of a nylon filter to the plate causes some of the phage DNA to transfer to the nylon. This can then be treated like a Southern blot and hybridised to a suitable probe to detect the plaque containing the cDNA of interest. The probe may be a short synthetic DNA molecule containing the predicted sequence of a part of the gene or a cDNA clone from a related gene or another species. In an expression library the probe may be an antibody. The nucleic acid sequence of the cDNA can be determined and from this the full amino acid sequence of the protein can be deduced (Fig. 1.18).

Gene tracking

Gene tracking is the technique of following mutated genes through families affected by the disease and relies on the concept of linkage. Consider two theoretical genes each with two alleles, i.e. each gene has two alternative forms. The first causes either black or brown hair, the second either a long or a short nose (these genes don't actually exist, this is just an example!). If the two genes are on different chromosomes there will be no relationship between inheritance of either phenotype. There will be no association between hair colour and nose length. The same will hold true if the two genes are on the same chromosome but some distance apart. The recombination that takes place between homologous chromosomes at meiosis will mix the alleles and there will be no association. If, however, the two genes are very close together on the same chromosome, recombination between them will rarely take place. In this case, in any particular family, one allele of one gene will usually be inherited with a particular allele of the other gene. So, for example, long-nosed individuals will tend to have black hair more often than would be expected by chance. In this situation these genes are said to be linked. The likelihood that recombination will occur between two genes is directly related to the distance between them. Genetic distance is measured in terms of recombination frequency. A distance within which recombination occurs in 1% of meioses is defined as 1 centimorgan. In general this cor-

responds to a physical distance of about 1 million base pairs but in some regions of a chromosome recombination occurs more or less frequently than in others and so genetic distance seems smaller or larger than physical distance.

Known examples of linked genes are far too few to be useful in linkage analysis so use is made of silent mutations usually within non-coding regions of the genome. A point mutation may create or destroy a recognition site for a restriction enzyme. If DNA is taken from an individual who is heterozygous for the mutation and digested with that enzyme, then that particular fragment of DNA will be of a different length in DNA from each of the two chromosomes. This *restriction fragment length polymorphism* (RFLP) can be detected on a Southern blot by using a gene probe complementary to a region of DNA adjacent to the mutation. The exact site of the RFLP on the chromosome can be found by hybridising the probe either to chromosome metaphase spreads or to Southern blots of panels of DNA from individuals with chromosome deletions. Linkage analysis is performed by following the inheritance of RFLP alleles in families with the disease under study. In general, there will be no relationship between inheritance of the disease and of the alleles of an RFLP. If the RFLP is not on the same chromosome as the disease gene they will segregate independently. If they are on the same chromosome but not close together, crossing over during meiosis will cause them to segregate independently. The RFLP is therefore not linked to the disease and that region of the chromosome can be excluded. With luck an RFLP will be found with which there is an association between inheritance of the disease and its alleles. In the same way that the statistical significance of a finding in a clinical trial depends upon the number of patients enrolled, so the significance of RFLP linkage depends upon the size of the family being studied. The larger the number of generations in the family and the larger the number of offspring, the higher the number of meiotic events. If an RFLP is found which appears to be linked it is possible that with a larger pedigree, and therefore more meiotic events, some recombination events will be found between it and the disease gene. Statistical analysis of gene tracking is complex and a number of computer programs are available for this purpose. Analysis is performed to determine the chance that the observed linkage is a statistically significant finding. If this exceeds odds of 1000 to 1 it is generally accepted as being a real result. To exclude linkage, odds of 1 to 100 are generally accepted. These odds are usually expressed as logarithms to base 10 (LOD score), in this case +3 and −2, respectively. In a suitably large pedigree, similar calculations can also be done when there are only a few recombination events between the RFLP and the gene which predict the genetic distance between the two. In this case the LOD score will be found to have a maximum value at a particular recombination frequency. A graph can be drawn relating the LOD score to the recombination frequency θ. θ will always lie between 0, complete linkage, no recombination, and 0.5, no linkage, 50% recombination. Once a linked RFLP has been found a search is made for new RFLPs closer to the gene. Eventually, when an RFLP has been identified very close on either side of the gene, other techniques are used to move in to identify the gene itself. Once the gene has been identified, techniques exist for elucidating the nucleic acid sequence. From this sequence the regulatory amino acid sequence coded by the gene can be deduced.

Polymerase chain reaction

Polymerase chain reaction (PCR) is a technique for the amplification, many million-fold, of specific regions of DNA from as little as one copy. It will amplify DNA from less than 100 to over several thousand base pairs in size but the sequence of the DNA, or at least of the ends of it, needs to be known. The reaction contains the template DNA, the four nucleotides, a DNA polymerase (*Taq polymerase*), and two oligonucleotide primers. The DNA polymerase is thermostable, isolated originally from bacteria (*Thermophylus aquaticus*) growing in hot springs, and has optimal activity at 72°C. The primers, usually around 20 bp in length are single-stranded molecules. One is complementary to the 5′ end of the sense strand of the template, the other is complementary to the other end of the anti-sense strand. The reaction is in-itially heated to 92°C. This denatures the template, forming single strands. The temperature then drops to below 65°C (the specific temperature depends upon the composition of the primers). At this lower temperature the primers anneal to the template at their complementary sites. Primer annealing is favoured over reformation of double-strand template because the primers are in great excess. The temperature is raised to 72°C when the *Taq* polymerase generates new complementary strands. There are now two double-stranded molecules for each original molecule of template. The cycle is repeated, and the number of molecules doubles again. In theory, after 30 cycles there would be over 500 million copies for each original template although in practice the final yield is limited by the availability of primers, nucleotides and the denaturation of the enzyme. It is usually necessary to optimise the reaction conditions for each set of primers (Fig. 1.19).

PCR has found widespread use in molecular biology. It has been used to amplify DNA regions from genomic DNA from blood, from single cells, from the DNA in Guthrie blood spots and from Egyptian mummies. It can identify the presence of minute quantities of viral DNA in epithelial scrapings or urine, identify carriers of disease genes from buccal scrapings and can be used to directly clone genes from mRNA without the need for cDNA libraries.

THE MOLECULAR BASIS OF INHERITED DISEASE

Any change in the sequence of DNA constitutes a mutation. Mutations within non-coding DNA are relatively common since they are unlikely to cause any effect. The large number of RFLPs that have been found throughout the genome are examples of such mutations. Mutations within genes usually alter or destroy their protein coding. Occasionally a mutation will not affect the protein coding because the new codon created codes for the same amino acid. These are silent mutations.

DNA mutation

There are three mechanisms for DNA mutation: substitution, deletion or insertion.

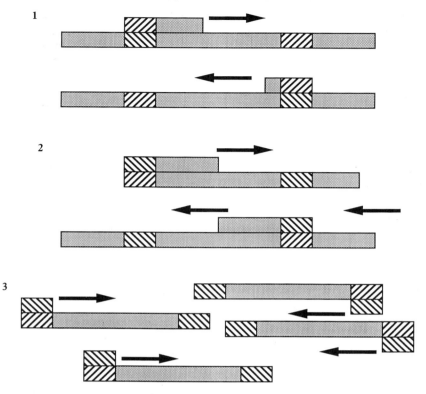

Fig. 1.19 The polymerase chain reaction. **1** The double-stranded template is denatured at 92°C. The temperature drops to allow the annealing of the primers ▨▨ and ◺◹◺ . Increasing the temperature to 72°C allows Taq polymerase to synthesize new complementary strands. The number of DNA molecules doubles. **2** Increasing the temperature again to 92°C causes the new double-stranded molecules to denature. The cycle repeats and the number of molecules doubles once more. **3** After several cycles, large numbers of DNA molecules have been generated, each of which can act as a template for new synthesis in the next and subsequent cycles.

Substitution is a single base change. If the substitution changes a codon the wrong amino acid will be incorporated into the growing protein chain. Even a single amino acid change may make a radical difference to the folding of a protein and destroy its function. Since the genetic code is degenerate not all substitutions lead to changes in the amino acid sequence. The best known example of a single base substitution is the sickle mutation. In this case the β-globin gene carries a single substitution of T for A, which changes a codon from GAG, coding for valine, to GTG, coding for glutamine. The single amino acid substitution changes the stereochemistry of β-globin to the form which sickles in conditions of low oxygen tension. This single base change also deletes a recognition site for the restriction enzyme MstII.

If genomic DNA is digested with this enzyme and a probe specific for the β-globin gene used on a Southern blot it will detect a band larger than usual if the sickle mutation is present. This can be used for DNA diagnosis of sickle disease (Fig. 1.20).

Deletions and insertions may be a single base, several bases or an entire exon or gene. A single base deletion or substitution will alter the entire reading frame. This *frameshift mutation* will code for a non-sense amino acid sequence until one of the stop codons is encountered. Deletion of a region of the gene which does not affect the reading frame, a deletion which is a multiple of 3 bp, may produce a protein which retains some of its original function. There is a variant of β thalassaemia caused by deletion of a 600 bp region of

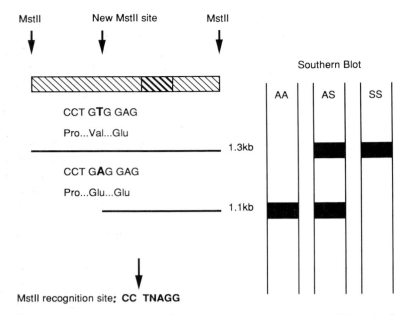

Fig. 1.20 Diagnosis of sickle cell disease using restriction analysis. Diagnosis of sickle disease using the restriction enzyme MstII. The point mutation creates a new MstII site. The β-globin DNA probe ▨▨▨▨ detects a 1.1 kbp fragment if this site is present or a 1.3 kbp fragment if it is absent.

the β-globin gene. This deletion shortens the distance between two BglII recognition sites. On Southern blotting, the β-globin gene probe detects a shorter fragment if this β-globin mutation is present. Unfortunately, there are a large number of other mutations which cause β thalassaemia which do not alter a restriction fragment and cannot be identified so simply.

Mutations outside the coding portion of a gene may also have profound effects upon transcription or translation of the gene. Mutations within the non-coding introns of a gene may prevent splicing of the intron portion from the mRNA. Such a splice mutation would disrupt the open-reading frame of the mRNA and prevent normal protein synthesis. Mutations in regulatory sequences of the gene may result in over or under expression of that gene. If the gene concerned regulates the function of other genes a single mutation might disrupt the function of several genes.

Patterns of inheritance

Genetic disorders may be classed in three groups.

1. Chromosomal abnormalities already have been discussed.
2. Genetic disorders where no recognisable abnormality of a chromosome exists, the condition being due to the genetic mutations we are now considering.
3. Mixed genetic/environmental abnormalities.

Genetic disorders where no chromosomal abnormality can be detected show two main types of inheritance — autosomal inheritance, the gene being on an autosome, and sex-linked inheritance when the gene is on one of the sex chromosomes. In autosomal inheritance the abnormality may be either dominant or recessive. Dominant gene anomalies are those in which the condition is clinically manifest when the abnormal gene is present on only one of the pair of homologous chromosomes. It is, therefore, clinically evident in the heterozygous state. On average, half the offspring of an affected individual are also affected whether they are male or female; unaffected individuals do not transmit the abnormality. However, if a dominant gene has only partial penetrance, it may occasionally appear to miss a generation, although the pattern of inheritance can be determined if the complete family tree is examined.

These are some examples of dominant conditions:

Achondroplasia
Dystrophia myotonica
Huntington's chorea
Marfan's syndrome (arachnodactyly, ectopia
  lentis)
Multiple exostoses
Multiple neurofibromatosis
Multiple polyposis of the colon
Multiple telangiectasia
Myotonia congenita
Osteogenesis imperfecta
Peutz's syndrome (multiple polyposis of
  intestine, circumoral melanin spots)
Tuberose sclerosis.

An autosomal recessive abnormality is one which is only clinically manifest in the homozygous individual who has the abnormal gene on each of the pair of homologous chromosomes. Both parents of an affected individual therefore must be carriers. On average two carrier parents will have one affected child, one normal child and two carrier children in four. Because the carriers reveal no clinical manifestation, the condition concerned may not appear in every generation of a family. When there is consanguinity between parents the likelihood that they share abnormal recessive genes is much increased.

Here are some examples of recessive conditions:

Amaurotic family idiocy
Congenital adrenal hyperplasia
Cystic fibrosis of the pancreas
Galactosaemia
Glycogen storage disease — all types
Morquio's disease (mucopolysaccharidosis
  type IV)
Phenylketonuria.

Sex-linked inheritance shows different characteristics. If the recessive gene exists on the X chromosome this will, in the female, be compensated for by the other normal X. In the male, however, the Y is unable to compensate in this way and the condition becomes clinically manifest.

Haemophilia and the Duchenne type of muscular dystrophy are good examples of such inheritance. An affected male cannot transmit the disorder to his sons since they will receive his Y chromosome which does not possess the genetic fault; all his daughters, however, will be carriers since they must receive the abnormal X. The carrier female would transmit the abnormal X on average to half her daughters who will be carriers and to half her sons who will be affected. The female herself will only be clinically abnormal if she is homozygous and such affected females are very rare indeed. An affected homozygous female would transmit the disorder to all her sons who would be certain to receive an abnormal X and all her daughters would be carriers.

Examples of X-linked conditions are:

Christmas disease (factor IX deficiency)
Duchenne muscular dystrophy (severe X-linked
  muscular dystrophy in boys)
Glucose-6-phosphate dehydrogenase deficiency
Haemophilia
Nephrogenic diabetes insipidus.

Y-linked genes are very rare. So also are X-linked dominant genes of which the best example is the Xg blood group.

Sex limitation of gene affects can sometimes mimic X-linked recessive inheritance. Sex-limitation may occur because a factor in the other sex prevents gene expression. These patterns of inheritance may be distinguished since an affected male can transmit to his son if the abnormality is sex limited but not if it is X linked. It may not be possible to distinguish the two modes of inheritance, however, if the patient is infertile. The condition of androgen insensitivity (testicular feminisation) is such an example since the sufferer is infertile.

Genetic/environmental interaction

A number of common malformations appear to have a pattern of inheritance which involves both genetic and environmental factors. These include major neural tube defects (spina bifida and anencephaly), congenital heart disease, talipes equinovarus and cleft lip and palate. The reasons for suspecting a combination of genetic and environmental factors in their causation comes from observations on twins. Abnormalities may be found, for example, on one or other of monozygotic twins, each of which could be expected to have been affected had a simple genetic basis for the abnormality existed. Unfortunately, we still lack knowledge of the genetic predispositions and the nature of the environmental factors which appear to spark off the abnormality.

2. Embryology

OOGENESIS, SPERMATOGENESIS AND ORGANOGENESIS

Oogenesis

The mature human oocyte is a surprisingly large cell developing to 120 μm diameter at the time of ovulation. Each mature oocyte develops in one of the 1–2 million primordial follicles which are present in the two ovaries at birth. These primordial follicles are scattered throughout the cortex of the ovaries, surrounded by interstitial connective tissue. Many of the oocytes become atretic by the time of puberty leaving only about 250 000 available in the reproductive phase of life.

The primordial follicular cells are flat initially but during the development of the primary follicle they become cuboid and are called granulosa cells. They surround the enlarging oocyte, separated from it by an amorphous shell, the zona pellucida. Microvilli extend from the plasma membrane of the oocyte through the zona pellucida to the granulosa cells and are intimately involved in the transfer of materials between the two. Thus the primordial follicle changes into a primary follicle.

A fluid-filled space, the antrum, develops between the granulosa cells, and as it enlarges it takes up most of the space of the secondary follicle. The oocyte itself is pushed to one side and is surrounded by two or three layers of tightly knit granulosa cells, the corona radiata.

During the final maturation of the follicle the corona cells become columnar and less tightly packed. The follicular wall becomes very thin in one area, and eventually bursts, allowing the gradual mucoid extrusion of the oocyte surrounded by loose coronal cells. This process of ovulation is a sticky ooze rather than an explosive ejection.

The mature ova originate as primordial germ cells which differentiate into oogonia by the 12th week of intrauterine life. Each oogonium gradually develops over the next few months into a primary oocyte containing a nucleus and cytoplasm, the latter rich in ribosomes and mitochondria. As the cytoplasm increases, a Golgi apparatus becomes apparent and many fat globules are seen amongst the mitrochondria.

The initial phase of the first reduction division commences before birth, and is called the prophase of the first meiotic division. The first meiotic division is arrested at this stage and does not go into completion until just before ovulation. It eventually results in two cells, the secondary oocyte and the first polar body. The nuclei of both contain 23 chromosomes, half of the original 46 chromosomes in the parent primary oocyte; however, the secondary oocyte takes virtually all the cytoplasm and is thus much larger than the polar body.

The second meiotic division begins as soon as the first meiotic division is complete. The secondary oocyte (containing 23 chromosomes) and the first polar body (containing 23 chromosomes) start to divide again, but once again the division is arrested, this time at the metaphase stage. Ovulation occurs at this time and the second meiotic division is not completed until the fertilising spermatozoon has penetrated the zona pellucida. Then the secondary oocyte completes division into the fertilised ovum and the second polar body. The first polar body also divides into two smaller bodies. Thus the original oogonium gives rise to a fertilised ovum and three polar bodies.

Spermatogenesis

By comparison with the mature ovum, the mature spermatozoon is very small, the head piece measuring only 4–5 μm in length.

Maturation of an ovum is a prolonged process starting in fetal life and involving two substantial resting phases before producing the definitive cell in the adult female. By contrast the spermatozoon is produced in 70–80 days in a continuous process of development and maturation, which only occurs after puberty in the male.

Spermatozoa develop from the basic germ cells of the male, the spermatogonia, which line the basal lamina of the seminiferous tubules interspersed with Sertoli cells. As the spermatozoa develop through the phases of primary spermatocyte, secondary spermatocyte, and spermatid (see Fig. 1.8, p. 10) they progress towards the lumen of the tubule into which the mature form is shed.

Spermatogenesis depends on the hormonal drive of the two principle gonadotrophins from the pituitary gland. Follicle-stimulating hormone (FSH) provides the impetus for the early development stages and the interstitial cell-stimulating hormone (ICSH) aids the later stages and also provokes the Leydig cells to produce testosterone. Spermatogonia constantly divide by mitosis providing an endless supply of stem cells, only some of which increase in size and develop into primary

spermatocytes each containing 46 chromosomes. Like the primary oocytes these primary spermatocytes undergo a reduction division, known as the first meiotic division, in which the two daughter cells receive 23 chromosomes and are known as secondary spermatocytes. Whereas the first meiotic division of the oocyte produces one secondary oocyte and one polar body, the same division in the male produces two equal secondary spermatocytes of the same size and cytoplasmic content (Fig. 1.8).

Each of the secondary spermatocytes undergoes a further meiotic division to form two equal spermatids, each with 23 chromosomes.

The various generations of spermatogonia, spermatocytes and spermatids are linked in small groups by cytoplasmic bridges possibly as an aid to nutrition and also to ensure synchronous development. The occasional occurrence of twinned mature sperm may represent failure of separation of these bridges.

The individual spermatids undergo substantial metamorphosis known as spermiogenesis in order to produce mature spermatozoa. The nuclear material migrates to form the dense sperm head covered by the acrosomal cap (Fig. 2.1). The acro-

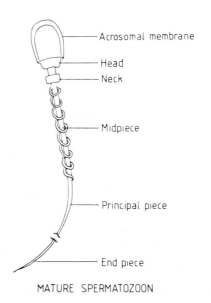

MATURE SPERMATOZOON

Fig. 2.1 Diagram of a mature spermatozoon showing its principal features.

somal cap is itself developed from vacuoles in the Golgi apparatus which fuse to form the acrosomal vesicle, which spreads out over the nucleus. The very important function of the acrosomal contents in penetrating the ovum is considered under fertilisation. The cytoplasm is gradually reduced leaving the head piece almost totally full of nuclear material. Meanwhile the centriole divides into two, from which the axial filament or flagellum develops. Most of the mitochondria form a sheath for the proximal part of the middle piece of the spermatozoon, whereas the tail piece develops a thin fibrous sheath.

The ripe spermatozoa are released into the lumen of the tubule together with the residual fragments of cytoplasm, mitochondria and Golgi apparatus which separate from the sperm and eventually degenerate. The mature spermatozoon thus consists of a head piece covered by an acrosomal membrane, and a tail divided into four sections, the neck, midpiece, principal piece and end piece. The DNA is confined to the nucleus in the head piece, and this alone penetrates the ovum at fertilisation. The remainder of the spermatozoon is responsible for its movement. The fully formed spermatozoa are passed through the tubules of the testis to the epididymis. Taken from this source they are known to have the capacity for fertilisation in vivo and in vitro. During ejaculation the spermatozoa are ejected through the vas deferens and prostatic urethra where they combine with local secretions to form the seminal fluid.

Early embryogenesis — fertilisation, transportation and implantation

The complicated process of fertilisation implies the union of the mature germ cells, the ovum, and spermatozoon.

In humans there is ready supply of spermatozoa constantly available from the normal healthy male after the age of puberty. An average ejaculate will consist of 2–5 ml of seminal fluid with an average sperm density of 60×10^6 per millilitre. It is true that the sperm density may decline if ejaculation is repeated more frequently than every 48 hours but this is seldom a factor in infertility.

By contrast the normal healthy female will only bring one ovum to maturity and ovulation in each 28-day cycle. Other follicles do develop partially in the same cycle but rarely will more than one reach full maturity. When it does it provokes the potential for binovular twinning.

The timing of ovulation is regulated by the cyclical release of gonadotrophins from the pituitary.

The ovum is released at the site of a slightly raised nipple on the follicle known as the stigma. As previously described, it oozes out in a sticky envelope of cumulus cells loosely packed around it. The fimbrial end of the ipsilateral fallopian tube gently folds over the ovary and comes to rest over the stigma so that the ovum is taken up into the tube directly. Although this is the normal pattern it is also possible for the ovum to move over the peritoneal surface of the pelvis behind the uterus to reach the fimbrial end of the contralateral tube.

Once inside the tube the ovum is wafted medially by the rhythmical action of the cilia which line the lumen. This movement is augmented by the finely tuned muscular activity of the fallopian tube which by a combination of peristalsis and shunting squeezes the contents towards the uterus. The whole process is temporarily halted for up to 38 hours when the ovum reaches the ampulla of the tube. There appears to be a physiological valve mechanism which prevents further passage of the ovum, and is possibly only released by the rising concentration of the progesterone from the newly formed corpus luteum. When the valve is released the ovum is moved on once again by the combination of cilial and muscular activity.

This temporary hold up of the ovum in the ampulla allows additional time for fertilisation, and means that sexual intercourse need not coincide precisely with ovulation. Furthermore, spermatozoa have the capacity to retain their potency in the tube for at least 48 hours after ejaculation with the implication that providing coitus occurs within 2 days before or after ovulation, fertilisation of the ovum is possible.

Sexual intercourse occurs at random in humans although the female may be more responsive at ovulation time, when the cervical glands produce a copious watery secretion which not only serves to lubricate the vagina but also assists the ascent of the spermatozoa. Normal ejaculation will occur into the upper vagina where the semen forms a coagulum for about 20 minutes before liquefying. The coagulum prevents immediate loss of fluid from the vagina after sexual intercourse. The surface cells of the vagina are rich in glycogen, especially when under the influence of oestrogen in the follicular phase of the menstrual cycle. Döderleins bacilli convert glycogen to lactic acid with the result that the vagina becomes weakly acidic and as such is hostile to spermatozoa. However, the seminal fluid is alkaline and acts as a buffer for the sperm until they can reach the cervical fluid, which is also alkaline. At midcycle the flow of cervical mucus will raise the pH of the upper vagina and facilitate the activity of the sperm.

The early progress of the spermatozoa is dependent on the propulsive effect of the tail piece which acts as a flagellum, thus poor motility of the sperm in the seminal sample is an important cause of male infertility. The acrosomal cap over the sperm head is capable of producing hydrolytic enzymes which aid the progress of the sperm through the cervical mucus.

In addition, the passage of the spermatozoa is aided by low-grade contractions of the uterus which produce a slight negative pressure in the cavity serving to draw the sperm upwards. Spermatozoa have the ability to pass through the uterus and fallopian tubes with amazing rapidity. It is possible to aspirate viable sperm from the pouch of Douglas within 30 minutes of artificial insemination in the upper vagina. Because the ovum is temporarily held up at the ampulla, the majority of fertilisations occur at that site. Experimental work in which the fallopian tubes have been cut into sections after insemination have defined the section of the tubes in which most newly fertilised ova are found.

Capacitation is an imprecise term coined to explain the concept of some indeterminate change which is said to occur to the sperm during the first six hours in the female genital tract, and without which fertilisation was thought to be impossible. With recent advances in extracorporeal fertilisation it is clear that spermatozoa have the ability to fertilise an ovum almost immediately, and without any contact with the genital tract.

When a spermatozoon reaches the cumulus around the ovum a quite definite change occurs in the acrosomal cap. The outer acrosomal membrane fuses with the plasma membrane surrounding the spermatozoon and, as they coalesce, fine pores open up with the release of various lytic enzymes which have the ability to break up the cumulus cells and penetrate the zona pellucida, through a narrow channel. The first spermatozoon to reach the cell membrane of the ovum fuses with it, and the head piece containing the nucleus passes into the cytoplasm of the oocyte, where it appears as the male pronucleus. It is easily discernable by light microscopy next to the nucleus of the oocyte which forms the female pronucleus. The tail piece of the spermotozoon is left behind outside the cell membrane of the oocyte.

As soon as the head piece has penetrated the oocyte a number of cortical granules appear around the perimeter of the egg, which apparently produce some change in the cell membrane which prevents further penetration by any other spermatozoa. Thus only one spermatozoon out of many million produced in a single ejaculation is needed for fertilisation; but, despite this fact, low density semen of less that 20 million per millilitre, is associated with relative infertility. In vitro, however, a much lower sperm density, even as low as 500 000 per millilitre, is compatible with fertilisation providing the motility and morphology are normal.

Following fertilisation the ovum continues to move towards the uterus aided as before by the muscle activity of the tube and to a lesser extent by the cilia which are sparser at the medial end of the tubes, where the glandular secretory cells are more numerous. The early development of the fertilised ovum depends on the nutrients derived from the secretions from these cells. It takes about 4 days to traverse the fallopian tube and reach the uterine cavity, which is also lined by a spongy secretory endometrium eager to encourage implantation of the blastocyst. The first 4 or 5 days after fertilisation produce the most remarkable series of changes in the oocyte, all of which have now been followed clearly during in vitro experiments. The second meiotic division of the oocyte is only completed after fertilisation, with the extrusion of the second polar body (see section on oogenesis). The male and female pronuclei each contain 23 chromosomes. They gradually migrate towards each other with eventual fusion when syngamy occurs as the chromosomes pair off producing the definitive 46 chromosomes in 23 matching pairs. The genetic features of the offspring are thus ordained.

Within 30 hours of fertilisation the first cell division occurs in which the fertilised ovum splits equally into two separate cells (Fig. 2.2). This process is known as cleavage, each of the daughter cells containing a nucleus with a full complement of 46 chromosomes. Within 12 hours a second cleavage occurs when each of the daughter cells divides into two again by mitotic division. Subsequent cleavage of successive generations of cells follows in quick succession and not always synchronously so that at any particular time there may be an uneven number of cells. The whole collection of cells is known as the zygote and the contained cells are called blastomeres. When the zygote contains so many blastomeres that they can no longer be differentiated it is known as the morula, Latin for a mulberry, which it resembles. The morula (Fig. 2.3) is a ball of cells which rolls

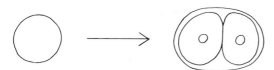

Fig. 2.2 Diagrammatic representation of the first cleavage division.

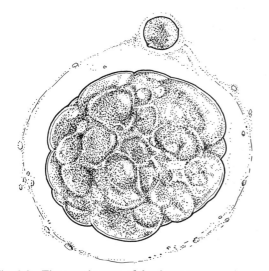

Fig. 2.3 The morula stage of development.

into the uterine cavity, at which stage a fluid-filled antrum develops between the cells in the centre of the ball. As the fluid increases the cells are pressed to the side, and the morula becomes a blastocyst (Fig. 22.2, p. 49).

The blastocyst is a symmetrical fluid-filled ball, the lining cells of which go on to form the trophoblast. On one area of the inner surface the trophoblast cells develop into a distinct group known as the inner cell mass, and it is from these cells that the embryo will form.

The blastocyst implants into the secretory endometrium of the uterus about 6 days after fertilisation. The trophoblast cells produce a proteolytic enzyme which allows invasion into the endometrium. As this occurs the basal cytotrophoblast divides rapidly, producing a more superficial syncitium of cells, the syncitiotrophoblast, which interlocks into the spongy network of the endometrium. By the end of 10 days the early embryo has burrowed into the endometrium to such an extent that it is completely covered. It extracts nutrients from the endometrial secretions and is already producing human chorionic gonadotrophin (hCG), which may be measured in the maternal serum or urine.

The trophoblast cells go on to form the placenta which is described later in this section.

Early development of the embryo

The few cells known as the inner cell mass which are heaped up on one wall of the trophoblast start a rapid development from the 10th day following conception. The mass is partially divided by a waist and takes on the shape of a cottage loaf (Fig. 2.23, p. 49). In the centre of each half of this inner cell mass a fluid cavity forms, that in the upper half is called the amniotic vesicle, later becoming the amniotic sac, and that in the lower half is called the endocervical vesicle, later becoming the yolk sac (Fig. 2.24, p. 49).

Only two layers of cells lie between the two fluid cavities of the amniotic sac and yolk sac. The layer of cells adjacent to the amniotic sac are tall columnar cells and form the embryonic ectoderm. From these few cells all the ectodermal tissues of the fetus develop, that is the skin and all its appendages, and also the neural tube and its derivatives (the brain, spinal cord, nerves, autonomic ganglia and adrenal medulla).

The layer of cells adjacent to the yolk sac form the embryonic endoderm, and from these few cells all the endodermal tissues of the fetus develop, that is the lining of the gut and the epithelial cells of the gut derivatives (the thyroid, parathyroid, trachea, lungs, liver and pancreas).

Between the ectoderm and endoderm a third layer of cells grows principally from ectodermal proliferation. This middle layer forms the embryonic mesoderm and, from it, all the mesodermal tissues of the fetus develops, that is the bones, muscles, cartilage and subcutaneous tissues of the skin.

Organogenesis

Development of the germ layers

The three layers of ectoderm, mesoderm and endoderm initially take the form of a flat circular sandwich, but later there is a disproportionate growth of the ectoderm at opposite poles so that the embryonic plate enlongates into an oval, each end of which curves towards the yolk sac thus forming the head fold and tail fold (Fig. 2.6). The amniotic sac enlarges until it completely surrounds the developing embryo and yolk sac.

On the dorsal or amniotic surface of the ectoderm a groove develops in the middle from the head to the tail of the embryo. Its edges grow over and eventually unite to change the groove into a tube, the neural tube, from which the nervous system will develop (Fig. 2.4). Meanwhile the mesodermal layer is growing laterally; that part nearest the midline becoming the paraxial mesoderm, that part further out becoming the intermediate cell mass, and that part which is most lateral becoming the lateral plate mesoderm (Fig. 2.4).

Growth of the endoderm is at first lateral and then ventral eventually folding round to form the gut tube. A portion of the yolk sac is incorporated in the foregut and also in the hindgut. At first the midgut is in direct continuity with the diminishing yolk sac but as the lateral folds of the embryo grow round they constrict the opening to the yolk sac which eventually becomes separated from the gut altogether and forms a tubular stalk, the vitello-

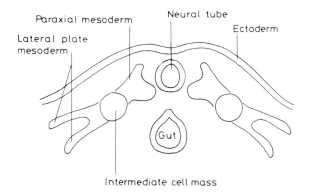

Fig. 2.4 Diagram to indicate the formation of the neural tube, the paraxial mesoderm, intermediate cell mass and lateral plate mesoderm.

intestinal duct. Occasionally, the connection with the gut may persist as Meckel's diverticulum.

The lateral plate of the mesoderm divides into the somatopleure, which remains adjacent to the ectoderm, and the sphenochnopleure, which grows round the developing gut. The space between the somatopleure and splanchnopleure forms the coelomic cavity (Fig. 2.5), later the pleural and peritoneal cavities.

The paraxial mesoderm and intermediate cell mass becomes segregated into discrete masses of cells, or somites, along the length of the embryo. The paraxial mesoderm somites develop into the vertebrae, dura mater and muscles of the body wall. The intermediate cell mass develops in a ventral direction towards the coelomic cavity and forms the origins of the urogenital system.

The limb buds develop from the lateral plate mesoderm, pushing out a covering of ectoderm. The nerve supply to the limb buds comes off the neural tube at the level at which they originate.

Much of the early development of the embryo is at the head end, where the coverings of the neural tube develop with the brain. Also a condensation of mesoderm occurs at the cranial end of the coelomic cavity, and this forms the pericardial cavity and the primitive heart tubes. A further accumulation of mesoderm caudal to the developing heart is called the septum transversum and is destined to become the centre of the diaphragm.

As the head fold grows more quickly on the dorsal surface than on the ventral surface it begins to curl round the developing heart and diaphragm (Fig. 2.6). The foregut also curves round behind the pericardium and reaches the surface at the pit between the forebrain and pericardium known as the stomatodoeum (Fig. 2.6). The thin buccopharyngeal membrane at this point breaks down at the 3rd week of embryonic life leaving a continuous channel between mouth, lined with ectoderm, and foregut or pharynx, lined with endoderm.

A small outpouch in the roof of the mouth grows up into the developing brain. This is Rathkes pouch, which develops into the anterior lobe of the pituitary gland.

The pharyngeal region. The lower part of the face (mandibles) and the whole of the neck region is developed from condensations of mesoderm into a series of symmetrical arches which grow round the sides of the pharynx and eventually meet ventrally in the midline thus becoming horseshoe shaped. In fishes these are the gill arches and the spaces between them are the gills, but in man the condensations of ectoderm and endoderm between

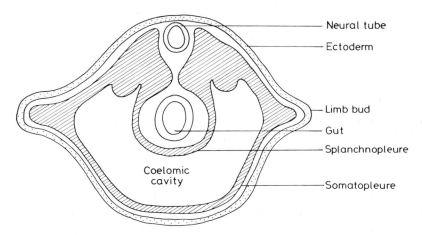

Fig. 2.5 Diagram showing division of the mesoderm into splanchnopleure and somatopleure to form the coelomic cavity.

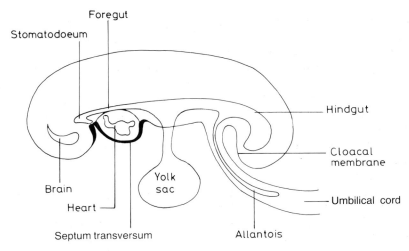

Fig. 2.6 Sagittal section of the early embryo to indicate the relationship of the various features referred to in the text.

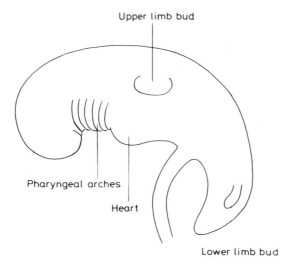

Fig. 2.7   Diagram showing embryonic development at the stage of preliminary pharyngeal arches.

the pharyngeal arches remain intact, and a very thick layer of mesoderm interleaves between them (Fig. 2.7). In each pharyngeal arch there develops a cartilage bar and surrounding muscle supplied by segmental blood vessels and nerves. Between the arches, a series of pharyngeal pouches develop.

Various structures develop from each of the pharyngeal arches and their adjacent pouches. Around the first arch the upper and lower jaws, the palate, the incus, maleus, anterior two-thirds of the tongue and muscles of mastication develop. The first pouch is extended laterally as the Eustachian tube and the middle ear.

The second pharyngeal arch structures include part of the hyoid bone, the stylohyoid ligament, the styloid process, and stapes, as well as the muscles of facial expression served by the seventh cranial nerve. The second pouch contributes to the tympanic cavity and forms the tonsil and supratonsillar fossa. The third pharyngeal arch gives rise to the lower part of the hyoid bone and stylopharyngeus muscle served by the ninth cranial nerve. The posterior third of the tongue and anterior part of the epiglottis are covered with mucous membranes derived from this arch. In the third pharyngeal pouch the inferior parathyroids and the thymus gland develop.

The fourth and sixth pharyngeal arches give rise to the laryngeal cartilages whilst the fifth arch

regresses. From the fourth pouch the superior parathyroid glands are formed.

Each of the pharyngeal arches has its own blood vessels and nerve supplying the structure derived from it. Each nerve divides into an anterior and posterior division, which in certain situations may supply the adjacent arch structures. Not all the pharyngeal arch arteries survive; the first and second regress apart from the small maxillary and stapedial arteries, and the fifth disappears altogether. The third arch arteries form part of the internal carotid artery, while the right fourth arch artery forms the right subclavian artery and the left fourth arch artery forms the arch of the aorta. The sixth arch arteries form the pulmonary arteries, and also the ductus arteriosus on the left side (Fig. 2.8). From the floor of the pharynx three important midline structures develop, the tongue, the thyroid and the respiratory system.

The muscles of the tongue develop from three occipital myotomes, but the connective tissue, lymph glands and mucosa are derived from the first and third pharyngeal arches, supplying the anterior two-thirds and posterior one-third respectively. Between the two components the thyroglossal duct exists in the fetus but is usually obliterated before birth. From the distal end of the duct grows the thyroid gland.

At the caudal end of the ventral aspect of the pharynx a fossa develops and this gradually grows away from the pharynx as the trachea. From this the bronchi and primitive lungs are derived. The cartilage of the fourth and sixth arches contribute to the bones of the larynx which border the opening to the trachea.

The development of the pharyngeal region, face and mouth is a complex one, sometimes occurring imperfectly. Amongst the more common developmental abnormalities which may arise are failure of fusion of the palate or maxillary processes giving rise to cleft palate or hare lip. Failure of occlusion of the second pharyngeal pouch may give rise to a branchial cyst, and failure of regression of the thyroglossal duct may produce thyroglossal cysts. At birth the ductus arteriosus normally closes, but occasionally fails to do so.

The cardiovascular system. Angiogenic tissue is recognisable in the very early presomite embryo, and will soon develop into the heart and blood

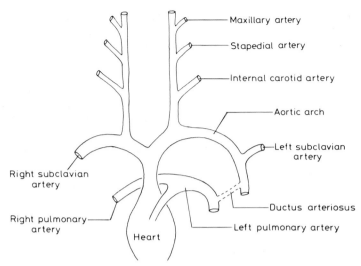

Fig. 2.8 The arterial development from the pharyngeal arch arteries as described in the text.

vessels of the fetus. A beating fetal heart tube can be recognised with ultrasound techniques by the 32nd day of intrauterine life.

The heart is formed as a pair of heart tubes developing from an accumulation of angiogenic cells in the area of the pericardial mesoderm. These left and right endocardial heart tubes fuse to form a single chamber within the pericardial mesoderm.

The caudal end of the tube receives blood from the confluence of the vitelline, umbilical, and cardinal veins which run into the left and right sinus venosus. The cranial end of the heart tube leads into the bulbus cordis and on to the newly formed aorta.

The two ends of the heart tube are soon fixed to the pericardium, so that further growth of the bulbus cordis and ventricle causes the tube to bend up on itself and form an S shape (Fig. 9.8, p. 261).

The atrium expands laterally and also moves up in front of, or ventral to, the bulbus cordis. The two lateral expansions become the left and right auricles. The atrium now receives blood through an opening on its dorsicaudal part from the sinus venosus. Blood leaves the atrium through an opening on the ventral surface, the atrial canal, which leads to the ventricle. Next, endocardial cushions appear on the dorsal and ventral surfaces of this atrial canal and eventually fuse, dividing the canal but leaving two small orifices, the atrioventricular canals. The division of the atrium into two cavities is brought about by the growth of two septa which eventually overlap and close the foramen ovale at birth. Throughout fetal life the foramen is patent conducting blood from right to left.

A more complex development of septa occurs in the ventricle and the truncus arteriosus, to form a left and right ventricle, and an aortic and pulmonary artery. Dorsal and ventral ridges arise on the walls of the ventricular cavity eventually fusing to divide the right and left ventricle. Failure of fusion leaves a patent interventricular foramen. The proximal bulbar septum is formed from right and left bulbar ridges and it divides the aorta from the pulmonary artery.

Finally, the heart valves are formed from endothelial projections at the atrioventricular orifices, and also at the distal end of the bulbus cordis at the pulmonary and aortic orifices.

The total development from heart tube to completion occurs between the 4th and 7th weeks of intrauterine life.

Fetal circulation. Oxygenation of fetal blood occurs in the placenta before it returns in the umbilical vein which joins the left branch of the portal vein. It bypasses the capillaries of the liver by going through the ductus venosus, which is obliterated after birth and becomes the ligamentum venosum. The oxygenated blood enters the inferior vena cava and is transported to the right atrium and thence through the patent foramen ovale to the left atrium and on to the left ventricle. From the left ventricle the blood flows into the aorta and through the fetal vascular network. Blood returning from the head of the fetus passes through the superior vena cava to the right atrium and straight on to the right ventricle and pulmonary artery. However, it does not enter the pulmonary circulation, being short circuited by the ductus arteriosus to the aorta. Aortic blood is carried via the umbilical arteries back to the placenta for reoxygenation (Fig. 9.9, p. 262).

At birth the three short circuits, the ductus venosus, foramen ovale and ductus arteriosus, close.

The alimentary system, the pulmonary and peritoneal cavities. The gut, which develops in continuity with the pharynx, may be subdivided into three sections each with its own blood supply.

The foregut extends as a tube, the oesophagus, to the stomach which forms as a sac at the 5th week of intrauterine life. Below the stomach the liver grows out from the ventral aspect of the foregut. At first it is a hollow diverticulum growing up into the septum transversum, but later it produces two solid buds of cells which form the left and right lobes of the liver. The foregut structures are supplied by blood from the coeliac artery (Fig. 2.9).

The midgut starts in the duodenum at the level of the entry of the bile duct. From it the pancreas develops initially as a ventral and dorsal part, the former arising from the bile duct and the latter from the duodenum itself. The two parts subsequently fuse and the two ducts form a common opening to the duodenum. The midgut extends down to the splenic flexure of the colon, and is supplied with blood from the superior mesenteric artery. This part of the gut grows far more rapidly than the vertebral column and therefore produces a large ventral loop held in place by an extensive dorsal mesentery, through which the blood vessels run. Fixation of folds in the lower part of the loop produce the characteristic position of ascending and transverse colon in the adult, whilst the ileum retains its mesentery, and mobility.

The hindgut forms the descending colon and rectum, and is supplied by the inferior mesenteric artery, although the anal canal is also supplied by a middle and inferior rectal arteries. The hindgut opens into the dorsal part of the cloaca.

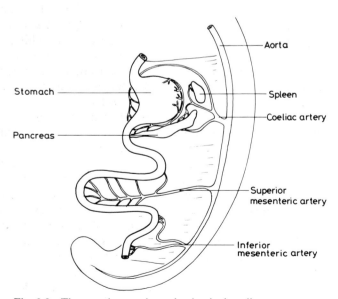

Fig. 2.9 The vascular supply to the developing alimentary system.

The spleen, which takes its blood supply from the splenic branch of the coeliac artery, arises from cellular islands in the coelomic epithelium, and is not a derivative of the foregut.

The respiratory organs. In the midline of the ventral surface of the primitive pharynx a groove appears at the fourth week of intrauterine life. The groove lengthens and becomes tubular as it grows away from the pharynx. From the growing end of the tube two lung buds develop, filling the pleural coeloms; these form the connective tissues of the bronchi and lungs. The lining of the respiratory passages is endodermal in origin.

The lung buds start to appear before the laryngotracheal groove is converted into a tube. They then subdivide into lobules, three on the right and two on the left, which in turn will form the lobes of the mature lungs. The airsacs do not appear until the 6th month of intrauterine life. Growth of the trachea and lung buds proceed in a caudal direction so that by full term the bifurcation of the trachea is at the level of the fourth thoracic vertebra.

The pleural coeloms form the pleural cavities, which are separated from the pericardial cavity by the pleuropericardial membrane, and from the peritoneal cavity by the developing diaphragm.

The diaphragm itself develops from the septum transversum, the pleuroperitoneal membrane, the costal margin, and the gastrohepatic ligament. There is a very small contribution from the dorsal mesentery behind the oesophagus, and from the mesoderm around the aorta.

The central nervous system. The cells of the central nervous system develop from the dorsal surface of the embryonic plate. A shallow neural groove develops in the primitive ectoderm and later becomes covered, thus forming the neural tube. The anterior end forms the forebrain limited by the lamina terminalis. The side walls of the foremost part of the neural tube develop into the hypothalamus, whilst the two cerebral hemispheres originate as two hollow diverticula, the cerebral vesicles. They grow forward and laterally from the hypothalamus. The cavities of the cerebral hemispheres form the lateral ventricles of the mature brain and interconnect through the interventricular foramen.

The midbrain, brain stem and cerebellum de-

velop by further cell proliferation at the cranial end of the neural tube whilst the caudal section develops into a spinal cord. When the neural tube closes over, a rapid proliferation of neural cells occurs throughout the length of the brain stem and spinal cord. These cells then undergo functional differentiation arranging themselves into distinct bundles to become the visceral and somatic, and efferent and afferent pathways.

As the tube closes, some neural cells are excluded on the dorsal aspect and form the neural crest between the spinal cord and the ectodermal surface. Some of these cells migrate laterally either side of the midline to become the cell bodies in the autonomic ganglia including the suprarenal medulla, and the posterior root ganglia (Fig. 2.10).

At the level of the brain stem the central canal is wider and flatter as it opens up into the fourth ventricle. The distribution of afferent and efferent pathways is similar to that in the cord but the afferent groups lie more laterally. In addition, special branchial afferent and efferent nerve cell groups appear supplying the pharygeal arch derivatives as the cranial nerves (Fig. 2.11).

Failure of closure of the neural tube on its dorsal aspect gives rise to the variety of neural tube defect abnormalities, most commonly seen at the caudal end as an open spina bifida.

The skeletal system. All the bones in the body are derived from embryonic mesenchyme. Some of the bones are preformed in cartilage before undergoing ossification, whilst others are ossified directly from membranous precursors.

The vertebrae are formed from the segmental sclerotomes around the notochord and neural tube. These sclerotomes are derived from the mesodermal somites. Each vertebra is preformed as a cartilagenous ring in which three centres of ossification appear, one for the body and one for each half of the neural arch. The process is complete by the 8th week of intrauterine life. The notochordal remnant eventually disappears in the centre of each vertebral body, but persists as the nucleus pulposus of the intervertebral discs.

The ribs are also preformed in cartilage and develop from the costal processes of the primitive vertebral arches. The sternum forms from two sternal plates which develop to link the central ends of the upper nine ribs on each side. The two

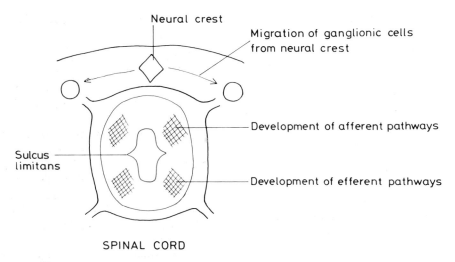

SPINAL CORD

Fig. 2.10   Early development of the spinal cord.

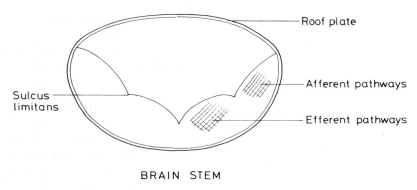

BRAIN STEM

Fig. 2.11   Diagram showing spinal cord development at the level of the brain stem.

plates pass through a cartilaginous phase before undergoing ossification and fusion to form the definitive single sternum.

The skull develops from the mesenchyme which envelops the cerebral vesicles. The vault of the skull and part of the base are ossified directly from membranous bone, whilst the major part of the base excluding the orbital part of the frontal bone and the lateral part of the greater wing, is preformed in cartilage.

The limbs appear as small limb buds at the end of the fourth week of intrauterine life (Fig. 2.7). The upper limb buds develop a little in advance of the lower ones. Each bud is derived from several primitive somites and carry with them the corresponding ventral rami of the spinal nerves.

The central mesenchyme forms the cartilaginous skeleton, which eventually ossifies to form the limb bones. The muscles pertaining to the skeleton are derived from the surrounding mesoderm.

The feet and hands appear very similar to start with, as flat extensions of the limb buds. Later the mesenchyme condenses into distinct digits, and failure of this phase gives rise to webbing of the fingers or toes.

The joints between bones evolve from the

residual core of mesenchyme which does not differentiate into membranous bone. This mesenchyme may develop into fibrous tissue as the fibrous joints between the skull bones, or it may become cartilaginous as in the cartilage joints. Synovial joints occur when the mesenchyme loosens out and a cavity forms in the centre, whilst some of the cells liquefy to fill the space.

Muscles, skin and appendages. It has already been observed that the muscles of the limbs develop from the mesenchyme of the limb buds, and the muscles of the head and neck develop from the mesenchyme of the pharyngeal arches.

The muscles of the trunk all develop from the dorsilateral part of the somites known as the dermomyotome. Spindle cells proliferate from it to form the muscle plate whilst the remainder forms the skin plate. The muscle plate or myotome divides into a dorsal part supplied by the dorsal ramus of the corresponding spinal nerve, and a ventral part supplied by the ventral ramus. The dorsal part develops into the muscle groups of the back, whilst the ventral part forms the muscles of the body wall.

Some of the myotome derivatives degenerate and disappear whilst others may fuse and form fibrous aponeuroses as seen in the anterior abdominal wall.

Involuntary muscles of the gut, ureters, bladder, and uterus are developed from the sphanchnopleuric mesoderm in situ.

The skin plate or dermatome develops into the true dermis, whilst the overlying ectoderm forms the epidermis, hairs, nails, sweat glands and sebaceous glands.

The dermis and subcutaneous areolar tissue develop towards the end of the 3rd month, and the dermal papillae appear in the 4th month. The primary nailfolds are also seen in the third month, and the sweat glands appear about 1 month later. The mammary glands develop as a collection of modified sweat glands at the cranial end of the milk ridge or nipple line. Occasionally, supernumerary nipples and even gland tissue may develop caudally in the same line. The epithelial lining of the ducts and glands are derived from the ectoderm, whilst the connective tissue and fat are developed from the underlying mesenchyme.

THE DEVELOPMENT OF THE GENITAL ORGANS

The genital organs develop in close association with those of the urinary tract. Both arise in the intermediate mesoderm on each side of the root of the mesentery beneath the epithelium of the coelom.

The pronephros, a few transient tubules in the cervical region, appears first and quickly degenerates. At the caudal end of the pronephros, however, an important duct develops which passes down the body to reach the cloaca. This is the mesonephric (Wolffian) duct and it will connect with some of the tubules of the mesonephros which appears next.

The mesonephros develops as a long bulge into the dorsal wall of the coelom in the thoracic and upper lumbar regions. It will later degenerate to a different extent in the two sexes (Fig. 2.12). Two important structures appear on the coelomic surface of the mesonephros: (1) the genital ridge from which the gonad will form; (2) the paramesonephric (Mullerian) duct.

The genital ridge appears as a swelling on the medial aspect of the mesonephros; at first it covers the whole extent of the latter, but later contracts to the central part only. The paramesonephric duct forms as a groove on the lateral aspect of the coelom which then sinks below the surface and becomes a tube. This occurs in embryos of some 10 mm crown-rump length (5–6 weeks).

The development of the uterus and tubes

The paramesonephric ducts on each side extend caudally to reach the dorsal wall of the urogenital sinus by about 9 weeks (Fig. 2.13). At that time the mesonephric and paramesonephric ducts are both present and capable of development (indifferent stage). From this point on in the female the paramesonephric duct continues to develop and the mesonephric one to degenerate; in the male the opposite occurs (Fig. 2.12). As the paramesonephric ducts progress caudally their lower portions come together in the midline and fuse; from this fused part the uterus and cervix develop and from the separate upper part the fallopian tubes develop.

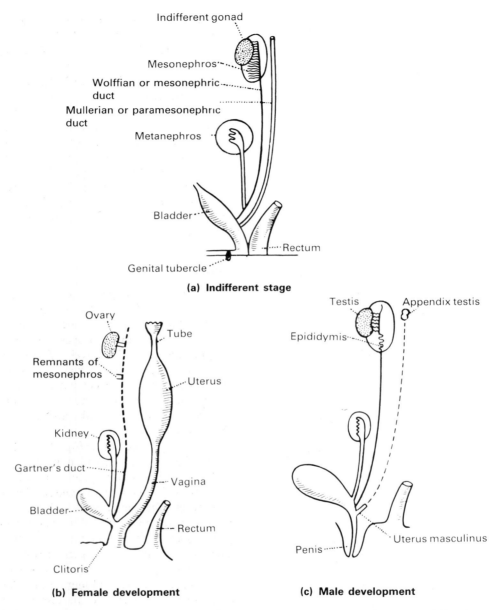

Fig. 2.12 Diagrammatic representation of genital tract development **a** Indifferent stage. **b** Female development. **c** Male development. (Reproduced with permission from Baillière Tindall.)

During the 4th month (12–16 weeks) proliferation of mesoderm around the fused lower parts of the ducts forms the muscular walls of the uterus and cervix.

The vagina

Vaginal development is more complex (Figs 2.14, 2.15). At the Mullerian tubercle, where the paramesonephric ducts reach the urogenital sinus, a

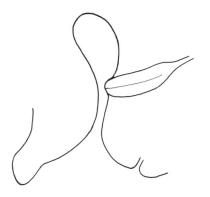

Fig. 2.13 The paramesonephric ducts which have reached the dorsal wall of the urogenital sinus by about 9 weeks.

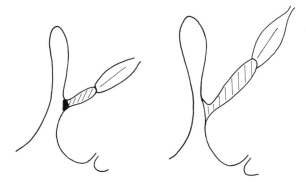

Fig. 2.14 Formation of the vaginal plate. This vaginal plate displaces the lower end of the fused Mullerian ducts cranially as indicated by the hatched areas.

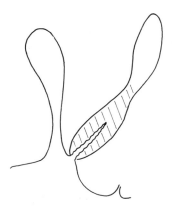

Fig. 2.15 The solid vaginal plate is beginning to break down to form the vaginal lumen around 16–18 weeks.

considerable growth of tissue occurs and the tubercle becomes obliterated. This tissue growth forms the vaginal plate (Fig. 2.14), which is thus composed of sinus epithelium and para-mesonephric ducts. The vaginal plate grows rapidly, pushing the remnants of the mesonephric duct, which had also reached the urogenital sinus, cranially. From this vaginal plate the vagina forms. At first it is a solid organ, but at about 16–18 weeks the central core begins to break down to form the vaginal lumen (Fig. 2.15). Because of the great growth of the plate it is not possible to be sure how much vagina is developed from the paramesonephric ducts and how much from the urogenital sinus.

External genitalia

About the 5 mm stage (4 weeks) the primitive cloaca becomes divided by a transverse septum into an anterior urogenital portion and a posterior rectal portion. From the upper part of the cloaca to approximately the level of the Mullerian tubercle this septum grows downwards; below that the septum grows inwards from each side. Shortly after division is complete the urogenital portion of the cloacal membrane breaks down.

Soon afterwards the urogenital sinus is seen to be made up of three parts (Fig. 2.16). In its lower portion there is an expanded phallic part above which is a deeper narrow pelvic part which reaches as far cranially as a point where the Mullerian ducts reach the sinus wall. Above this is the vesico-urethral part which is connected on its upper aspect with the allantois. On the external surface of the embryo the genital tubercle can be seen, which is a conical projection encircling the anterior part of the cloacal membrane; the tubercle can be seen before cloacal division is complete (6 weeks). On either side of the urogenital sinus may be seen two pairs of eminences — a medial pair called the genital folds and a lateral pair called the genital swellings. These are formed by the proliferation of mesoderm around the lower por-tion of the sinus. Until approximately 10 weeks the external appearances of the male and female are similar and it is not possible to determine the sex of a child. Then differentiation occurs. The

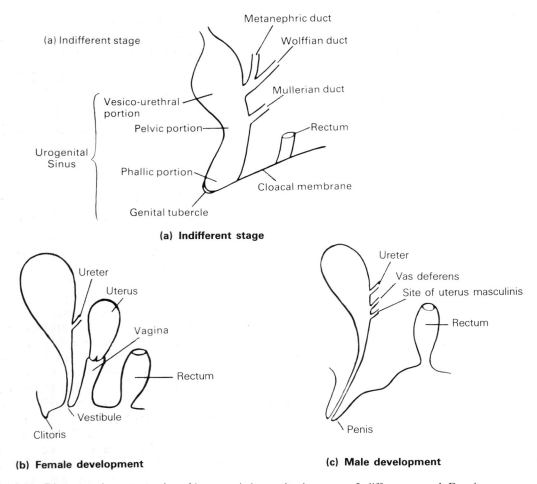

Fig. 2.16 Diagrammatic representation of lower genital tract development. a Indifferent stage. b Female development. c Male development. (Reproduced with permission from Baillière Tindall.)

bladder and urethra are formed from that part of the vesico-urethral division of the urogenital sinus whilst the pelvic and phallic portions become shallow and, ultimately, form the vestibule (Fig. 2.16b). The genital tubercle remains small and becomes the clitoris; the genital folds form the labia minora and the genital swellings enlarge to become the labia majora. In males the genital tubercle enlarges to become the penis; the genital folds fuse to form the phallic portion of the male urethra and the genital swellings enlarge and fuse to form the scrotum.

Finally, proliferating mesoderm spreads ventrally around the lower part of the body wall uniting with its fellow from the opposite side to complete the development of the clitoris or penis and the anterior surface of the bladder and anterior abdominal wall below the umbilicus.

The development of the gonads

The first sign of a primitive gonad may be seen at about 5 weeks.

The gonad has a triple origin from:

1. The coelomic epithelium of the genital ridge
2. The underlying mesoderm
3. The germ cells which enter it from an extragonadal source.

We have seen that the gonad begins as a bulge on the medial aspect of the mesonephric ridge. First there is proliferation of the coelomic epithelium at that point and further proliferation of the mesenchyme beneath that epithelium. By 5–6 weeks, cords of coelomic epithelium can be seen projecting into the substance of the developing gonad and breaking up the mesenchyme into loose strands. Rapid development of these cords follows and in the deeper layers they become branched and complex. During these early stages, primitive germ cells can be seen lying between the cords. These germ cells have originated from beneath the epithelium of the yolk sac, from which site they migrate through the root of mesentery to enter the genital ridge. They can be seen in the region of the genital ridge at approximately 4 weeks. At this stage, therefore, the sex cords which have developed from the coelomic epithelium, the primitive mesenchymal tissue and the primitive germ cells all lie together in the developing gonad which is at its indifferent stage.

Gonadal differentiation can be seen first in the testis about 7 weeks. There is then great development of the sex cords and a decrease in number and size of the cells of the outer cellular layer from which primitive germ cells disappear. The cells of this outer zone later become differentiated into spindle-shaped fibroblasts and ultimately form the tunica albuginea. The rete testis and the straight and seminiferous tubules arise from the sex cords whilst the interstitial cells develop from the mesenchyme.

The ovary cannot be identified until some time later. The outer zone remains more cellular and it is possible to distinguish three groups of cells — the larger primitive germ cells, the supporting cells, which may now be called pregranulosa cells, and more spindle-shaped cells which have formed from the mesenchyme of the genital ridge. This is a phase of tremendous growth and, in particular, the germ cells increase markedly in number and become smaller in size. By 20 weeks they have almost reached 7 million in number, after which many become destroyed by various processes.

By 20–24 weeks, follicle formation can be seen, the germ cells being surrounded by pregranulosa cells, outside of which is an increasing quantity of supporting stromal cells which have grown out-wards from the deeper layers of the gonad. An interesting feature is that those germ cells which do not succeed in surrounding themselves with a protective layer of pregranulosa cells are destroyed by the advancing stroma. This destruction along with atresia of some follicles, which have passed into the early stage of development, results in many germ cells being eliminated, so that perhaps only 1–2 million remain at birth.

DEVELOPMENT OF THE PLACENTA

The ovum is fertilised in the fallopian tube and enters the uterine cavity as a morula which rapidly sheds its surrounding zona pellucida and converts into a blastocyst. The outer cell layer of the blastocyst then proliferates to form the primary trophoblastic cell mass (Fig. 2.17a) from which cells infiltrate between those of the endometrial epithelium: the latter degenerate and the trophoblast thus comes into direct contact with the endometrial stroma, this process of implantation being complete by the 10th or 11th postovulatory day. In the 7-day ovum the trophoblast forms a peripheral plaque which rapidly differentiates into two layers, an inner layer of larger clear mononuclear cytotrophoblastic cells with well-defined limiting membranes and an outer layer of multinucleated syncytiotrophoblast (Fig. 2.17b), this latter being a true syncytium. That the syncytiotrophoblast is derived from the cytotrophoblast, not only at this early stage but also throughout gestation, is now well established for, even when trophoblast is growing rapidly, DNA synthesis and mitotic activity occur only in the nuclei of the cytotrophoblastic cells. It would appear that the syncytiotrophoblast is formed by fusion of cytotrophoblastic cells for, though no intercellular membranes can normally be seen in the syncytial layer, remnants of such membranes can occasionally be found on electron microscopy. Cells with a cytoplasmic complexity intermediate between that of cytotrophoblast and syncytiotrophoblast can also be identified by electron microscopy: these intermediate-type cytotrophoblastic cells appear to be ones which are beginning to differentiate into syncytiotrophoblast but have not yet lost their limiting plasma membranes.

Between the 10th and 13th postovulatory days a series of intercommunicating clefts, or lacunae, appear in the rapidly enlarging trophoblastic cell mass (Fig. 2.18): these are probably formed as a result of engulfment within the trophoblast of endometrial capillaries. The lacunae soon become partially confluent to form the precursor of the intervillous space and as maternal vessels are progressively eroded this becomes filled with maternal blood: at this stage the lacunae are incompletely separated off from each other by trabecular columns of syncytiotrophoblast which, between the 14th and 21st postovulatory days, tend to become radially orientated and come to possess a central cellular core that is produced by proliferation of cytotrophoblastic cells at the chorionic base. These trabecular columns are not true villi but serve as the framework from which

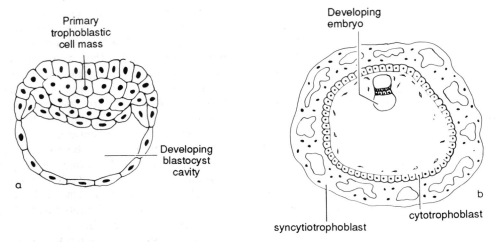

Fig. 2.17 Diagrammatic representation of **a** formation of primary trophoblastic cell mass and **b** the differention of this into cytotrophoblast and syncytiotrophoblast.

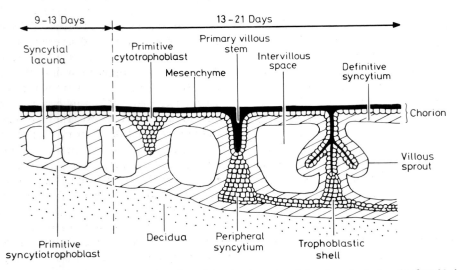

Fig. 2.18 Diagrammatic representation of the development of the placenta during the first 21 days of gestation.

the villous tree will later develop, the placenta at this stage being a labyrinthine rather than a villous organ and the trabeculae being therefore best known as primary villous stems. Continued growth of the cytotrophoblast leads to its distal extension into the region of decidual attachment and, at the same time, a mesenchymal core appears within the villous stems, this being formed by a distal extension of the extraembryonic mesenchyme. Later the villous stems become vascularised, the vessels arising from the mesenchyme within the core and not, as previously thought, being formed as a downward extension of the chorioallantoic arteries. In due course the vessels within the stems establish functional continuity with others differentiating from the body stalk and inner chorionic mesenchyme.

The distal part of the villous stems is formed almost entirely by cytotrophoblast which is not invaded by mesenchyme and not vascularised but which is anchored to the decidua of the basal plate. These cells, which form the cytotrophoblast cell columns, proliferate and spread laterally to form a continuous cytotrophoblastic shell which splits the syncytiotrophoblast into two layers, the definitive syncytium on the fetal aspect of the shell and the peripheral syncytium between the shell and the decidua. The definitive syncytium persists as the limiting layer of the intervillous space but the peripheral syncytium eventually degenerates and is replaced by a layer of fibrinoid material (Nitabuch's layer). The establishment of the trophoblastic shell is a mechanism to allow for rapid circumferential growth of the developing placenta and this leads to an expansion of the intervillous space into which sprouts extend from the primary villous stems. These offshoots consist initially only of syncytiotrophoblast but as they enlarge they pass through the stages previously seen during the development of the primary villous stems, i.e. intrusion of cytotrophoblast, formation of a mesenchymal core and eventual vascularisation. These sprouts form the primary stem villi and, as these are true villous structures, the placenta is by the 21st day of gestation a vascularised villous organ. The primary stem villi grow and divide to form secondary and tertiary stem villi and these latter eventually break up into the terminal villous tree.

During the early weeks of gestation, cytotrophoblastic cells from the trophoblastic shell break through the peripheral layer of syncytiotrophoblast and spread into the underlying decidua, many going on to colonise the adjacent myometrium where they often fuse to give the typical multi-nucleated giant cells of the placental bed; the function of, and the role played by this interstitial extra-villous trophoblast is currently unknown. Groups of cytotrophoblastic cells also grow, however, into the lumen of the spiral arteries and extend as far as the deciduomyometrial junction: these cells which form the endovascular trophoblast, replace the endothelium and invade the walls of the intradecidual portion of the spiral vessels and appear to destroy the muscular and elastic tissue of the media, the vessel wall eventually being replaced by fibrinoid material which appears to be derived partly from fibrin in the maternal blood and partly from proteins secreted by the trophoblastic cells. Because the walls of the intradecidual portions of the spiral vessels are markedly weakened as a result of this process of trophoblastic invasion these vessels dilate considerably under the pressure of the maternal blood (Fig. 2.19), this being an important factor in allowing for a greatly augmented blood flow.

Between the 21st postovulatory day and the end of the 4th month of gestation those villi orientated towards the uterine cavity degenerate and form the chorion laeve whilst the thin rim of decidua covering this area gradually disappears to allow the chorion laeve to come into contact with the parietal decidua of the opposite wall of the uterus. The villi on the side of the chorion towards the decidua basalis proliferate and progressively arborise to form the chorion frondosum which develops into the definitive placenta. During this period there is some regression of the cytotrophoblastic elements in the chorionic plate and in the trophoblastic shell where the cytotrophoblastic cell columns degenerate and are largely replaced by fibrinoid material (Rohr's layer): clumps of cells remain, however, as the cytotrophoblastic cell islands. Although there is cytotrophoblastic regression in the basal plate, during the 4th month of gestation a further proliferation of endovascular cytotrophoblast occurs, a wave of these cells moving

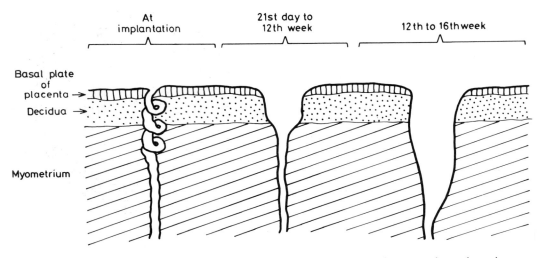

Fig. 2.19   Diagrammatic representation of the conversion of the spiral arteries into uteroplacental arteries.

in retrograde direction to involve the intra-myometrial segments of the spiral vessels where again they replace the endothelium, invade and destroy the medial muscular and elastic tissue and lead to deposition of fibrinoid material in the wall: these changes extend almost to the origin of the spiral vessels from the radial arteries and, when complete, result in the transformation of the coiled spiral arteries of the placental bed into dilated, funnel-shaped flaccid uteroplacental arteries which can accommodate the progressively increasing blood flow to the placenta (Fig. 2.19).

The placental septa appear during the 3rd month of gestation: they protrude into the inter-villous space from the basal plate and divide the maternal surface of the placenta into between 15 and 20 lobes. These septa are simply folds of the basal plate, being formed partly as a result of regional variability in placental growth and partly by the pulling up of basal plate into the inter-villous space by anchoring columns which have a poor growth rate. As the basal plate is formed principally by the remnants of the cytotrophoblas-tic shell embedded in fibrinoid material it follows that the septa will have a similar composition, though some decidual cells may also be carried up into the folds. The septa are therefore simply an incidental by-product of the architectural refashioning of the placenta and have no physio-logical or morphological importance.

The lobes between the septa are not functional or structural subunits of the fetal placenta, this role being played by the lobules: each placental lobule is derived from a single secondary stem vil-lus which breaks up just below the chorial plate into tertiary stem villi which sweep down towards the basal plate to form a hollow globular structure; the terminal villous tree, derived from the tertiary stem, is mainly in the outer shell of the hollow globule and the centre of the lobule is relatively empty and villus free. The term cotyledon, if used at all, is best defined as that part of the villous tree which has arisen from a single primary stem villus: such a primary stem villus may give rise to a vary-ing number of secondary stem villi and hence the number of lobules in a cotyledon varies from two to five.

Each fetal lobule is supplied by a single utero-placental artery, this being not coincidental but due to the preferential formation of the lobules in relationship to the opening of a maternal vessel. The blood from the uteroplacental artery, driven by the maternal head of pressure, flows up, rather like a fountain, in the central hollow core of the lobule towards the chorial plate (Fig. 2.20). Towards the apex of the lobule the driving press-ure force becomes dissipated and the blood disperses laterally to flow back towards the basal plate in the outer shell of the lobule. Hence, it is only in the outer shell of the lobule that the ma-

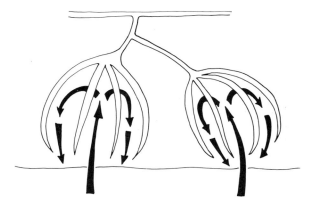

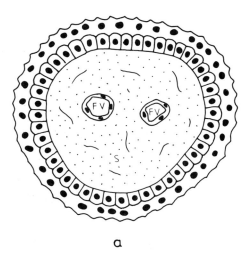

a

Fig. 2.20 Diagrammatic representation of the flow of maternal blood (black arrows) through the fetal lobule.

ternal blood comes into contact with the terminal villi and only here is there a true physiological intervillous space, this being probably of capillary dimensions throughout.

By the end of the 4th month of gestation the placenta has achieved its definitive form and undergoes no further anatomical modification. Growth continues, however, until term and this is due principally to continuous arborisation of the villous tree and formation of fresh villi. This continuing growth is accompanied by a progressive alteration in the morphological appearances of the most distal villi of the tree, these being the only villi which are concerned with maternofetal transfer. In the first trimester the villi are large and have a regular circumferential mantle of trophoblast which consists of an inner layer of cytotrophoblastic cells and an outer layer of syncytiotrophoblast: the villous stroma is formed of loose mesenchymal tissue in which, towards the end of the first trimester, small centrally placed fetal vessels are present (Fig. 2.21). During the second trimester the villi are smaller, the trophoblastic covering is less regular and the cytotrophoblastic cells less numerous: more collagen is present in the stroma and the fetal vessels are becoming larger in diameter and are beginning to move towards the periphery of the villus. In the third trimester the villi are much smaller in diameter, the trophoblastic layer is irregularly thinned and the cytotrophoblastic cells are few and inconspicuous: much of the trophoblastic

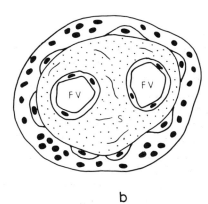

b

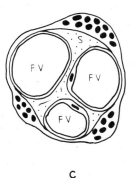

c

Fig. 2.21 Diagrammatic representation of the histological appearances of the placental villi in **a** the first trimester **b** the second trimester and **c** at term. FV, fetal vessels; S, villous stroma.

irregularity is due to the formation of thinned anuclear areas of syncytiotrophoblast; these, the vasculosyncytial membranes, being areas of trophoblast specially differentiated for gaseous transfer. The fetal villous stromal vessels are sinusoidally dilated and occupy most of the cross-sectional area of the villus: they have moved peripherally and lie in an immediately sub-trophoblastic position. These villous changes represent a form of functional maturation and are not an indication of aging: the net result of these intermediate changes is to increase the surface area of trophoblast in contact with the maternal blood in the intervillous space, to approximate the fetal and maternal circulation, to increase the maternofetal concentration gradient and to provide optimal conditions for maternofetal transfer.

The placental bed

The term placental bed is applied to the decidua and myometrium which directly underlie the placenta. As previously described, the placental bed is extensively colonised by extravillous cytotrophoblastic cells during the early stages of gestation. The intravascular component of this extravillous trophoblastic cell population plays a crucial role in converting the spiral arteries of the placental bed into uteroplacental vessels whilst the interstitial component intermingles with the basal decidual cells and infiltrates between the myometrial fibres.

In the past the magnitude of this trophoblastic invasion of the placental bed was markedly underestimated, largely because on simple light microscopy it is difficult to distinguish decidual from cytotrophoblastic cells; these two cell populations can, however, be differentiated by staining for cytokeratins, the decidual cells reacting negatively and the trophoblastic cells giving a positive reaction. The use of cytokeratin stains has shown that a high proportion of the apparent decidual cells in the placental bed are, during early pregnancy, extravillous trophoblast: the number of these cells does, however, diminish as pregnancy progresses and at term relatively few trophoblastic cells survive in the placental bed, these commonly being fused into multinucleated cells.

The function of the interstitial trophoblastic cells in the placental bed is unknown but their principal secretory product is, unlike villous trophoblast, human placental lactogen rather than human chorionic gonadotrophin. The extravillous trophoblastic cells also differ from their villous counterparts in their ability to express a class 1 major histocompatibility antigen, which is, however, of an unusual nature and not necessarily functioning as a transplantation antigen.

The maternal component of the placental bed includes decidualised endometrial stromal cells and two leucocytic populations, macrophages and granular lymphocytes. The macrophages are prominent throughout pregnancy and may well play an immunological role whilst the granular lymphocytes are most conspicuous in the early months of gestation and may be of importance in the processes of implantation and placentation.

Residual endometrial glands are present in the placental bed but are usually attenuated or compressed into slits and only identifiable with epithelial markers.

DEVELOPMENT OF THE MEMBRANES AND FORMATION OF AMNIOTIC FLUID

The membranes

The conversion of the early morula to a blastocyst is accomplished by the formation of a central fluid-filled cavity. This largely separates the primary trophoblastic cell mass, from which the placenta and extraplacental chorion develop, from those cells which give rise to the embryo and contribute to the formation of the yolk sac and amnion: these latter cells form the eccentrically situated inner cell mass which remains in contact with the cytotrophoblast on the inner aspect of the blastocyst wall (Fig. 2.22). During the 8th and 9th postovulatory days the inner cell mass arranges itself into a bilaminar disc, the inner layer (i.e. that facing the blastocyst cavity) forming the primitive embryonic endoderm and the outer, which is in contact with the cytotrophoblast, forming the primitive embryonic ectoderm. The amniotic cavity first appears as a slit-like space between the embryonic ectoderm and the adjacent cytotrophoblast: this enlarges to form, by the 12th postovulatory day, a small cavity, the base of which is formed by embryonic ectoderm and the walls and roof of which are formed of cytotrophoblast (Fig. 2.23). At the same time endodermal cells migrate out from the deeper layer of the embryonic disc to line the blastocyst cavity and thus form the primary yolk sac. Extraembryonic mesenchyme subsequently appears (Fig. 2.24), possibly derived from the trophoblast, and separates off the primary yolk sac from the blas-

tocyst wall: the extraembryonic mesenchyme also intrudes between, and largely separates off, the roof of the amniotic sac and the trophoblast of the chorion. A connection between the two is, however, maintained for a time by the persistence of a column of cells, the amniotic duct, which provides a pathway for the continuing migration of cells of trophoblastic origin into the amniotic

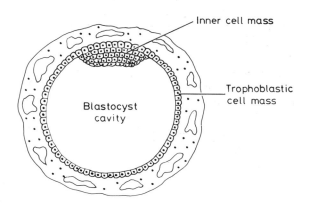

Fig. 2.22 Diagrammatic representation of the blastocyst and inner cell mass.

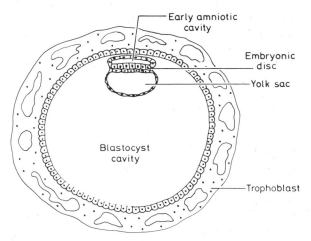

Fig. 2.23 Diagrammatic representation of early stage in the formation of the amniotic cavity.

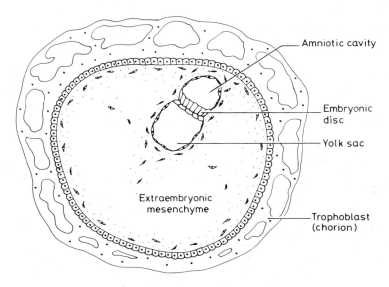

Fig. 2.24 Diagrammatic representation of relationship between developing amniotic cavity and extraembryonic mesenchyme.

epithelium. Mitotic activity at the margin of the embryonic ectodermal disc suggests that the ectoderm is also a continuing source of supply of amniotic epithelial cells.

The extraembryonic mesenchyme forms a loose reticulum in which small cystic spaces appear: these gradually enlarge and fuse to form the extraembryonic coelom which splits the extraembryonic mesenchyme into two layers, one opposed to the trophoblast and also covering the amnion (the parietal extraembryonic mesenchyme) and the other covering the yolk sac (the visceral extraembryonic mesenchyme (Fig. 2.25)). The progressively enlarging extraembryonic coelom also separates the amnion away from the inner aspect of the chorion, except at the caudal end of the embryo where an attachment of extraembryonic mesenchyme persists to form the body stalk from which the umbilical cord will eventually be derived.

Subsequently the amniotic space enlarges at the expense of the extraembryonic coelom and the developing embryo bulges into the expanding amniotic cavity (Fig. 2.26). Meanwhile the yolk sac becomes partially incorporated into the embryo where it gives rise to the gut: that part of the yolk sac remaining outside the embryo communicates with the primitive gut but this communicating channel gradually becomes elongated and attenuated to form the vitelline duct, the extraembryonic yolk sac becoming progressively removed further away from the embryo to be eventually incorporated into the lower end of the body stalk.

Further expansion of the amniotic sac leads to more or less complete obliteration of the extraembryonic coelom with eventual fusion of the extraembryonic mesenchyme covering the amnion with that lining the chorion. At the same time the extraplacental chorion (the chorion laeve) ceases to produce syncytiotrophoblast and the cytotrophoblastic component undergoes a partial regression. Hence the single fused amniochorionic membrane is now fully formed and will consist of, from fetal to maternal side, amniotic epithelium, condensed extraembryonic mesenchyme, a loose reticular layer which possibly represents the vestige of the extraembryonic coelom, extraembryonic mesenchyme and trophoblast.

Amniotic fluid

Amniotic fluid volume can now be measured by ultrasound techniques, although measurements were achieved previously by dilution studies. At

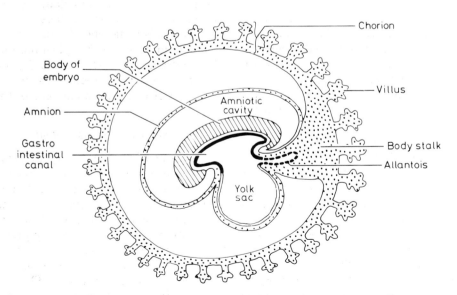

Fig. 2.25 Diagrammatic representation of the relationship between the expanding amniotic cavity and the developing embryo.

varying amount of fat. In its lower part it can separate into superficial and deep layers, between which lie superficial vessels, nerves and the superficial inguinal lymph nodes. These drain the abdominal wall below a line drawn upwards and laterally from the umbilicus. The superficial fatty layer continues into the thigh, labia majora and perineum. The membranous deeper layer is attached to the linea alba and symphysis pubis.

Fascia deep to the abdominal wall. The deep aspect of the transversus is covered by the transversalis fascia, thick below, thinning above, where it continues into the diaphragmatic fascia, which is firmly attached to the under surface of the diaphragm. The psoas and iliacus are covered anteriorly by the iliac fascia, which is attached above to the medial arcuate ligament, laterally along the outer border of the psoas, the iliac crest lateral to the origin of the iliacus and the outer third of the inguinal ligament. Here it adjoins the transversalis fascia. Its medial attachment to the pelvic brim means that the iliac vessels are anterior to it, the nerves of the lumbar plexus behind. There remains the fascia covering the quadratus lumborum, which is the anterior layer of the lumbar fascia (Fig. 3.1c).

In the inguinal region the iliac fascia covers the iliopsoas and receives attachment to the iliopectineal eminence. Lying behind the femoral sheath it passes into the thigh, the femoral nerve deep to it. The transversalis fascia passes into the inguinal canal, of which it forms the posterior wall, and also reaches the thigh anterior to the femoral vessels.

Anterolateral group

Transversus abdominis. This muscle arises from the inner aspect of the lower costal cartilages (interdigitating with the muscular origin of the diaphragm), the lumbar fascia, anterior two-thirds of the iliac crest and the lateral third of the inguinal ligament. An aponeurosis is formed which contributes to the rectus sheath and ends in the linea alba. From the inguinal origin, fibres arch medially and are joined by part of the internal oblique, the resulting falx inguinalis (conjoint tendon) being inserted at the crest and pecten pubis, there lying behind the superficial inguinal ring.

Nerve supply is from the lowest six thoracic and first lumbar spinal nerves.

Obliquus externus abdominis. Eight fleshy slips arise from the outer surfaces and lower borders of the eight lowest ribs in a line which extends downwards and backwards, the slips interdigitating with the origins of the serratus anterior and latissimus dorsi. The most posterior slips pass downwards to insert in the iliac crest, producing a free posterior border to the muscle. Successively higher slips are directed downwards and forwards, ending in an aponeurosis which ends in the linea alba and whose lowest part is attached to the pubic crest as far as the pubic tubercle.

That part of the aponeurosis between the anterior superior iliac spine and the pubic tubercle is strong, thick and recurved with a grooved upper surface. It is the inguinal ligament.

The muscle is supplied by the ventral rami of the lowest six thoracic spinal nerves and the first lumbar spinal nerve.

Inguinal ligament (Fig. 3.2). This forms the floor of the inguinal canal on which run the round ligament and ilio-inguinal nerve. From its lateral two-thirds arise fibres of the internal oblique and its outermost third gives origin to part of the transversus abdominis. From the back of the medial part of the ligament a triangular sheet passes horizontally backwards to the pecten pubis. This lacunar ligament (the pectineal part of the inguinal ligament) is attached at its apex to the pubic tubercle, its base forming the medial border of the femoral ring. From its pubic attachment there extends laterally along the pecten pubis a strong fibrous band, the pectineal ligament.

The superficial inguinal ring, a triangular gap in the external oblique aponeurosis, extends upwards and laterally from the crest of the pubis. Its lateral margin is that part of the inguinal ligament attached to the pubic tubercle, whilst the fibres of the medial margin are inserted into the front of the symphysis pubis.

Opposite the superficial ring the posterior wall of the inguinal canal is strengthened by insertion of the conjoint tendon (falx inguinalis) whose fibres have arched above the contents of the canal as its roof.

The inguinal canal lies obliquely along the recurved surface of the inguinal ligament between

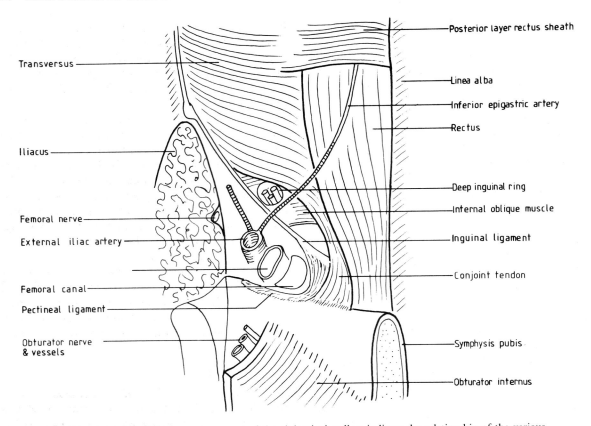

Fig. 3.2 Representation of the posterior aspect of the abdominal wall to indicate the relationship of the various structures described in the text.

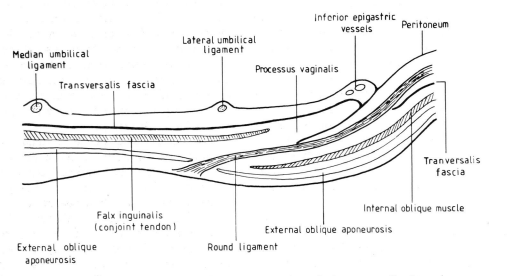

Fig. 3.3 Representation of the arrangement of the muscles, aponeuroses, fascia transversalis, the peritoneum and the round ligament at the level of the inguinal canal.

the deep ring (lateral to the inferior epigastric vessels) and the superficial ring. The origin of the internal oblique strengthens the anterior wall opposite the deep ring and the external oblique forms the rest of the anterior wall (Figs 3.2 and 3.3).

Obliquus internus abdominis. Thinner than the external oblique, this has a continuous muscular origin from the upper surface of the inguinal ligament in its outer two-thirds, the iliac crest and the lumbar fascia. The fibres from the inguinal ligament end in the falx inguinalis (conjoint tendon), the posterior fibres are inserted into the lowest ribs. The remaining fibres end in an aponeurosis which ends in the linea alba and at the costal margin behind the rectus. The nerve supply is from the ventral rami of the lower six thoracic and first lumbar spinal nerves.

Posterior muscles

The lumbar fascia has three layers: posterior, middle and anterior (Fig. 3.1c).

The posterior layer attaches to the spines and supraspinous ligaments of the lumbar vertebrae, lying behind the erector spinae muscles. The middle arises from the tips of the lumbar transverse processes and intertransverse ligaments behind the quadratus lumborum and is attached below to the iliac crest and above to the lower border of the 12th rib and lumbocostal ligament. The anterior layer extends in front of the quadratus lumborum behind the margin of the psoas major, fusing with the periosteum of the front of the lumbar transverse processes, and being fixed below to the iliolumbar ligament and iliac crest; above it forms the lateral arcuate ligament (from the first lumbar transverse process to the 12th rib) (Fig. 3.1c).

At the outer border of the erector spinae the middle and posterior layers fuse, to be joined at the lateral border of the quadratus lumborum by the anterior layer. The completed structure provides the aponeurotic origin of the transversus abdominis (Fig. 3.1c).

Psoas major (Fig. 3.1c). This is a posterior relation of many abdominal structures and leaves the abdomen behind the inguinal ligament with the iliacus lateral to it. Its origins are from the lumbar transverse processes, by five muscular slips from adjoining borders of contiguous vertebrae from the 12th thoracic to fifth lumbar and the intervening discs, and by tendinous arches between these slips. It enters the abdomen behind the medial arcuate ligament, which may be regarded as a thickening of the iliac fascia behind which the muscle lies.

Quadratus lumborum. This lies between middle and anterior layers of the lumbar fascia. It is attached to the iliolumbar ligament and posterior part of the iliac crest below, the lumbar transverse processes and the medial half of the lower border of the last rib. It is supplied by the 12th thoracic and upper four lumbar ventral rami and probably fixes the last rib, so increasing diaphragmatic efficiency. It is overlapped by the psoas major and, above, by the diaphragm.

Iliacus. This triangular muscle lies outside the iliac fascia, which separates it from extraperitoneal tissue; it fills the iliac fossa as it sweeps from a wide peripheral attachment to leave the abdomen lateral to the psoas behind the inguinal ligament.

The diaphragm

The diaphragm (Fig. 3.4), the main muscle of inspiration, is a domed sheet separating the thorax and abdomen. It is generally convex upwards but its central area is lower than the summits of the lateral areas or cupulae. Muscular slips arise from the back of the xiphisternum, the inner aspect of the lowest six ribs and cartilages, the medial and lateral arcuate ligaments and by the right and left crura from the anterolateral parts of the first three and first two lumbar vertebral bodies respectively. They converge on a thin trifoliate aponeurosis (central tendon) which is nearer the front than the back, lying immediately below the pericardium, with which it fuses.

The aortic aperture is strictly behind the diaphragm between the crura at the lower border of the 12th thoracic vertebral body and transmits the aorta, thoracic duct, descending lymphatic trunks and occasionally the azygos and hemiazygos veins. The oesophagus, vagi, sympathetic nerves and ascending branches of the left gastric vessels are transmitted by the oesophageal opening at the level of the 10th thoracic vertabra to the left and in front of the aorta. The oesophagus is attached to the diaphragm by elastic connective tissue.

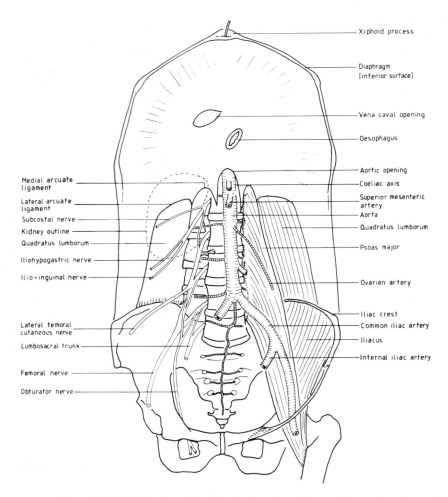

Fig. 3.4 View of the posterior wall of the abdomen and pelvis showing the relative positions of muscles, arteries and nerves.

Still higher lies the vena caval opening at the level of the eighth to ninth thoracic vertebra in the central tendon, the vein being·attached to its fibrous margins.

Other transmitted structures penetrate the crura (greater and lesser splanchnic nerves), lie behind the medial arcuate ligament (sympathetic trunk), or pass between sternal and costal origins (superior epigastric vessels).

Much of the lower diaphragmatic surface is covered with peritoneum and is related to the liver, gastric fundus and spleen. Part of the liver, oesophagus, kidneys and suprarenal glands are in direct contact, no peritoneum intervening. The upper surface is covered by the right and left pleural sacs with the pericardium between.

Peripheral sensory supply is from the lower six or seven intercostal nerves, the phrenic nerve (C3–5) being motor. Before expulsive efforts, deep inspiration with glottic closure allows the diaphragm to provide additional thrust.

The bowel in the abdomen

The abdominal portion of the oesophagus

Having pierced the diaphragm at the level of the 10th thoracic vertebra, the oesophagus lies in the upper part of the lesser omentum and passes forwards and to the left, lying in the oesophageal groove on the liver. Its anterior and left aspects are covered by peritoneum, which is reflected onto the diaphragm as part of the gastrophrenic ligament in which lie branches of the left gastric artery. The cardiac notch separates the left oesophageal margin from the gastric fundus but its right margin runs into the lesser curve, the oesophagus thus widening as it approaches the stomach. Vagal trunks lie on the front and back surfaces of the organ.

The stomach

A distensible muscular sac continuous with the oesophagus at the cardiac orifice proximally and with the duodenum at the pylorus, the stomach forms much of the anterior wall of the omental bursa. In front of it from right to left are the liver, abdominal wall and diaphragm. The organ is invested with peritoneum. This leaves it as the lesser omentum along its superomedial border or the lesser curve, which runs from the medial edge of the oesophagus above, to the upper border of the duodenum below and to the right. The opposite border is five times as long — the greater curve. Starting at the cardiac notch it passes upwards to outline the gastric fundus then runs along the body, pyloric antrum and pyloric canal to the lower border of the first part of the duodenum. Barium outlines the curvatures at radiography. Peritoneum from the posterior and anterior surfaces of the body and pyloric region leaves the stomach along the greater curvature, uniting to form the anterior leaf of the greater omentum. If the line of reflection is traced upwards to the left, it leaves the greater curve, passing to the back of the stomach and up to the cardia at the left border of the oesophagus. During its ascent, the double fold changes its name successively from the gastrosplenic ligament to the gastrophrenic ligament. The posterior aspect of the organ above and to the right of the line of reflection is part of the anterior wall of the omental bursa but the whole of the remainder is covered by peritoneum of the greater sac. This includes the posterior aspect of the stomach to the left of the attachment of the gastrosplenic ligament, which is related to the spleen, separated by a recess of the greater sac (Fig. 3.5).

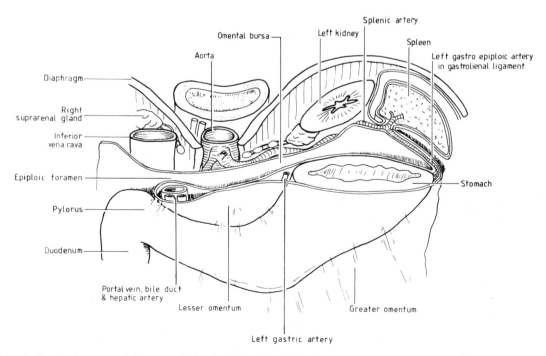

Fig. 3.5 A view of the upper abdomen at the level of the epiploic foramen to show the omental bursa in relation to surrounding structures.

Along the lines of attachment of the lesser and greater omentum run the right and left gastric and gastro-epiploic vessels respectively.

The stomach bed (Fig. 3.6). The omental bursa intervenes between the stomach and its bed except over a small triangular area near the oesophagus. Here it is in contact with diaphragm and the left suprarenal, the left gastric vessels passing forwards at its right margin to reach the lesser curve.

The remainder of the bed behind the posterior wall peritoneum of the lesser sac has the body of the pancreas running across it, with the diaphragm, left suprarenal and upper part of the left kidney above it. The splenic artery courses along the upper edge of the pancreas, whose lower border provides attachment to the transverse mesocolon and posterior leaf of the greater omentum, which separates the stomach from the duodenojejunal flexure and jejunum.

Arteries to the stomach from the coeliac trunk itself (left gastric), the common hepatic artery (right gastric and gastroepiploic) and the splenic artery (left gastroepiploic and short gastric), anastomose freely within and upon the organ. Veins, in general, follow the arteries, ending in the splenic, superior mesenteric and portal veins. Sympathetic nerves from the coeliac and hepatic plexuses together with parasympathetic vagal fibres provide innervation.

Small intestine

The small intestine occupies the greater sac below the transverse mesocolon, behind the greater omentum and usually between the ascending and descending colon. It wends a convoluted way from the pylorus to the ileocaecal opening, becoming slightly narrower as it does so, and is some 5 m long. Some loops fall into the pelvis and may be contained in an enterocele.

Duodenum (Figs 3.6 and 3.7). The proximal portion, the duodenum, has no mesentery and is

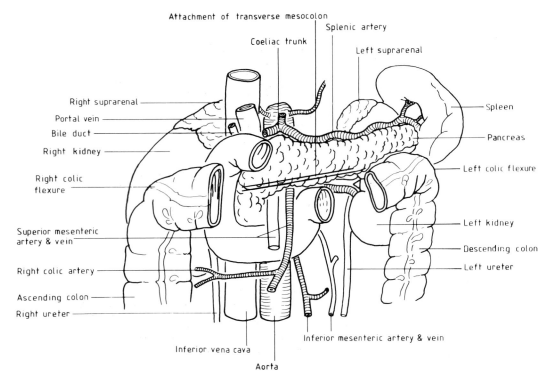

Fig. 3.6 Further view of the upper abdomen to show the relative positions of the pancreas, duodenum, spleen, kidneys and other important structures.

the shortest, widest and most fixed part, its C-shape embracing the head of the pancreas. Its first (superior) part, 5 cm long, runs upwards, backwards and to the right to the neck of the gall bladder. Anteriorly it is covered with peritoneum, separating it from the liver and gall bladder. The lesser omentum is attached to its upper border and the greater omentum to the lower border of its proximal half, making the peritoneal posterior surface of the duodenum at this point a part of the anterior wall of the omental bursa. More distally the duodenum forms the floor of the epiploic foramen and here the posterior surface has no peritoneum. Below and beneath it are the head and neck of the pancreas (Fig. 3.7) and behind it run the bile duct, portal vein and gastroduodenal artery.

The descending (second) part of the duodenum is twice as long as the first. It has medial to it the head of the pancreas and bile duct. This, having joined the main pancreatic duct, opens into the medial side of the second part halfway down it. Posteriorly the second part lies directly on the right kidney and renal vessels near the hilum and on the inferior vena cava, descending to the level of the lower part of the third lumbar vertebra to continue as the third or horizontal part. To its right is the right colic flexure, the transverse colon crossing it anteriorly, areolar tissue intervening. Above and below the colon the anterior surface is covered with peritoneum, separating it from the liver above, and the colon and coils of jejunum below.

The horizontal (third) part, again 10 cm long, passes slightly upwards from right to left to end in front of the aorta as the ascending part. It is covered anteriorly by peritoneum except near its end where the root of the mesentery and superior

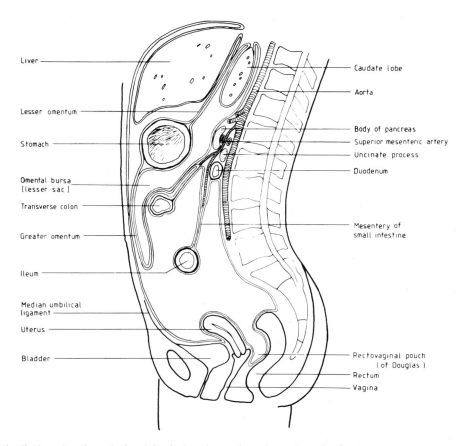

Fig. 3.7 Longitudinal section through the abdominal cavity to show the peritoneal reflections.

mesenteric vessels cross it. Above is the head of the pancreas, below are coils of the jejunum. Posteriorly it rests on the right ureter, psoas major, ovarian vessels, inferior vena cava and aorta at the origin of the inferior mesenteric artery.

The ascending (fourth) part, only 2.5 cm long, runs up alongside or upon the aorta to turn sharply forwards at the duodenojejunal junction immediately to the left of the root of the mesentery. Behind it lie the left sympathetic trunk, psoas major, left renal and left ovarian vessels and the inferior mesenteric vein. To its left are the kidney and ureter, above is the body of the pancreas. Anteriorly the transverse mesocolon hangs in front of it and must be lifted to reveal it.

Duodenal blood supply is from branches of the coeliac axis, venous drainage being to the splenic, superior mesenteric and portal veins, whilst the coeliac plexus provides the nerve supply.

Jejunum and ileum. The transition is gradual but, arbitrarily, the jejunum comprises three-fifths of the remaining small gut, the whole of which is invested with peritoneum. This leaves it along a mesenteric border as a double layer (the mesentery) which attaches the intestine to the posterior abdominal wall, its vessels, lymphatics and nerves running between the layers (Fig. 3.7). The jejunum is thicker and more vascular than the ileum and, when palpated between the finger and thumb, thick mucosal folds are felt. Its upper folds lie in front of the lower pole of the left kidney behind the transverse mesocolon. When traced distally the bowel becomes narrower, thinner and paler, mucosal folding no longer being felt. It hangs in coils into the pelvis, finally ascending in front of the right iliac vessels and psoas muscle to end by opening at the ileocaecal valve where the caecum and ascending colon meet.

In 2–3% of patients and from 20–100 cm proximal to that valve a Meckel's diverticulum (ileal diverticulum) occurs. Projecting from the antimesenteric border of the ileum as a blind pouch about 5 cm long, its end is usually free. A fibrous band (remains of the vitello-intestinal duct) may run from the tip to the umbilicus or, rarely, to another piece of the gut. Within the diverticulum may occur heterotopic gastric, jejunal or colonic mucosa and, very rarely, pancreatic tissue, but it is usually typical ileum.

Jejunal and ileal branches of the superior mesenteric artery are accompanied by autonomic nerves and tributaries of the superior mesenteric veins. At the root of the mesentery are found numerous lymph nodes.

The mesentery of the small intestine arises along an almost straight line, the root of the mesentery, which passes downwards and to the right from the duodenojejunal flexure to the upper part of the right sacroiliac joint, crossing successively the horizontal part of the duodenum, aorta, inferior vena cava, right ureter, right ovarian vessels and right psoas major. Short at either end, the mesentery is longest at its central part (about 20 cm) and is therefore fan shaped, its intestinal border being pleated at its attachment to the coils of jejunum and ileum. Between its two peritoneal surfaces lie the jejunal and ileal branches of the superior mesenteric artery, accompanying veins, nerve plexuses, lymphatics, mesenteric lymph nodes, connective tissue and fat. In the upper part, fat-free translucent areas adjoin the jejunum but the lower portion of the mesentery contains more fat and this extends from the root to intestinal border. At the gut attachment the peritoneal layers separate to invest the intestine (Fig. 3.7).

At the root of the mesentery the right peritoneal layer passes laterally to cover the ascending colon and at a higher level can be followed into the inferior layer of the transverse mesocolon, whilst the left peritoneal layer of the mesentery passes over the posterior abdominal wall to cover the descending colon.

The large intestine

The large intestine begins in the right iliac fossa as the caecum, runs up to the inferior surface of the right lobe of the liver lateral to the right kidney as the ascending colon before turning sharply to the left at the right colic flexure. The succeeding transverse colon is directed generally upwards and to the left, although, because of its mesocolon, it is mobile and is curved in two planes, being convex forwards and also downwards. The left colic flexure is tucked between the lower part of the spleen and tail of the pancreas above and in front of the diaphragm and left kidney, at a higher level

At the anterior extremity of the visceral surface a flattened impression is related to the left colic flexure and phrenicocolic ligament. Between it and the hilum the spleen may be in contact with the pancreas which lies in the lienorenal ligament. The splenic surfaces are separated by a superior border, notched and slightly convex, the rounder inferior border, a blunt posterior end and a sharper anterior margin.

Except at the hilum the organ is invested with peritoneum of the greater sac which fuses with its capsule. The spleen has developed as a protrusion to the left from the original dorsal mesogastrium, expanding the left-hand leaf of that two-leaved structure to invest it.

The double fold in the adult forms the left-hand boundary of the omental bursa, separating it from the left subdiaphragmatic recess of the greater sac. Its two layers are peritoneum of the lesser and greater sacs respectively. Confusingly, that part posterior to the spleen, carrying splenic vessels and the terminal pancreas, is called the lienorenal ligament. That between the spleen and stomach, carrying the short gastric and left gastroepiploic vessels, is the gastrosplenic ligament. Above the

spleen the same structure is the gastrophrenic ligament. Below the spleen the two layers continue along the left wall of the lesser sac as the gastrocolic ligament to run into the left margin of the greater omentum.

The liver (Fig. 3.10)

Firm to the touch, this red-brown wedge-shaped organ weighs about 1.5 kg, is very vascular and easily lacerated. It occupies the right hypochondrium, much of the epigastrium and the left hypochondrium to the left lateral line.

An inferior (visceral) surface is separated from the anterior aspect of the liver by the sharp inferior border. This becomes rounded when traced to the right, to separate the visceral surface from its lateral aspect. The notch for the ligamentum teres is just to the right of the midline, a second notch 4–5 cm further right indicating the fundus of the gall bladder.

To the right of the gall bladder the inferior border follows the costal margin. Traced to the left it crosses the epigastrium to the tip of the left eighth costal cartilage, thereafter ascending sharply to

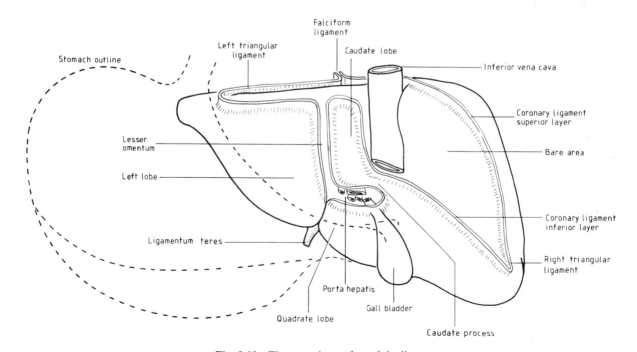

Fig. 3.10 The posterior surface of the liver.

merge into the thin left margin. This separates the superior and visceral surfaces of the left lobe.

A diaphragmatic surface is formed by the superior, anterior and lateral aspects of the liver between which are no definable borders.

A posterior surface is also recognised, though the peritoneum-covered right extremity of this is best included with the diaphragmatic surface with which it is continuous.

The diaphragmatic surface. The superior aspect follows the under surface of the diaphragm closely; it separates the convex right and left portions from the corresponding pleura and lung. Between these the pericardium and ventricles cause a shallow cardiac impression. Except for a small triangular area where the layers of the falciform ligament diverge, the whole aspect is covered with peritoneum which is continued into that which covers the anterior aspect.

Triangular in shape, most of the anterior aspect is in contact with the diaphragm which separates it from the pleura and ribs 6–10 with cartilages on the right and cartilages of ribs 7 and 8 on the left. In the midline are the xiphoid and anterior abdominal wall.

The lateral (right) aspect of the diaphragmatic surface is also covered with peritoneum. The diaphragm separates it from the lung and pleura in its upper third, the pleura of the costodiaphragmatic recess in the middle third and costal arches below this. Continuity of the diaphragmatic surface is completed by the peritoneum-covered part of the posterior surface which lies to the right of the bare area.

The posterior surface is moulded over the forward convexity of the vertebral column, is wide and convex to the right, narrow on the left. The inferior vena cava occupies a groove (or tunnel) in which it is joined by the hepatic veins, the groove being the medial border of a triangular area (the bare area) free of peritoneum. Its other boundaries are the upper and lower layers of the coronary ligament. It is attached to the diaphragm by areolar tissue and its lowest part lies in front of the right suprarenal gland and upper pole of the right kidney.

To the left of the groove for the inferior vena cava the peritoneum invests the caudate lobe which projects to the left into the upper recess of the omental bursa, its inferior surface (the caudate process) forming the roof of the epiploic foramen and its anterior surface the posterior wall of the fissure for the ligamentum venosum. This deep fissure contains the two layers of the lesser omentum and separates the caudate lobe from the left lobe proper.

The remainder of the surface is covered by peritoneum and is related to the oesophagus and fundus of the stomach. The visceral (inferior) surface, directed downwards, backwards and to the left, is covered with peritoneum except at the porta hepatis, fossa for the gall bladder and fissure for the ligamentum teres. This, the obliterated left umbilical vein of the fetus, runs from the notch in the inferior border of liver to the left end of the porta hepatis. It there joins the left branch of the portal vein opposite the attachment of ligamentum venosum. From its notch the ligamentum teres runs to the umbilicus in the free margin of the falciform ligament.

To the right of the fissure for the ligamentum teres lies the quadrate lobe bounded on the right by the fossa for the gall bladder. The pylorus and first part of the duodenum are related to the anterior part of the quadrate lobe, the free border of the lesser omentum and its contained structures to the posterior part. To the left of the lobe the visceral surface is in contact with the stomach and lesser omentum and merges into the gastric and oesophageal impressions of the posterior surface. To the right of the gall bladder fossa near the inferior border, the visceral surface is related to the right colic flexure whilst the right kidney and suprarenal gland lie posteriorly, their upper portions extending above the reflection onto the kidney of the lower layer of the coronary ligament. Between the colon and kidney lies the duodenum, which produces its impression on the liver.

The accurate demarcation of hepatic lobes and segments is important to those planning resection and is based on the distribution of hepatic ducts (accompanied by hepatic artery branches and portal vein tributaries). Unfortunately the hepatic venous tributaries are at variance with these. The gynaecologist in describing the external features of the organ is content with the demarcation into lobes by the attachment of the falciform fold and the fissures for the ligamentum teres and ligamentum venosum.

The gall bladder lies in its fossa on the visceral surface of the liver, its fundus projecting just below the inferior border. It passes backwards across the first part of the duodenum to the porta hepatis as the cystic duct, there joining the hepatic duct to form the common bile duct. Separated from its bed by connective tissue, the organ is elsewhere covered with peritoneum and is in relation to the transverse colon.

The common bile duct lies in the right free margin of the lesser omentum with the hepatic artery and portal vein. It then passes behind the first part of the duodenum, between the second part and head of the pancreas, is joined by the pancreatic duct and opens on a papilla halfway down the posteromedial aspect of the second part of the duodenum.

Peritoneal arrangements

The general peritoneal cavity (greater sac)

This potential space, lined with moistened mesothelium, allows abdominal and pelvic organs to adjust their relative positions during respiration, peristalsis, filling and emptying. It is converted to an actual space at laparotomy by a pneumoperitoneum or by ascites. Though divided by convention into parietal and visceral components, the peritoneum forms a continuous sheet. This is reflected from the parieties directly on to a viscus, e.g. the anterior abdominal wall to the bladder, the diaphragm to the upper aspect of the liver, the margins of the ascending and descending colon to the posterior wall. Elsewhere, the peritoneum is reflected from a line of attachment on the abdominal wall as a double fold or mesentery between whose layers vessels and nerves travel before they separate to invest the viscus (e.g. the mesentery of the small bowel, transverse mesocolon or broad ligament) (Figs 3.7 and 3.11).

Visceral peritoneum fuses with the connective tissue of the invested organ. Parietal peritoneum is more loosely attached to the abdominal wall by extraperitoneal connective tissue except along the linea alba and under the diaphragm where the at-

tachment is firm. Extraperitoneal connective tissue may contain fat, especially near the kidneys.

The general configuration of the greater sac is best understood if one starts at the attachment of the transverse mesocolon along the anterior border of the pancreas. This line, the ascending colon and the descending colon, outline a posteroinferior part of the space, largely occupied by loops of the small bowel. It extends into the pelvis in front of the sacral promontory, is crossed obliquely by the root of the mesentery and communicates on either side in front of the colon with the paracolic gutters.

Lateral to the ascending and descending colon are the right and left paracolic gutters, which also communicate freely below with the pelvic cavity. When traced upwards each continues into a subdiaphragmatic space bounded above by peritoneum of the under surface of the diaphragm. The right is made irregular in shape by the protrusion of the right lobe of the liver, that on the left is similarly modified by the presence of the spleen.

It can be seen that malignant cells or pus can spread readily from the pelvis to the upper abdomen and subdiaphragmatic spaces.

The remaining greater sac lies above and in front of the greater omentum, stomach, lesser omentum and liver. Its upper portion is divided into unequal parts by the falciform ligament. This double fold runs from the liver forwards to the left to a midline attachment from the umbilicus as far as the undersurface of the diaphragm.

Its free lower border carries the obliterated left umbilical vein (ligamentum teres) and at its upper end the layers separate. On either side of the falciform fold the upper anterior part of the general peritoneal cavity communicates freely with the corresponding subdiaphragmatic space. Below, it runs into the posteroinferior part at the lower free border of the greater omentum.

The greater omentum contains much fat and hangs like an apron in front of the transverse colon and small bowel. It has, in theory, an anterior and a posterior leaf which become continuous along its inferior right and left lateral free borders, being separated between by a downward extension of the omental bursa. Each leaf has an outer layer of greater sac peritoneum and an inner layer which

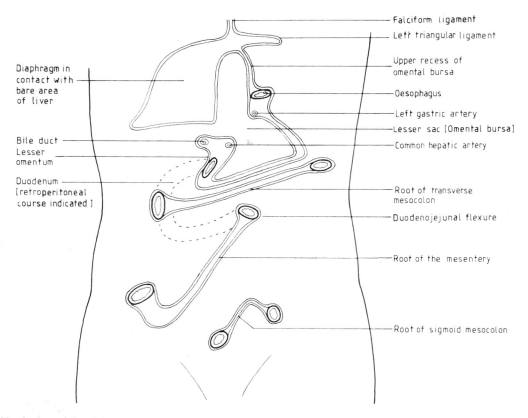

Fig. 3.11   A view of the abdomen to show the reflections of the peritoneum from the posterior abdominal wall.

lines the lesser sac. The layers of the anterior leaf are attached to the stomach and diverge to cover it. The left margin is continuous with the gastrocolic ligament. When traced upwards the layers of the posterior leaf diverge just above the root of the transverse mesocolon — the inner continuing upwards over the stomach bed, the outer passing downwards, soon to be again reflected forwards as the upper layer of the transverse mesocolon.

In practice, the extension of the lesser sac between the leaves is minimal, the layers are observed only where they diverge and the posterior leaf is usually attached to the transverse colon and the upper surface of its mesocolon along an avascular plane of cleavage.

The omental bursa (lesser sac) (Fig. 3.5)

This potential space lined with peritoneum lies behind the lesser omentum, posterior wall of the stomach and anterior leaf of the greater omentum where it leaves the stomach. Traced downwards this leaf turns at the free margin of the greater omentum to run upwards as the posterior leaf in front of the small intestine and transverse colon. It then adheres to the upper surface of the transverse mesocolon and at its root the layers of the posterior leaf of the omentum separate. The lower leaf is reflected forwards immediately as the upper layer of transverse mesocolon whilst the upper leaf turns upwards onto the anterosuperior pancreatic surface as the posterior wall of the omental bursa. The continuity of the omental bursa is completed by reflection forwards of this peritoneum to make the posterior layer of the lesser omentum, so leading the peritoneum back to the posterior wall of stomach.

To its left the space is closed below by fusion of the anterior and posterior leaves of the greater omentum and at a higher level by the confusingly named gastrocolic, gastrosplenic, lienorenal and gastrophrenic ligaments.

The right side is also closed below by the continuity of the anterior and posterior leaves of the greater omentum at its right border, higher up by reflection backwards of the peritoneum from the back of the first part of the duodenum and higher still by reflection of the peritoneum from the liver onto the posterior abdominal wall.

Between the duodenal and hepatic reflections is the aditus to the omental bursa (epiploic foramen), its only communication with the greater sac. This slit lies behind the right free margin of the lesser omentum (with its contained portal vein, hepatic artery and bile duct) above the fixed portion of the first part of the duodenum, below the caudate process of the liver and in front of the inferior vena cava. At the epiploic foramen the peritoneum of the greater and lesser sacs becomes continuous. The caudate lobe of the liver projects into the right-hand border of the space and is almost completely invested with peritoneum of this superior recess of the lesser sac.

Abdominal blood supply

The aorta (Fig. 3.12)

This enters the abdomen behind the diaphragm, between its crura, in front of the 12th thoracic vertebra. It runs slightly to the left in front of the first four lumbar vertebral bodies to the end of the midline by dividing into the common iliac arteries.

From above downwards it lies behind the omental bursa, the body of the pancreas, the splenic vein, the left renal vein, the third part of duodenum, the root of the mesentery and the peritoneum of the greater sac. To its right are the inferior vena cava and sympathetic trunk, to the left the sympathetic trunk.

Three groups of branches are described, in addition to the terminal divisions. They may be dorsal, lateral or ventral (Table 3.1).

Posterior branches. These supply the diaphragm (inferior phrenic arteries), muscles of the back and abdominal wall (lumbar arteries) and the front of the sacrum and back of the rectum (median sacral artery). The lumbar and median sacral branch to supply the vertebrae, vertebral canal and nerves therein.

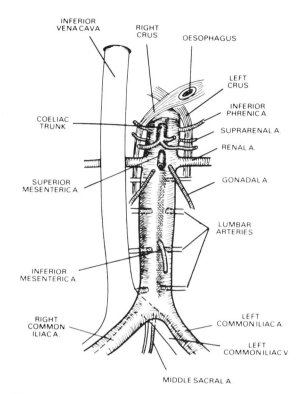

Fig. 3.12 The aorta and its branches. (Reproduced with permission from Professor J. Joseph and Macmillan Press.)

Table 3.1 Branches of the aorta

Group	Name	Structures supplied
Dorsal	Lumbar	Muscles, nerves, vertebrae
	Median sacral	Nerves, sacrum
Lateral	Inferior phrenic	Diaphragm
	Middle suprarenal	Suprarenal
	Renal	Kidney, ureter
	Ovarian	Ovary, tube, uterus, ureter
Ventral	Coeliac trunk	Oesophagus, stomach, duodenum, liver, gallbladder, pancreas, spleen, ureter
	Superior mesenteric	Bowel to transverse colon
	Inferior mesenteric	Bowel from transverse colon to rectum

Lateral branches. The middle suprarenal arteries are small and arise near the superior mesenteric artery, the right passing behind the inferior vena cava.

The renal arteries arise immediately below the superior mesenteric. The right passes behind the inferior vena cava, the right renal vein, the head of the pancreas and the descending part of the duodenum. The left lies behind the left renal vein, pancreas, splenic vein and inferior mesenteric vein.

The ovarian arteries. The ovarian arteries arise anterolaterally just below the renal, running retroperitoneally to leave the abdomen by crossing the common or external iliac artery in the infundibulopelvic fold. They cross the corresponding ureter and may supply twigs to it but have no other abdominal branches. The right artery crosses the inferior vena cava and is crossed by the middle colic vessels, the caecal, terminal ileal and ileocolic veins. The left is crossed by the left colic and sigmoid branches of the inferior mesenteric vessels and the descending colon. Lymphatics and veins accompany the arteries, the left vein ending in the left renal vein and the right in the inferior vena cava.

Ventral branches. The coeliac trunk arises just below the aortic opening, behind the lesser sac and juts forward for 1 cm just above the pancreas and splenic vein, surrounded by the coeliac plexus. It divides into the left gastric, common hepatic and splenic arteries.

The left gastric artery is small, runs upwards and to the left in front of the suprarenal gland, supplies the oesophageal and cardiac branches and curves forward lateral to the lesser sac to run along the lesser curve between the layers of the lesser omentum to anastomose with the right gastric artery.

The common hepatic artery is larger, passing below the epiploic foramen above the first part of the duodenum where it gives off the right gastric artery. Just above or behind the duodenum arises the gastroduodenal artery, which passes downwards to the right of the peritoneal reflection from the back of the duodenum, at the lower margin of which it supplies a branch for the head of the pancreas, bile duct and descending part of the duodenum. Its larger terminal branch, the right gastroepiploic artery, runs about 1 cm from the greater curve between the layers of the anterior leaf of the greater omentum. It supplies the omen-

tum and stomach and anastomoses with the left gastroepiploic.

The main vessel, now the hepatic artery proper, crosses in front of the portal vein to run in the free margin of the lesser omentum to the left of the bile duct. In the porta hepatis arise terminal right and left branches. From the former, the cystic artery arises, although its origin and course are variable.

The largest terminal branch of the coeliac trunk, the splenic artery, is invested by the splenic plexus, is tortuous and lies above its vein. Running behind the lesser sac along the upper border of the pancreas, it crosses the left suprarenal and kidney, enters the lienorenal ligament and ends in five segmental branches at the splenic hilum. It supplies pancreatic branches, five or six short gastric arteries which run in the gastrosplenic ligament, a posterior gastric branch in the gastrophrenic fold and the left gastroepiploic artery, a large branch which runs near the greater curve to anastomose with the right vessel. It gives off large tortuous branches to the greater omentum.

Superior mesenteric artery (Fig. 3.13). This arises 1 cm below the coeliac trunk, behind the body of the pancreas and splenic vein. It crosses in front of the left renal vein, which separates it from the aorta. Passing down and forwards in front of the uncinate process and the horizontal part of the duodenum, it curves downwards to the right near the root of the mesentery, in front of the psoas and crossing in turn the inferior vena cava and right ureter. It is surrounded by the superior mesenteric plexus and its vein lies to its right. It ends by anastomosing with the ileal branch of the ileocolic artery.

Its first branch, the inferior pancreaticoduodenal, passes upwards to the right. Just below the pancreas the middle colic artery springs from the front of the superior mesenteric, runs in the transverse mesocolon and ends in arches 3–4 cm from the colon by anastomosing with the right and left colic arteries. This last is a branch of the inferior mesenteric artery.

The right colic artery arises separately halfway down the superior mesenteric or from a common stem with the ileocolic and runs to the right. Ascending and descending branches are formed

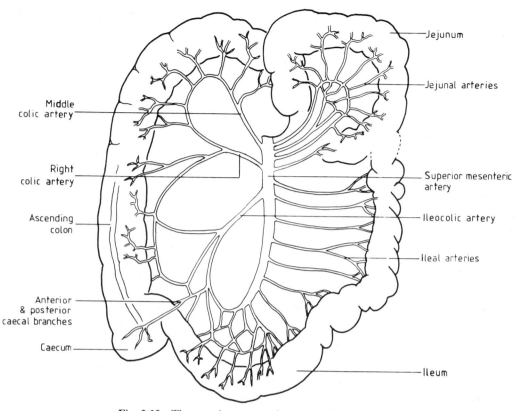

Fig. 3.13 The superior mesenteric artery and its branches.

which anastomose with the middle colic and ileocolic respectively, arches being formed from which blood reaches the colon.

The lowest branch from the right side of the superior mesenteric, the ileocolic artery, runs across the right ureter, ovarian vessels and psoas to the right iliac fossa. There, a superior branch anastomoses with the right colic whilst an inferior branch runs to the ileocaecal junction. It gives the ascending colic, anterior and posterior caecal, and appendicular branches, then ends as an ileal branch which follows the ileum to anastomose with the end of the superior mesenteric trunk itself. The appendicular artery runs behind the terminal ileum in the free border of the meso-appendix, making contact with the appendix towards its tip. A recurrent branch anastomoses with a branch of the posterior caecal artery near the base of the appendix.

From the left side of the superior mesenteric spring 12–15 branches which run parallel to one another in the mesentery. Each divides into two, which form arcades with neighbouring branches. Further series of arches are formed from branches of the first, up to six arcades being found where the mesentery is longest. Straight arteries from the terminal arcade supply the gut, jejunal straight arteries being longer and less numerous than ileal ones.

Inferior mesenteric artery (Fig. 3.12). Smaller than the superior mesenteric, this arises just behind the lower border of the horizontal part of the duodenum 4 cm above the aortic bifurcation. Lying retroperitoneally it lies in front of then to the left of the aorta, descending to cross the left common iliac artery medial to the ureter, so entering the pelvis in the sigmoid mesocolon as the superior rectal artery.

In the abdomen it gives off the left colic artery. This runs upwards to the left, behind the peritoneum in front of the psoas, ureter and ovarian vessels. It divides into an ascending branch, which crosses the left kidney and enters the transverse mesocolon, and a descending branch, which anastomoses with the highest sigmoid artery.

The sigmoid (inferior left colic) arteries, three in number, run downwards to the left, forming a marginal artery as they supply descending and sigmoid colon. They anastomose above with the left colic and below with the superior rectal artery. The superior rectal artery anastomoses with the middle rectal from the internal iliac and the inferior rectal from the internal pudendal artery.

Common iliac arteries (Fig. 3.4). From their origin at the left side of the fourth lumbar vertebral body, the common iliac arteries run towards a point midway between the anterior superior iliac spine and symphysis pubis. They end anterior to the sacroiliac joint at the level of the lumbosacral intervertebral disc by dividing into internal and external iliac arteries, the latter continuing the line of the parent vessel.

The right common iliac (5 cm long) is 1 cm longer than the left. Lying retroperitoneally, crossed by fibres of the superior hypogastric plexus and at its termination by the ureter, it passes across the fifth lumbar body, the sympathetic trunk and the union of the common iliac veins intervening. Laterally the right common iliac vein and inferior vena cava separate the vessel from the psoas major. Deep to this muscle, between it and the fifth lumbar body, the lumbosacral trunk, obturator nerve and iliolumbar artery are posterior relations.

The anterior relations of the left artery are similar but in addition it is crossed by the superior rectal vessels. Its vein is medial to and partly behind the artery. Laterally lies the psoas and the deep posterior relations are similar to those of the right. Branches supply the areolar tissue and structures with which they are in contact, including the ureter.

The external iliac artery becomes the femoral artery as it enters the thigh beneath the inguinal ligament. It lies, with lymph nodes anteriorly and on both sides, on the medial border of the psoas major, the bulk of which lies lateral to the vessel.

The corresponding vein is medial to its lower part and partly behind its upper part. In front and medially it is covered by peritoneum and extraperitoneal tissue, being crossed near its origin by the ovarian vessels and near its end by the genital branch of the genitofemoral nerve, the deep circumflex iliac vein and the round ligament.

In addition to small branches to the lymph nodes and psoas, there are two main branches, the inferior epigastric and deep circumflex iliac, which arise immediately above the inguinal ligament from its anterior and lateral aspects respectively. The former passes forwards, upwards and medially, passing below and medial to the deep inguinal ring, pierces the transversalis fascia to run upwards behind the rectus muscle in its sheath to anastomose with the superior epigastric and lower posterior intercostal branches. It has a pubic branch which enters the pelvis to anastomose with the obturator artery, this branch occasionally being very large and sometimes replacing the obturator artery. The deep circumflex iliac runs upwards and laterally to the anterior superior iliac spine.

Blood supply of the pelvis (Fig. 3.14)

The internal iliac artery (4 cm long) ends at the upper margin of the greater sciatic foramen by dividing into a posterior and an anterior trunk. The former passes backwards, gives an ascending

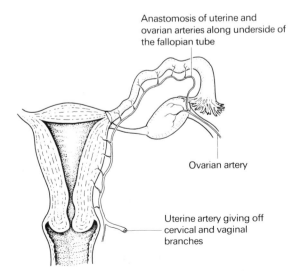

Anastomosis of uterine and ovarian arteries along underside of the fallopian tube

Ovarian artery

Uterine artery giving off cervical and vaginal branches

Fig. 3.14 The divisions of the anterior branch of the internal iliac artery and the ovarian artery in the pelvis.

branch (iliolumbar), the superior and inferior lateral sacral and the superior gluteal artery, which runs to the buttock above the pyriformis. The anterior trunk continues the line of the main vessel towards the ischial spine and provides visceral branches as follows:

The superior vesical artery supplies the lower ureter and upper bladder then continues as the obliterated umbilical artery to the umbilicus.

The inferior vesical artery often arises with the middle rectal, supplying the ureter and bladder base.

The middle rectal artery supplies muscle of the lower rectum, anastomosing with the superior and inferior rectal arteries.

Vaginal arteries may also arise direct from the anterior trunk.

The uterine artery runs medially on the levator ani and above the transverse cervical condensation above and in front of the ureter and above the lateral vaginal fornix. Having supplied the ureteric and vaginal branches it runs up the side of the uterus in the broad ligament supplying the uterus and anastomoses with the ovarian artery.

The parietal branches of the anterior trunk are, from above down, the obturator, internal pudendal and inferior gluteal. The obturator runs with its nerve above and vein below to the obturator canal and its anastomosis with the pubic branch of the inferior epigastric is important surgically. This may be a large vessel and can run lateral to, across or medial to the femoral canal.

External iliac veins. The right iliac vein is first medial to its artery at the inguinal ligament then behind it, medial to the psoas major. The left vein is entirely medial to its artery. Each ends in front of the sacroiliac joint by uniting with the internal vein iliac to form the common iliac. Tributaries are the inferior epigastric and deep circumflex iliac. A pubic branch connects the external iliac and obturator veins accompanying the pubic branches of the inferior epigastric artery and, like it, may replace the normal obturator vein.

Internal iliac vein. Formed by confluence of veins behind and medial to its artery, the tributaries of this vein correspond with branches of the artery, though the iliolumbar vein usually enters the common iliac direct.

Common iliac veins. These begin by union of the external and internal iliac veins and join to

form the inferior vena cava to the right of the fifth lumbar vertebra. The shorter right vein ascends vertically behind then lateral to its artery, the right obturator nerve crossing obliquely behind it. The left vein, longer and more oblique, is first medial to its artery then behind the right common iliac artery, being crossed by the root of the sigmoid mesocolon and superior rectal vessels. It receives the iliolumbar, lateral sacral and median sacral veins. Very rarely the left common iliac vein may ascend to the left of the aorta as high as the kidney, receive the left renal vein and cross in front of the aorta to join the inferior vena cava.

The inferior vena cava (Fig. 3.15). Formed behind the right common iliac artery by union of the common iliac veins, it runs upwards to the right of the aorta. Having received renal veins it passes forward to the inferior caval opening in the diaphragm.

Behind it are the three lowest lumbar vertebrae, the right psoas major and sympathetic trunk. The right renal, middle suprarenal, and inferior phrenic arteries cross behind it and the lumbar arteries pass behind the medial border. Higher up,

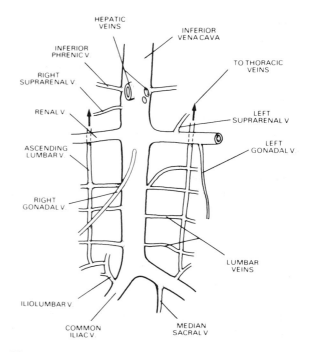

Fig. 3.15 The inferior vena cava and its branches. (Reproduced with permission from Professor J. Joseph and Macmillan Press.)

the coeliac ganglion and right suprarenal gland separate it from the right crus.

Its lowest part is retroperitoneal, being crossed by the root of the mesentery, iliolumbar, ovarian and right colic vessels. Passing behind the third part of the duodenum, it lies behind the head of the pancreas and splenic vein at the origin of the portal vein. This vessel and the bile duct lie between it and the first part of the duodenum. The vena cava is next covered anteriorly by peritoneum of the posterior wall of the lesser sac at the aditus, this opening separating it from the free edge of the lesser omentum and its contents. Still ascending, the vessel occupies its groove on the liver, through the floor of which it receives hepatic veins.

To its right at some distance are the ureter, the descending part of duodenum, the medial border of kidney and the right lobe of liver. On its left, below is the aorta, above are the right crus of the diaphragm and the caudate lobe of the liver.

Numerous lumbar and inferior phrenic tributaries are received but the main branches are the right ovarian, right and left renal, right suprarenal and hepatic. The left suprarenal drains to the left renal vein, as also does the left ovarian vein.

Azygos vein. At or below the level of the renal vein the lumbar azygos springs from the back of the inferior vena cava, ascends in front of the vertebrae and enters the thorax through, behind or medial to the right crus. In the aortic opening it has the cisterna chyli to its left. It is joined by a large vessel formed by the union of the ascending lumbar and subcostal vein then passes upwards to end in the superior vena cava above the roof of the right lung.

The hemiazygos vein begins similarly on the left side and joins the azygos vein by crossing at the eighth thoracic body.

External and internal vertebral venous plexuses complete a rich intercommunicating network, posteriorly along which emboli or clumps of tumour cells may travel.

The hepatic portal system

Venous drainage from the spleen, pancreas, gall bladder and gut from the lower oesophagus to the rectum is to the liver by the portal vein. Permeating the sinusoids it then leaves by the hepatic veins to enter the inferior vena cava.

The portal vein

The portal vein is 8 cm long and starts in front of the inferior vena cava, behind the neck of the pancreas at the second lumbar vertebral level by union of the splenic and superior mesenteric veins. It passes upwards slightly to the right behind the first part of the duodenum, bile duct and gastroduodenal artery, then in the right free border of the lesser omentum in front of the epiploic foramen to the right end of the porta hepatis where its right branch receives the cystic vein. The longer left branch supplies the caudate and quadrate lobes before it finally enters the left lobe. Just before its entry it is joined anteriorly by the ligamentum teres (obliterated left umbilical vein) and is connected to the vena cava by the ligamentum venosum (obliterated ductus venosus).

The splenic vein

Straighter than its artery, the vein runs below it behind the pancreas in front of the left renal hilum, the renal vein separating it from the sympathetic trunk, crus of the diaphragm and abdominal aorta. The superior mesenteric artery runs down between the splenic and renal veins in front of the aorta. The splenic tributaries are the splenic, pancreatic, short gastric and left gastroepiploic and the inferior mesenteric, which runs behind or above the duodenojejunal flexure to enter it behind the pancreas.

Inferior mesenteric vein. This lies to the left of its artery and may run in the free edge of a paraduodenal fold, where such exists.

Superior mesenteric vein. Starting by union of appendicular, caecal and ileal branches, this lies to the right of its artery having similar relations and ends at the origin of the portal vein. Its tributaries correspond to the arterial branches plus the right gastroepiploic and pancreaticoduodenal veins.

Portal and systemic communication. This is as follows: (1) lower oesophagus; (2) anal canal and rectum; (3) umbilicus — along ligamentum teres;

(4) retroperitoneally — lumbar veins with veins which leave the colon posteriorly.

Abdominal lymphatics

Cisterna chyli

The cisterna chyli, when present, is a saccular dilatation 5–7 cm long in front of the first two lumbar vertebral bodies to the right of the aorta and to the left of the azygos vein. It lies behind the edge of the right crus. It is joined by the right and left lumbar trunks from the lateral aortic nodes and by an intestinal trunk. Lumbar trunks drain the lower limbs, walls of the pelvis and deep abdomen, pelvic viscera, kidneys, suprarenal and spleen. The intestinal trunk receives from the gut, pancreas, spleen and lower anterior parts of the liver. At the lower border of the 12th thoracic body the thoracic duct begins and is joined by descending branches from the lower thorax.

The lymph nodes of the abdomen

Lumbar lymph nodes (Fig. 3.16)

Preaortic nodes correspond to the ventral branches of the aorta and may be grouped according to the related artery, further nodes being found along its peripheral course, e.g. the colon has very small epicolic, more numerous paracolic nodes near the border of the gut, intermediate nodes along the right, middle, left colic and sigmoid vessels and, finally, terminal nodes near the main arterial trunks.

Lateral aortic nodes cluster round lateral and dorsal aortic branches, some outlying members becoming retroaortic. They drain by the lumbar trunk of each side.

Traced downwards, the lateral aortic nodes continue as four to six common iliac nodes on each side. They lie lateral and medial to and in front of the artery, the lateral chain being the most important. This contrasts with the 8–10 nodes along the external iliac artery where the medial group is the most important, lateral and anterior groups being present also.

Inferior epigastric and circumflex iliac nodes are outlying members of the external iliac group.

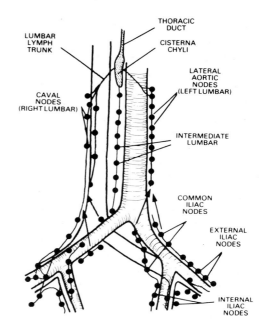

Fig. 3.16 Lymphatic nodes and vessels of the lateral pelvic wall and posterior abdomen. (Reproduced with permission from Professor J. Joseph and Macmillan Press.)

Finally, the internal iliac group is in relation with that artery having outlying sacral, gluteal and obturator nodes.

Lymph drainage of individual organs

Ureter:
Renal or lateral aortic nodes
Common iliac nodes
Internal and external iliac nodes.

Bladder:
External iliac nodes.

Urethra:
Internal iliac nodes.

Ovaries:
Along vessels to lateral aortic and preaortic nodes.

Tube and fundus uteri:
Mainly with ovaries:
 With round ligament to superficial inguinal nodes
 Some to external iliac nodes.

Lower body of uterus:
Mainly with cervix
External iliac nodes.

Cervix uteri:
Parametrial:
  External iliac nodes
  Internal iliac nodes
  Rectal and sacral nodes
  Occasionally obturator nodes.

Liver:
Deep drainage:
  Nodes around inferior vena cava
  Nodes around hepatic artery
Superficial:
  Nodes around inferior vena cava
  Nodes at porta hepatis
  Coeliac nodes
  Paracardiac nodes near the oesophageal
  opening.

Vagina:
Highest portion — with cervix
Middle — internal iliac nodes
Lowest, i.e. below hymen — with vulva and
perineum.

Abdominal wall:
Superficial:
  Below a line upwards and laterally from the
  umbilicus — superficial vaginal nodes
  Above this line — axillary and parasternal
Deep:
Follow lumbar arteries to lateral aortic nodes
Upper anterior — superior epigastric arteries to
parasternal nodes
Lower anterior — along the appropriate artery
to external iliac nodes.

Autonomic nerve supply of the abdominal and pelvic organs

The sympathetic supply is from the thoracolumbar
outflow relays in ganglia at a distance from the effector (e.g. ganglia of the sympathetic trunk).
Terminals release noradrenalin. Adrenergic postganglionic effectors in the gut and urogenital
tract are controlled by sympathetic preganglionic
efferents. Parasympathetic cranial outflow in the
vagus is distributed as far as the left side of the

transverse colon, ganglia being near to or in
the wall of the viscera and terminals, producing
acetylcholine. The sacral outflow S2–S5 supplies the remaining gut, bladder, generative organs
and pelvic blood vessels.

In general the parasympathetic nervous action
increases glandular and peristaltic action, the
sympathetic action contracting sphincters and les-
sening peristalsis. In the bladder the sympathetic
has no motor function, affecting only blood vessels
of the organ.

Lumbar sympathetic trunk

This continues on each side of the thoracic trunk,
passing down behind the medial arcuate ligament
along the medial border of the psoas anterolateral
to the vertebral bodies in front of the lumbar vessels and behind the inferior vena cava on the right.
The trunks pass behind the common iliac vessels
to run medial to the anterior sacral foramina before
meeting in front of the coccyx. There are four
ganglia which receive white rami from the lumbar
loci L1 to L3 and give grey rami to all lumbar
nerves.

From the ganglia arise four lumbar splanchnic
nerves — the upper two joining the plexuses round
the aorta and its named branches along which they
are distributed, others passing in front of and
behind the common iliac vessels to the superior
hypogastric plexus.

The splanchnic nerves

In addition to the lumbar splanchnic nerves there
are three which arise from the thoracic trunk
and descend to the plexuses around the upper abdominal aorta. They are the greater (thoracic ganglia T5–T10), lesser (thoracic ganglia
T9 + T10 or T10 + T11) and lowest splanchnic
nerves (last thoracic ganglion, T12).

The abdominal autonomic plexuses (Fig. 3.17)

1. Coeliac. A dense network surrounding the
coeliac and superior mesenteric origins and distributed along their branches by correspondingly
named secondary plexuses. It receives the greater
and lesser splanchnic and branches from the vagus
and phrenic nerves and is densest laterally (coeliac

cupied by a single fluid-filled cavity containing a serous albuminous fluid rich in oestrogen, the liquor folliculi. The follicle epithelial cells, several layers thick, lining the cavity are known from their appearance as the granulosa cells. Those immediately surrounding the zona pellucida are called the corona radiata from their radial arrangement, and the small mound of cells covering the ovum and projecting into the cavity, the cumulus ovaricus. The stroma cells immediately surrounding the follicle differentiate into an internal covering layer with a rich capillary network, the theca interna, and an outer more fibrous layer, the theca externa. About midcycle, 14 days before the next menstruation, ovulation takes place. The ovum, the zona pellucida and surrounding granulosa cells become detached and are extruded into the peritoneal cavity near to the fimbrial end of the tube due to rupture of the follicle. Following ovulation the follicle collapses, the granulosa cells enlarge and multiply taking on a yellow pigment, lutein, and fatty material, to form the corpus luteum (Fig. 3.20). The granulosa–lutein cells become arranged in pleats or folds surrounding a cavity containing a clotted mass into which oozing of blood takes place. On the outside the theca interna forms similar theca–lutein cells, and disappearance of the basement membrane brings them and their blood vessels into intimate contact with the granulosa–lutein cells. Ingrowing fibroblasts organise the internal clot. In the event of

fertilisation and embedding of the ovum the corpus luteum continues to grow until it is 2–3 cm in diameter. It is known as a corpus luteum of pregnancy and although it persists as a grey body for about 6 months, it gradually ceases to function after 3 months. If fertilisation does not take place the corpus luteum of menstruation remains about 15 mm in diameter. It functions for rather less than 2 weeks before some bleeding takes place inside, the lutein cells degenerate and connective tissue replaces it, forming a pale corpus albicans.

In the course of normal sexual activity only about 400 follicles go through the cycle described above. The vast majority of primordial follicles degenerate into atretic follicles and disappear through phagocytosis. The same fate overtakes the corpora albicantes and also the maturing follicles which do not ovulate. It follows that a section of the adult ovary will show a mixture of primordial, atretic, maturing and degenerating follicles in accordance with what has taken place in it so far.

The fallopian tube

Each fallopian tube is a hollow fibromuscular cylinder lined by epithelium extending outwards and backwards for about 10 cm from the uterine cornu to the ovary. It lies in the two peritoneal layers of the broad ligament which form a mesentery, the mesosalpinx. At the medial end, the uterine ostium, it opens into the uterine cavity

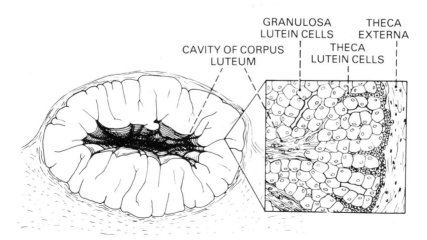

Fig. 3.20 Diagram of corpus luteum. (Reproduced with permission from Edward Arnold and the editors of *Ten Teachers Gynaecology*.)

and at the outer end, the abdominal ostium, it opens into the peritoneal cavity. The lateral part of the uterine tube is in close contact with the upper pole of the ovary, curling down the free posterior border and coming to rest on the medial surface.

Each tube is divided into four parts:

1. The interstitial, about 0.7 mm wide and 2.5 cm long, which runs a slightly tortuous course within the uterine wall
2. The isthmus, about 1.0 mm wide and 2.5 cm long
3. The ampulla, about 6 mm wide and 5 cm long
4. The infundibulum, the dilated trumpet-shaped outer end about 10 mm wide.

The mucous membrane lining the tube occurs in folds which become more elaborate as they approach the abdominal ostium. These folds fill the lumen, almost obliterating it, and are continued through the abdominal ostium as a number of fine projections or fimbriae.

Histology

The microscopic appearance of the tube differs according to which part is being examined (Fig. 3.21). All parts have an outer peritoneal covering, which is incomplete inferiorly where the two layers of broad ligament come together to form the mesosalpinx, a muscle coat of inner circular and outer longitudinal smooth muscle fibres and a folded mucous membrane lining of epithelial cells. In the isthmus the lumen is narrow, the muscle layers are prominent and a few longitudinal folds of the mucous membrane project into the lumen, which tends to be star shaped. The epithelial lining cells are low columnar, some ciliated. In the ampulla the lumen is wide but it is occupied by a labyrinthine system of branching and secondary branching folds of mucous membrane. The muscle layers are relatively thin and vascular. Ciliated cells predominate and thin peg cells with an elongated deeply staining nucleus are seen. Morphological changes in the epithelium are slight during the menstrual cycle. The cells are said to be taller at midcycle, lower at other times and in pregnancy. Decidual cells are found in the epithelial tunica propria and also in the outer layers of the tube in pregnancy, especially when it is ectopic. Atrophic changes occur in the tube after the menopause.

The uterus

The uterus (Fig. 3.22) is a pear-shaped hollow organ 7.5 cm long, 5 cm wide at the fundus and

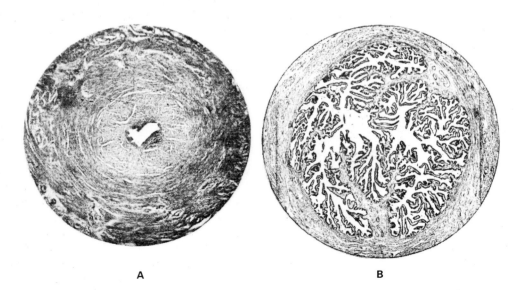

Fig. 3.21 Sections of uterine tube: **A** through isthmus; **B** through ampulla.

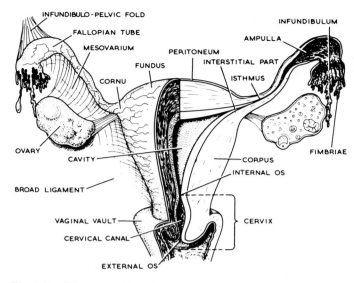

INFUNDIBULO-PELVIC FOLD

FALLOPIAN TUBE

MESOVARIUM

FUNDUS

CORNU

PERITONEUM

INFUNDIBULUM

AMPULLA

INTERSTITIAL PART

ISTHMUS

OVARY

CAVITY

BROAD LIGAMENT

FIMBRIAE

CORPUS

INTERNAL OS

VAGINAL VAULT

CERVICAL CANAL

CERVIX

EXTERNAL OS

Fig. 3.22 Diagram to show the uterus, tubes and ovaries from behind. (Reproduced with permission from H. K. Lewis and the authors of *Gynaecological and Obstetrical Anatomy*.)

2.5 cm from front to back. Its walls are 1–2 cm thick. It lies between the bladder in front and the recto-uterine pouch and the rectum behind. The lumen is connected to the peritoneal cavity by the uterine tubes above and to the exterior by the vagina below. It is divided into a triangular body (or corpus) above and a fusiform cervix below, joining at the isthmus. The part of the uterine body between the uterine tubes is known as the fundus. The cavity of the body has a smooth lining and is triangular in shape, but because the anterior and posterior walls are in apposition the cavity on sagittal section is seen only as a cleft. The cavity of the cervix is fusiform in shape. It joins the cavity of the body at the internal os and the vagina at the external os. The lining is thrown into oblique folds running into vertical folds in the midline in front and behind like the branches and stem of a tree, called the arbor vitae because of the belief in ancient times that the sperm climbed up on their way into the uterus.

The size of the uterus varies at different time. Before puberty and after the menopause it is much smaller than during active sexual life. In infancy the cervix is larger than the body. Anteflexion is acute in childhood and the uterus is said to be cochleate. By adulthood the body has grown to occupy two-thirds of the uterus. The nulliparous uterus weighs between 40 and 50 g and the parous uterus between 50 and 70 g. The external os of the cervix is small and round in the nullipara, larger and slit shaped in the multipara with slight dilation of the lower end of the canal. The uterus grows enormously during pregnancy and by full term it measures about 35×25 cm weighing about 900 g. After delivery it gradually shrinks to normal size by a process of autolysis and phagocytosis.

Relations (Figs 3.23 and 3.24)

The uterus is tilted forwards on the vagina (anteversion) and it is bent forwards at the isthmus (anteflexion). In this way the superior surface over the fundus is directed forwards, the posterior convex surface looks directly upwards at the top and upwards and backwards toward the recto-uterine pouch lower down. The anterior surface is flat, and directed downwards and forwards; it is in direct relation to the uterovesical pouch of the peritoneum and the bladder, which pushes the uterus backwards as it fills. Laterally the uterus is in relation from above down to the tubes, the round and ovarian ligaments, the broad ligament and the uterine vessels and the parametrium. The

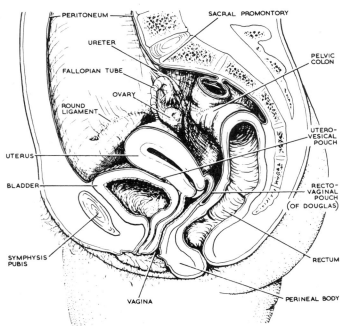

Fig. 3.23 Sagittal section through the female pelvis to show relation of the uterus to the bladder, vagina and rectouterine pouch. (Reproduced with permission from H. K. Lewis and the authors of *Gynaecological and Obstetrical Anatomy*.)

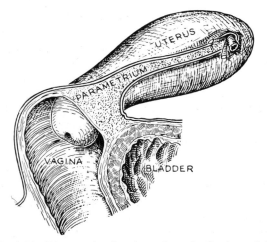

Fig. 3.24 Diagram showing the peritoneal reflections of the uterus and the vaginal fornices. (Reproduced with permission from H. K. Lewis and the authors of *Gynaecological and Obstetrical Anatomy*.)

ureter, which is an important lateral relation to the cervix at its junction with the vagina, turns obliquely forwards and medially beneath the uterine

vessels into the base of the bladder about 1.5 cm from the lateral vaginal fornix. The left ureter tends to enter the bladder nearer to the midline than the right, which makes it more liable to injury at hysterectomy.

The peritoneum is reflected from the bladder on to the anterior aspect of the uterus at the level of the isthmus to form the uterovesical pouch. It is loosely attached to the uterus inferiorly for about 1 cm, but above this level is firmly adherent to the uterine musculature. From the lateral borders of the uterus a double layer of peritoneum passes laterally to the pelvic wall to form the broad ligament, containing the fallopian tube, the round ligament and the ovarian ligament. Behind the uterus the peritoneum passes down to cover the back of the cervix and the posterior aspect of the upper quarter of the vagina. It is then reflected onto the anterior aspect of the rectum, forming the recto-uterine pouch (or pouch of Douglas). Lateral indentations of peritoneum cover the uterosacral ligaments running from the cervix backwards to the sacrum to form the uterosacral folds. The pararectal fossa is found on each side

component of the levatores ani, which run backwards from the posterior aspect of the pubis to the anorectal junction and the anococcygeal raphe. This part of the pubococcygeus forms a U-shaped sling round the upper end of the anus and is known as the puborectalis. At a more superficial level is the external sphincter consisting of a deep circular involuntary portion, which surrounds the internal sphincter and fuses with fibres of the puborectalis; a superficial portion which runs from the coccyx to the perineal body; and a subcutaneous portion which runs from the anococcygeal ligament to the perineal body.

The bladder

The bladder is a hollow, muscular pelvic organ whose principal functions are to:

1. Act as a reservoir for urine
2. Actively discharge its contents clear of the body at an appropriate time and place.

Embryology

The lining of the bladder is endodermal in origin, whilst the musculature is mesodermal.

About the 4–7th week of intraembryonic life, a mesodermal ridge (urorectal septum) grows downwards into the cloaca dividing the angle between the allantois and the hindgut.

About the 7th week the urorectal septum fuses with the cloacal membrane dividing the cloaca into a ventral urogenital sinus and dorsal hindgut.

The pelvic portion of the urogenital sinus becomes tubular and forms the urethra. The upper portion of the urogenital sinus becomes saccular and forms the bladder. The allantois eventually becomes obliterated to form the median umbilical ligament.

The ureteric buds arise from the distal end of the mesonephric duct, grow cranially into the metanephric blastema (the future kidney).

Mesonephric ducts atrophy and their caudal portions become incorporated into the wall of the bladder in the trigone.

Between the 7th and 12th weeks the single-layered endodermal epithelium becomes transitional in nature.

At about the 8th week the local mesenchyme, together with the mesenchyme which has migrated from the primitive streak, becomes incorporated to form the bladder musculature (deficiency in the development of this ventral wall mesenchyme results in the formation of an ectopia vesicae and/or an epispadias of the urethra).

Histology

The bladder is lined by folds of transitional waterproof epithelium whose cells have scalloped margins with complex interdigitations to allow alteration in shape. Mucous glands are absent in this layer and under normal circumstances there is no passage of solutes in either direction.

Except at the trigone there is a loose layer of areolar elastic tissue lying beneath the transitional cells to allow expansion of their folds during bladder filling.

The smooth involuntary musculature (the detrusor) is a dense meshwork of fibres with no obvious stratification except at the bladder outlet where there is an inner longitudinal layer, a middle circular layer and an outer longitudinal layer. This musculature is both embryologically and histochemically separate from the musculature of the urethra.

The upper surface of the fundus of the bladder has a firmly adherent covering of pelvic peritoneum, and the rest of the bladder is surrounded by loose areolar tissue.

The urethra

The urethra is a musculoelastic tube draining the bladder. In the adult female the urethra is 3–4 cm in length. It is endodermal in origin and arises from the pelvic portion of the urogenital sinus. It is lined with transitional epithelium in its proximal half and stratified squamous epithelium in its distal half. The latter portion, like the vaginal epithelium, is sensitive to oestrogen and progesterone. This portion also contains small rudimentary mucous glands (Skene's glands) homologous to the prostate. The submucosa contains an extensive plexus of veins and many arteriovenous anastomoses. In addition, there is an abundance of elastic tissue which occludes the urethral lumen at rest.

The urethral musculature has two components:

1. An inner poorly developed longitudinal smooth muscle which shortens the urethra during micturition and is separate from the detrusor.

2. An outer well developed voluntary striated component which is made up of circularly orientated muscle fibres lying at the level of the urogenital diaphragm and circular or obliquely directed periurethral fibres which arise from the latter and are inserted midway between the urogenital diaphragm and the bladder neck. This voluntary musculature serves as a secondary defence mechanism in stress incontinence, can halt urine flow during micturition and empties the urethral lumen at the end of micturition.

A continuous layer of collagen separates this musculature from that of the pelvic floor.

Innervation of the bladder and urethra

The bladder is principally under the control of the parasympathetic nervous system. There is an abundance of acetylcholinesterase activity on histochemical staining in the detrusor and profuse cholinergic nerve fibres can be demonstrated on electron microscopy. Cholinergic drugs stimulate muscular contraction and anticholinergic drugs reduce the vesical pressure and increase the bladder capacity. The sacral reflex arc is mediated through the nerve roots of S2–S4 with S3 being the main root for the detrusor muscle.

The sympathetic innervation of the bladder is poorly understood. There are very few noradrenergic fibres and minimal catecholamine activity is seen on fluorescent staining. There are, however, few efferent fibres arising from T11 to L3 which pass by the hypogastric nerves to the bladder base and urethra and experimental stimulation of these nerves cause a rise in intra-urethral pressure, which is abolished by α blockade (phentolamine). Histochemical analyses suggest that the sympathetic fibres form peri-cellular plexuses around the parasympathetic ganglia and thus may regulate and integrate ganglionic activity.

The smooth muscle of the urethra is predominantly innervated by the parasympathetic splanchnic nerves, which cause a rise in intra-urethral pressure on stimulation that is blocked by atropine.

The striated voluntary component of the urethral musculature is innervated by the somatic fibres of S2–S4, which are railroaded to the urethra by the pelvic plexus. Unlike the striated musculature of the pelvic floor, the pudendal nerve plays no part in its innervation.

Blood supply and lymphatic drainage

The arterial blood supply to the bladder arises from the anterior trunk of the internal iliac artery by means of the superior and inferior vesical arteries. A few branches are, in addition, derived from the uterine and vaginal arteries.

The veins from the bladder drain into a vesical plexus at its base and communicate with veins in the base of the broad ligament, draining on each side to the internal iliac veins.

The lymphatic channels follow the course of the blood vessels and drain to nodes mostly in the internal iliac group.

The urethra is supplied by branches of the inferior vesical artery as well as the internal pudendal artery. The venous drainage is to the vesical plexus and the lymph channels pass mainly to the internal iliac nodes with a few in the region of the external urethral meatus draining to the superficial inguinal nodes.

Anatomical relations

Bladder	Urethra
Anteriorly:	
The retropubic space (cave of Retzius), pubic bone and anterior abdominal wall musculature.	Pubic arch and the cave of Retzius.

Bladder	Urethra
Posteriorly:	
Pubocervical fascia and anterior vaginal wall. Supravaginal cervix and uterovesical pouch.	Anterior vaginal wall.
Superiorly:	
The reflection of pelvic peritoneum. Loops of small intestine.	The bladder.
Laterally:	
The levator ani muscle. The ureters and pubocervical ligaments.	The bulbus cavernosus muscle, the urogenital diaphragm and inferior pubic ramus.

The supports of the uterus, vagina and the pelvic floor

The normal positions of the uterus and vagina in the pelvis depend on the supports given to each organ. The axis of the uterus is at right angles to the vagina with the fundus at the level of the pelvic brim and the cervix at the level of the ischial spines. The supports can be classified as follows:

1. Upper supports: the anteverted position of the uterus; the round and broad ligaments.
2. Middle supports: the transverse cervical ligament (also known as the cardinal ligament or Mackenrodt's ligament); the pubocervical ligament; and the uterosacral ligaments.
3. Lower supports: the pelvic floor, consisting of the levatores ani and coccygeus muscles; the urogenital diaphragm and the superficial and deep perineal muscles; and the perineal body.

The upper supports. The round ligament is a fibrous cord about 12 cm long which runs laterally between the layers of the broad ligament from the body of the uterus just below and in front of the insertion of the fallopian tube through the internal inguinal ring to the labium majus. On its way to the internal inguinal ring it crosses the psoas muscle and the external iliac artery and vein. It hooks round the inferior epigastric artery, enters the internal inguinal ring, traverses the inguinal canal, comes out of the external inguinal ring and breaks up into strands in the labium majus. Medially it has some smooth muscle fibres from the uterus and terminally some striated fibres from the internal oblique and transversalis muscles as they arch over it in the inguinal canal. These fibres correspond to the cremaster muscle in the male. In the fetus the round ligament is surrounded by a tube of peritoneum, the processus vaginalis. This is usually obliterated at birth, but may remain patent as the canal of Nuck.

The broad ligament is a double fold of peritoneum extending from the uterine tube above to the pelvic floor below, from the uterus medially to the pelvic wall laterally. Its lateral border forms the infundibulopelvic ligament containing the ovarian vessels. Running outwards from the uterus in the layers of the broad ligament below the fallopian tube are the round ligament in front and the ovarian ligament behind. Attached laterally to the posterior layer of the broad ligament is the mesovarium of the ovary. These structures play a small part in supporting the uterus and are not as important as the middle and lower supports.

The middle supports. The endopelvic fascia is continuous with the fascia tranversalis lining the abdominal cavity. The parietal layer is attached to the capsule of the sacroiliac joint and lines the obturator internus muscle. A thickened band of fascia over the obturator internus gives rise to the origin of the levatores ani from the back of the pubis to the ischial spine. It is known as the white line. The parietal pelvic fascia ensheaths the levator ani. The lower layer lines the ischiorectal fossa as the anal fascia; the upper layer passes medially to form the visceral layer of pelvic fascia which surrounds the bladder and urethra, the uterus and the vagina, and the rectum and anal canal. Between the peritoneum above and the levatores ani and pelvic fascia below is a layer of extraperitoneal connective and adipose tissue known as the pelvic cellular tissue. That part in relation to the vaginal vault and supravaginal cervix at the base of the broad ligament is known as the parametrium.

Extending between the pelvic viscera and the pelvic wall are thickened bands in the pelvic fascia and in the pelvic cellular issue which are reinforced by voluntary muscle fibres from the levatores ani and by smooth muscle fibres derived from the adjacent viscera. They form important supports to the bladder, uterus, vagina and rectum. Extending forwards from the cervix and vagina to the bodies of the pubic bones supporting the bladder and urethra is the pubocervical ligament. Extending laterally to the parietal fascia on the pelvic wall from the vaginal vault and supravaginal cervix are the transverse cervical (cardinal or Mackenrodt's) ligaments. And passing backwards from the cervix to the second sacral vertebra are the uterosacral ligaments, which are almost vertical when the woman is standing upright. By pulling the cervix backward they not only support the uterus and vagina but also maintain the uterus in an anteverted position. In common with other pelvic organs they hypertrophy during pregnancy and atrophy after the menopause.

The lower supports: the pelvic floor. The pelvic floor is a muscular diaphragm or shelf formed by the levatores ani and the coccygeus muscles,

the urogenital diaphragm and the superficial and deep perineal muscles. Each levator ani muscle arises peripherally and runs backwards and medially to blend in the midline with the muscle of the opposite side. It arises from the posterior aspect of the body of the pubis, from the white line of the parietal pelvic fascia on the obturator internus muscle and from the ischial spine. There is a gap anteriorly, bridged by the urogenital diaphragm, for the passage of the urethra and vagina; and another gap behind the perineal body for the anus. The main part of the levator ani muscle is the pubococcygeus (Fig. 3.28). It arises from the back of the pubis and the part of the white line which lies in front of the obturator canal. Its fibres sweep backwards to form U-shaped loops round the urethra, vagina and anorectal junction. Its most medial fibres blend with the upper urethra and a few of them surround it. Intermediate fibres form a loop round the vagina, which on contracting close its lower end. They are inserted into the perineal body. Lateral fibres form a loop round the anus, being inserted into the lateral and posterior walls of the anal canal between the internal and external anal sphincters, into the anococcygeal ligament and into the lateral

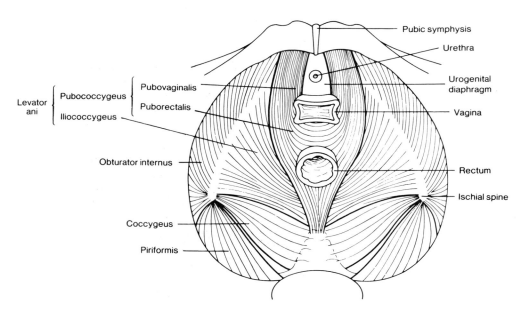

Fig. 3.28 The pelvic floor as seen from above. (Reproduced with permission from the authors of *Illustrated Textbook of Gynaecology* and W. B. Saunders.)

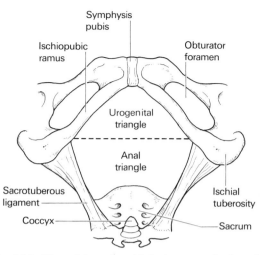

Fig. 3.36 The pelvic outlet with its important land marks.

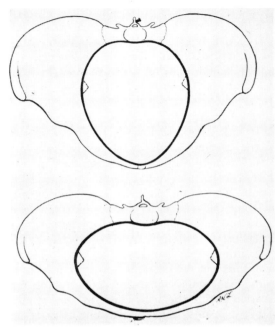

Fig. 3.38 Diagrammatic representation of the anthropoid pelvis (upper) and platypelloid pelvis (lower).

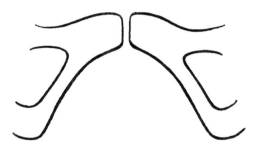

Fig. 3.37 Diagrammatic view of the subpubic arch.

Beneath the symphysis pubis is the subpubic arch which has an angle of roughly 85°, although since its walls are curved (Fig. 3.37) this cannot be measured accurately.

There are a number of variations of the pelvic shape and size in females in addition to the characteristics of the normal gynaecoid pelvis just described. Other types include the anthropoid (in which the pelvic brim is longer anteroposteriorly than from side to side) and android (in which the brim is heart shaped and the pelvis funnels from above downwards) and the platypelloid (in which the pelvic brim is a good deal wider in the transverse measurement than anteroposteriorly, giving the brim a kidney-like shape (Figs 3.38 and 3.39).

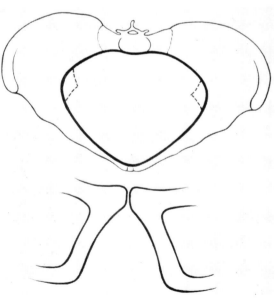

Fig. 3.39 Diagrammatic representation of the android pelvis. Note the heart-shaped brim, the prominent ischial spines and the acute subpubic angle.

There are a number of important true ligaments of the pelvis (as distinct from the structures such as the broad ligament, round ligament, etc., already described). The sacrospinous ligament runs from the lateral aspect of the sacrum to the ischial spine and the sacrotuberous ligament from the same area of the sacrum to the inner aspect of the ischial tuberosity (Figs 3.32 and 3.33). It will be seen from Fig. 3.32 that the sacrospinous ligament and the greater sciatic notch form the greater sciatic foramen whilst the sacrospinous ligament and the lesser sciatic notch form the lesser sciatic foramen. The strong posterior sacro-iliac ligament runs from the medial surface of the ilium to the sacrum and the smaller iliolumbar ligament from the iliac crest posteriorly to the transverse process of the fifth lumbar vertebra.

Movement at the pelvic joints is minimal in the non-pregnant state, but there is considerable joint relaxation during pregnancy and, in some women, instability results. Such movement as does take place at the symphysis pubis precipitates delivery.

THE BREAST

In the human the breasts are bilateral apocrine glands whose function is principally to provide nutrition by lactation for the newborn. For a consideration of lactation see page 222.

Embryology

The breast is ectodermal in origin.

About the 6–7th week of intra-embryonic life, a 4–6 cell layer thickening appears in the thoracic region of the galactic band (which extends from the axilla to the groin).

By 8 weeks the layer of cells becomes condensed and invaginates to invade the underlying mesenchyme.

Around 15 weeks, sprouting takes place with 16–25 epithelial strips radially penetrating the underlying dermis to become the future lactiferous ducts.

Between the 20th and 26th weeks, secondary and tertiary sprouting occurs with progressive canalisation taking place up to the 9th month. In association with this, there is increased vascularisation and deposition of fat.

At term, mesodermal proliferation takes place beneath the nipple causing its eversion. In addition, maternal prolactin may stimulate colostrum secretory activity which appears soon after delivery.

Breast development at puberty

Breast duct growth is primarily stimulated by oestrogens and the alveolar cells and sebaceous glands are stimulated by progesterone. In addition, maturation of the breast is promoted by growth hormone, parathyroid hormone, thyroid hormone, cortisol and insulin.

Secondary breast growth in the female commences between the ages of 9 and 12 years (thelarche) and is usually complete by the age of 17–20 years.

Changes in the breast during pregnancy

In the first trimester of pregnancy, the sex hormones promote intense sprouting and branching of the ducts, increased alveolar and lobular formation and increased areolar pigmentation. In addition, there is a marked increase in vascularity and dilatation of the superficial veins.

During the second trimester, colostrum formation commences with increased lymphocytic activity, and prolactin secretion from the anterior pituitary increases three- to five-fold.

In the third trimester, fat droplets accumulate in the aveolar cells and colostrum formation becomes further increased.

Overall, the weight of the breast increases two- to three-fold and the blood supply is doubled.

Milk synthesis takes place following the withdrawal of a blockade caused by the sex steroids on prolactin activity about the 3–5th day following delivery. Breast weight further increases by approximately 200 g, one-third of this volume being due to milk secretion and storage.

Macroscopic anatomy

In the adult female the breasts are hemispherical, dome-like eminences, lying in the superficial fascia of the anterior thoracic wall. They occupy an area between the second and sixth rib vertically and the parasternal margin to the midaxillary line horizontally. They are commonly somewhat unequal in size. Their weight varies from person to person. The non-pregnant weight is approximately 200 g, that in pregnancy, 400–600 g, and during lactation, 600–800 g.

The nipple is a conical prominence overlying the fourth intercostal space in the midclavicular line. It measures approximately 10 mm in diameter. It consists of 15–25 orifices of the lactiferous ducts, has a rich nerve supply and is capable of erection.

The areola is a pigmented circular area surrounding the nipple, the diameter being approximately 35 mm. It contains numerous large sebaceous glands (Montgomery's glands) which become prominent in pregnancy and secrete a bactericidal lubricant onto the surface. This region contains collagen and elastic tissue fibres as well as smooth muscle but is free of fat.

The breast consists of 15–25 lobes, each of which drain 20–40 lobules, into which 10–100 alveoli drain. The diameter of the alveolus is approximately 0.12 mm, the lactiferous ducts, 2 mm, and the lactiferous sinuses, which are terminal expansions of the ducts serving as reservoirs for milk beneath the areola, are approximately 5–8 mm in diameter.

Fibrous tissue invests the entire surface of the mammary gland and sends down septa between the lobes connecting them together. Fibrous strands (the suspensory ligaments of Astley–Cooper) extend from this fibrous tissue to the overlying skin and provide support for the breast. They are responsible for the dimpling appearance seen when there is underlying oedema, as in carcinoma of the breast, causing a peau d'orange appearance.

Histology

In the non-pregnant state, the alveolus is small and filled with a mass of granular polyhedral cells. These enlarge during pregnancy and at the commencement of lactation they have a short columnar appearance with spherical nuclei lying close to the basement membrane. Fat secretion accumulates in the superficial parts of the cells and droplets are discharged by apocrine secretion into the central lumen. Around these alveoli there is a layer of myoepithelial cells, which are contractile.

The ducts are lined by columnar epithelium and surrounded by longitudinal and transverse elastic fibres as well as inner longitudinal and outer circular smooth muscle fibres.

Blood supply

Arteries

Five anterior perforating branches of the internal mammary artery supply the medial part of the breast (60%). The lateral thoracic artery arises from the axillary artery and supplies the lateral half of the breast (30%). Anterior and lateral branches of the intercostal arteries supply the lower lateral quadrants of the breast (5–10%). In addition, the pectoral branch of the acromiothoracic artery, the external mammary artery and the superior thoracic artery supply 1–5%.

Veins

These form an anastomotic circle around the base of the nipple and drain mainly to the internal mammary and axillary veins.

Lymphatics

These drain the interlobular spaces and the walls of the lactiferous ducts. The superficial lymphatics drain into the axillary glands on the same side of the body although some lymphatics on the medial side of the breast cross the midline, entering the other breast and drain to the opposite axilla. A few lymphatics drain the inferior quadrants of the breast on the rectus sheath.

The central part of the mammary gland beneath the areola forms a subareolar plexus on the pectoralis major, which drains to the anterior axillary nodes. Deep lymphatic drainage is mostly to the anterior axillary nodes although the medial part of the breast may drain into the internal mammary nodes and the subdiaphragmatic nodes.

Nerve supply

The upper quadrants of the breast are innervated by the supraclavicular nerves (C3 and C4). The rest of the breast is innervated by medial and lateral cutaneous branches of the intercostal nerves (T4–T6).

Anatomical relations

The breast lies within the superficial fascia and is separated from the deep fascia overlying the pectoralis major in its medial two-thirds by the submammary space in which the lymphatics run. The outer one-third of the breast overlies the deep fascia covering the serratus anterior muscle.

4. Pathology, microbiology and immunology

PATHOLOGY

Inflammation

The inflammatory response is probably the most important of the body's natural defence mechanisms, and is, simply, the body's response to tissue injury. It is initiated by numerous agents or stimuli and occurs in any part of the body, but its basic character is always the same, whatever the cause or site. The suffix *-itis* indicates inflammation, e.g. appendicitis.

Traditionally, inflammation is divided into acute and chronic, but, in practice, both may appear together.

Acute inflammation

These are the initial or early changes, occurring over hours or days, and represent the body's attempt to destroy or neutralise the causative agent.

Causes. Common causes are summarised in Table 4.1; the commonest is undoubtedly bacterial infection.

Macroscopic features constitute the cardinal signs attributed to Celsus and comprise tumor (swelling), rubor (redness), calor (excess local heat) and dolor (pain).

Table 4.1 Causes of acute inflammation

Organisms	Bacteria
	Viruses
	Parasites
Mechanical trauma	Cutting
	Crushing
Chemicals	Inorganic
	Strong acids
	Strong alkalis
	Organic
	Extravasated body fluids
	(e.g. bile and urine)
Radiation	Ionising
	Ultraviolet
Extremes of temperature	Cold
	Heat
Deprivation of blood supply	Infarction
Immunological reactions	Immune complexes
	Sensitised lymphocytes

Local events, seen microscopically, relate to dynamic changes in blood vessels, blood flow and leucocytes. They usually occur sequentially:

1. Transient arteriolar constriction, probably due to a local neurogenic reflex, may develop, but lasts only for a few minutes. It is rapidly followed by prolonged   (*contd on p. 104*)

2. Arteriolar dilatation. There is therefore

3. Increased local blood flow (hyperaemia) and local capillary dilatation.

4. Increased capillary permeability is due to two main factors. Firstly, arteriolar dilatation raises the capillary hydrostatic pressure, promoting greater outflow of water and solutes into the interstitial fluid. Secondly, capillary and venular endothelial permeability is increased, allowing larger molecules, especially albumin, to enter interstitial tissues. These molecules alter local osmotic pressures and attract more water.

This accumulation of interstitial fluid ('inflammatory oedema') (Fig. 4.1) produces

5. Slowing of capillary blood flow and intravascular haemoconcentration, followed by

6. Loss of normal axial blood flow. Normally, blood cells flow in the centre of the capillaries, with relatively cell-free plasma in contact with the endothelium. In acute inflammation, circulating white cells, initially neutrophil polymorphs and later monocytes (see below), move towards to produce

7. Margination of leucocytes (pavementing of endothelium) and

8. Central 'sludging' of red cells, forming rouleaux.

9. Adhesion of leucocytes to capillary endothelium then occurs, followed by

10. Active emigration into perivascular tissues. Once outside, they migrate by

11. Chemotaxis towards higher concentrations of chemical substances (chemotaxins). This produces

12. Aggregation of numerous leucocytes. This aggregation, so easily seen microsopically, is the main criterion for the histopathological diagnosis (Fig. 4.1).

13. Phagocytosis, the main function of leucocytes in acute inflammation, involves ingestion, digestion and disposal of unwanted foreign particulate matter, especially bacteria and damaged host cells.

Leucocytes in acute inflammation. Only two types are important. Initially, the majority are neutrophil polymorphs; they are highly motile, contain many lysosomes for digesting bacteria and effete cells, and are relatively short lived. Later, macrophages (derived from circulating mono-

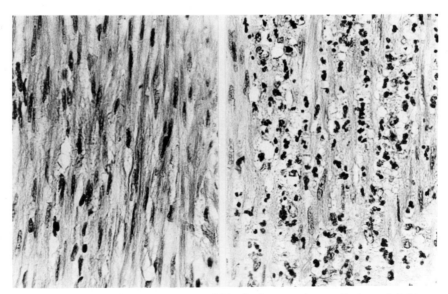

Fig. 4.1 Normal appendix and acute appendicitis. In the normal appendicular wall (left), parallel smooth muscle fibres are closely packed; in acute appendicitis (right), the muscles fibres are separated by inflammatory oedema and an infiltrate of polymorphs.

cytes) predominate; they are less motile, contain fewer lysosomes and remove debris, including dead polymorphs, bacteria and fibrin.

The acute inflammatory exudate comprises fluid, proteins and cells. The fluid is in constant exchange with plasma; it may contain drugs (including antibiotics), and dilutes local irritant substances and toxins. The proteins include albumin, globulins (possibly effecting humoral-mediated immunity) and fibrinogen. Fibrin (polymerised fibrinogen) helps to prevent bacterial invasion, unites severed tissues and promotes phagocytosis. The cells are described above. With considerable local vascular damage, red cells may accumulate.

Mediators. Many have been proposed but few proven. Histamine, predominantly from local mast cells, is the principal mediator of the immediate response, and mainly produces arteriolar dilatation. The kinins (e.g. bradykinin) are derived from the circulation by a cascade system and are largely responsible for increased vascular permeability; they also maintain vasodilatation. Other possible mediators include biologically active complement cleavage products (e.g. C3a, C5a and C567), extracts released from dead polymorphs (e.g. lysosomal enzymes), prostaglandins and fibrin products (see the section on the innate immune system below).

Results. If the inflammatory response destroys or neutralises the causative agent without significant local tissue damage, resolution (i.e. total restoration of normality) occurs. With tissue destruction, there will be regeneration or organisation (see the section on 'wound healing' below).

Suppuration (pus formation) may develop, with collections of pus-producing abscesses. If the agent persists, chronic inflammation will supervene.

Chronic inflammation

These changes, occurring over weeks, months or years, indicate a prolonged or persistent insult, and represent the body's attempt to localise the causative agent and to repair the resulting damage.

Causes. It may follow acute inflammation (see above) or arise *de novo*; common causes are summarised in Table 4.2.

Table 4.2 Causes of chronic inflammation

Organisms	Bacteria, especially
	    Mycobacteria
	    Treponema (syphilis)
	Fungi
	Parasites (e.g. *Schistosoma spp.*)

Foreign material	Industrial
	    Silica
	    Asbestos
	Sutures
	Talc

Cell-mediated hypersensitivity	Tuberculosis Sarcoidosis Autoimmune diseases
Poor blood supply (e.g. varicose ulcers)	
'Chemical' (e.g. peptic ulcers)	

Cells involved may be from blood or local tissues (Fig. 4.2).

Blood cells are mononuclear (cf. polymorphonuclear in acute inflammation). Lymphocytes and plasma cells provide local cellular and humoral immunological defence reactions (described elsewhere). Macrophages, as in acute inflammation, remove local tissue debris; sometimes they form multinucleated giant cells, either by fusion or incomplete cell division. Occasionally, eosinophils are also present.

Tissue cells: proliferating fibroblasts and capillaries (granulation tissue) represent repair by organization (see the section on 'wound healing' below).

Granulomatous chronic inflammation is a variant where macrophages predominate in multiple, small, discrete, concentric aggregates (granulomata) (Fig. 4.3). They are usually associated with hypersensitivity reactions, fungal infection, parasitic infestation or aseptic foreign material. They consist largely of an avascular mass of macrophages, some of which form multinucleated giant cells, at the centre of which may be the causative agent or cellular necrosis. Around this is a cuff of lymphocytes, often with granulation tissue and, in older lesions, fibrosis.

Results. Scar tissue is usually beneficial — it limits the causative agent and ultimately repairs local tissue deficiencies. Occasionally, excess fibrosis causes deformity, obstruction or immobilisation of organs and tissues.

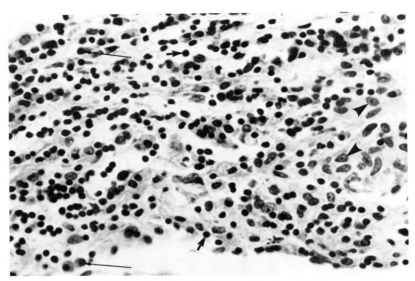

Fig. 4.2 Chronic inflammation. A typical non-specific chronic inflammatory cell infiltrate containing lymphocytes (small, dark cells with scanty cytoplasm — short arrows), plasma cells (dark cells with eccentric nuclei — long arrows) and occasional macrophages (larger, paler-staining cells — arrowheads).

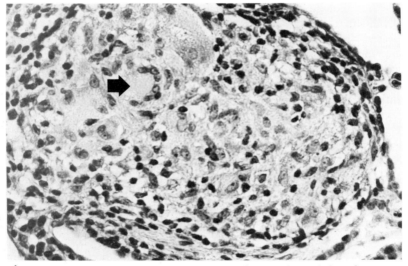

Fig. 4.3 Granulomatous chronic inflammation. A granuloma consisting of numerous, pale-staining macrophages, some of which are forming a multinucleated giant cell (arrow), surrounded by a cuff of smaller, darker-staining lymphocytes.

Wound healing

This is the replacement of dead cells or tissue by living cells or fibrous tissue, and occurs by regeneration or organisation; the ultimate result depends on the local balance between these two factors.

Regeneration is the replacement by proliferating similar, adjacent, undamaged parenchymal cells.

Cellular regeneration capacity is related to normal mitotic activity — thus, some (e.g. epidermis and gastrointestinal epithelium) invariably regenerate, others (e.g. liver, renal tubule epithelium and thyroid) regenerate under favourable circumstances, whilst some (e.g. neurones) are incapable of regeneration.

Organisation is replacement by fibrosis. It occurs not only in wounds, but also in fibrinous acute inflammatory exudates and chronic inflammation (see elsewhere), and in infarcts and thrombi. The process begins with digestion and removal of debris by macrophages and growth into the necrotic area of capillary loops with prominent lining endothelial cells and large, plump fibroblasts (granulation tissue) from the adjacent connective tissue; some inflammatory cells, both acute and chronic, are also usually present. As healing progresses, fibroblasts lay down collagen and ground substance, and cellularity is reduced by the gradual disappearance of inflammatory cells, fibroblasts and capillaries. Ultimately, only avascular and acellular collagenous scar tissue remains.

Skin wound healing

Exact changes depend on whether the edges are in apposition.

Primary union (healing by first intention) occurs when skin edges are in contact, as when held by sutures following surgical incisions. Immediate haemorrhage produces a fibrin-rich blood clot in the small gap and a mild acute inflammatory reaction is initiated. Macrophages and granulation tissue soon invade the area, the former to remove debris including fibrin, the latter to begin the process of organisation, which continues rapidly until a relatively small scar is produced. Meanwhile, the adjacent overlying epidermis proliferates until continuity is restored.

Secondary union (healing by second intention) occurs with extensive local tissue loss. The wound contains fibrin and tissue debris, and may initially be covered by a scab. A brisk acute inflammatory reaction develops and granulation tissue begins to grow into the area from the periphery. Organisation progresses slowly until ultimately a large, irregular scar is produced. Simultaneously, the overlying epidermis proliferates below the scab until regeneration is complete; rete ridges and skin appendages do not reappear.

Factors delaying wound healing may be local or general. Local factors include poor local blood supply, persistence of infection, retention of foreign materials and repeated local movement or trauma. General factors: collagen formation is defective in generalised states of vitamin C, zinc or protein (especially sulphur-containing amino acid) deficiency. Excess glucocorticosteroid hormones suppress repair.

Neoplasia

Neoplasia is an abnormal, uncontrolled proliferation of cells. Although not strictly correct, the terms 'neoplasm' and 'tumour' are invariably used synonymously.

Two distinct aspects are always considered — firstly, whether the tumour is benign or malignant and secondly, its cell of origin (histiogenesis).

Benign or malignant?

Five major differences exist:

Local growth. Benign tumours grow by expansion, compress adjacent tissues and are often surrounded by a fibrous tissue capsule: malignant tumours expand, but also show direct invasion (infiltration) of local tissues including blood vessels and lymphatics.

Growth rate. Benign tumours usually grow slowly and ultimately may stop growing or even regress.

Distant spread (metastasis). Benign tumours never metastasise. The spread of malignant cells may be via lymphatics (primarily to regional lymph nodes), blood vessels (commonly to lungs and liver) or body cavities (transcoelomic spread through peritoneum, pleura or pericardium).

Histological appearances. Benign tumours are very similar histologically to their cell of origin (i.e. they are very well differentiated); with malignant tumours, there is a spectrum, ranging from well differentiated to anaplastic (undifferentiated), where no histological features exist to indicate the cell of origin.

Clinical effects. Benign tumours are relatively harmless, but may cause problems by local pressure or hormone production: most malignant tumours will ultimately kill the patient, especially if untreated, by local and distant spread.

These features help to distinguish benign and malignant tumours, but benign tumours may undergo subsequent malignant change; with some (e.g. colonic adenomatous polypi) transformation is quite common, but with others (e.g. uterine leiomyomata) it is very rare.

Histiogenesis

Tumours may be subdivided into epithelial, connective tissue and 'others'.

Epithelial

1. *Surface epithelium*. Benign tumours here are papillomas, with the term qualified by the epithelial type involved (e.g. squamous cell and transitional cell); characteristically, they project from epithelial surfaces as finger-like processes (papillae). Malignant tumours are carcinomas and, again, qualification by epithelial type is added.

2. *Glandular epithelium*. Benign tumours are adenomas. They are usually solid, but occasionally may show excessive secretion and cyst formation (cystadenomas), and epithelial papillae may project into these cysts (papillary cystadenomas). Their malignant counterparts are, respectively, adenocarcinomas, cystadenocarcinomas and papillary cystadenocarcinomas.

3. *Chorionic epithelium*. Benign proliferation produces a hydatidiform mole; the corresponding malignant tumour is the choriocarcinoma. An intermediate lesion (penetrating or invasive mole) exists, where extensive local invasion occurs without metastases.

Connective tissue. Usually, the suffix implies behaviour; thus benign tumours end in -ma whilst malignant ones have -sarcoma, and the prefix indicates the connective tissue of origin, e.g. fibro- (fibro tissue, i.e. fibroblasts), lipo- (fat), chondro- (cartilage), osteo- (bone), leiomyo- (smooth muscle), rhabdomyo- (striated muscle), haemangio- (blood vessels) and lymphangio- (lymphatics). Occasionally, no stromal features exist to suggest the connective tissue of origin; such tumours are usually designated spindle cell sarcomas.

'Other'. These cannot be classified satisfactorily in either group above:

1. *Teratomas*. These are complex mixed tumours, probably derived from germ cells, which incorporate tissues derived from all three primitive germ layers. Many, especially in the ovary ('dermoids'), are benign, and show recognisable but randomly arranged organoid development of such structures as hair, teeth, cartilage, bone or brain tissue. Others, especially in the testis, are malignant; they may contain similar organoid structures, but always show features of malignancy in one or more elements, and extrafetal tissues (e.g. trophoblast or yolk sac) may also be seen.

2. *'Embryonal' tumours*. These growths are malignant, usually arising in infancy or early childhood. They are derived from residual immature embryonic tissue, and bear the suffix -blastoma, e.g. nephroblastoma, neuroblastoma and medulloblastoma.

3. *Central nervous system tumours*. Many unique types are found: only two are common. Gliomas (e.g. astrocytomas, ependymomas and oligodendrogliomas) show variable differentiation and are malignant; all invade locally but never metastasise outside the central nervous system. Meningiomas are derived from the arachnoid; most are benign.

Leukaemias and lymphomas. Classifications, particularly of the latter, are still being defined and remain controversial.

MICROBIOLOGY

Bacteria

Introduction

Bacteria are the smallest organisms that contain all the machinery required for growth and self-replication from exogenous foodstuffs. They are morphologically more simple than the cells of higher organisms although biochemically they are just as complex. Bacteria are designated as 'prokaryotic' because they lack the organised nucleus, with the nuclear membrane and mitotic apparatus, of higher 'eukaryotic' cells. Other characteristics of prokaryotic cells include the absence of steroids, the presence of a unique cell wall and, in some cases, obligate anaerobiosis. While the internal structure of bacteria is less complex than that of animal or plant cells, bacteria have a more complex surface structure with a rigid cell wall surrounding the cytoplasmic membrane. All true bacteria, but not chlamydiae, rickettsiae, mycoplasmae or viruses, possess a cell wall consisting of an N-acetyl muramic acid/N-acetyl glutamic acid backbone (NAM–NAG) to which may be attached polypeptides, polysaccharides, lipids and, in the case of Gram-positive bacteria, either ribitol or glycerol teichoic acids. The cell wall is responsible for many of the taxonomically significant features of bacteria: for example, their shape, their major division into Gram-positive and Gram-negative organisms, the antigenic specificities that are important in classification and the interactions of pathogens with the host.

Morphology

Most bacteria are larger than 1 μm in diameter and can therefore be seen by the light microscope (resolving power, 0.2 μm). The light microscope cannot reveal any internal detail and as a result bacteria were long regarded as essentially bags of enzymes lacking any interesting organisation. The electron microscope revealed the distinctive architecture of the prokaryotic cell, which is diagramatically represented in Figure 4.4. The nucleus consists of a single 1 nm long, tightly coiled and packed ribbon of double-stranded deoxyribonucleic acid (DNA), in the form of a closed circle, which carries the genetic information of the cell. The nucleus replicates by growth and simple fission, not by mitosis. Bacteria may contain other units of DNA (plasmids) unassociated with the chromosome which may code for non-essential features of the organism. They are important medically because many of the genes coding for antibiotic resistance are carried on plasmids — 'plasmid-mediated' as distinct from 'chromosomally mediated' resistance. The ability of bacteria to transfer plasmid or chromosomal DNA, including genes coding for antibiotic resistance to bacteria of other species and genera is also of importance medically.

Some bacteria have capsules, microcapsules or loose slime outside the cell wall. Most motile strains of bacteria possess filamentous appendages called flagellae. The arrangement of flagellae around the cell is characteristic of the bacteria concerned. Their presence is usually inferred from the observation of motility. Fimbriae or pili are similar to flagellae but they are shorter, thinner, straighter and more numerous.

Some species, notably of the genus *Bacillus* (aerobic) or *Clostridium* (anaerobic), develop a highly resistant resting phase or endospore. Spores are important in the medical context because they are far more resistant to physical and chemical destruction than vegetative cells. Once formed they may remain viable in an adverse environment for many years. The temperature and pressure used to sterilise medical equipment is determined by the conditions necessary to destroy the most resistant bacterial spores.

Bacilli that are comma shaped are known as vibrios. The spirochaetes are corkscrew-like spirals. Actinomycetes are known as 'higher bacteria' because they are thought to represent a more advanced state of evolution, although they are still prokaryotes. In forming branched filaments the actinomycetes resemble fungi and are known as filamentous bacteria. Lactobacilli, although they are not filamentous bacteria, also produce this filamentous appearance, which on occasion results in confusion when cytology smears are being examined.

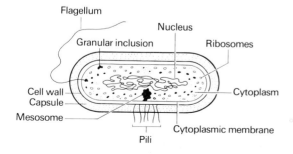

Fig. 4.4 Diagram of prototype bacterial cell.

Classification of bacteria

The classification of bacteria is even more complex than that of plants and animals. In the absence of reliable criteria for phylogenetic relationships, the classification that has developed is primarily useful as a determinative key. That is, a key for identifying an unknown organism and relating it to previously described organisms. Many properties are used for this purpose: morphology (rod or coccus), staining characteristics (Gram positive or Gram negative), motility, biochemical properties (fermentation of sugars), growth requirements, atmospheric requirements, the presence of characteristic surface macromolecules, the ability to parasitise higher organisms and cause disease, etc. By consulting published descriptions of such features and by reference to collections of 'type culture', that is, standard strains that are maintained nationally, bacteriologists can communicate meaningfully with each other. Bacteriology follows the Linnean tradition of zoology and botany by using an official Latin binomial, with a capitalised genus (e.g. *Staphylococcus*) followed by an uncapitalised species (e.g. *aureus*) designation. The major groups containing pathogenic or medically important bacteria are shown in Table 4.3.

The bacterial species is far less well defined than species of higher organisms and as a result usually includes a continuum of organisms with a relatively wide range of properties. This is particularly so in groups such as the Enterobacteriaceae which appear to undergo considerable genetic recombination in nature. Each species thus represents a cluster of biotypes more or less resembling the parent strain but without the sharp boundaries that we are accustomed to in higher organisms. Bacteria share antigenic components not only with other bacteria that may be taxonomically quite distinct but also with their mammalian or plant hosts. For example, the surface polysaccharide of *Escherichia coli* type O86 cross reacts with blood group substance B of human cells, and strains of *Neisseria meningitidis* have antigenic similarities with components of human brain cells.

Bacterial replication

Bacteria reproduce by binary fission in which one cell enlarges and then divides into two ap-proximately equal cells, following the formation of a septum. The division is preceded by simple replication of the nuclear ring without the polarised mitosis that is characteristic of higher organisms. Bacteria are divisible into large groups according to the morphology of the bacterial cells (Table 4.3). Cells that are spherical or nearly so are called cocci, those occurring in pairs such as *Streptococcus pneumoniae* are referred to as diplococci. Repeated division in the same plane produces chains, e.g. streptococci; division in two or three planes at right angles produces regular packets of four, eight or more cells; and division without any definite orientation produces irregular clusters, e.g. staphylococci. The bacilli or rods are elongated cylindrical forms, e.g. *Escherichia coli*. Replication is in a single plane longitudinally (corynebacteria) or laterally (enteric Gram-negative rods). The organisms may be straight or slightly curved, with ends that are rounded, square, pointed or sometimes swollen to form clubs.

Antigenic structure

Most of the protein and polysaccharide components of bacterial cells are antigenic and show a very high degree of specificity. Thus more than 50 lipopolysaccharide antigens have been recognised in a single species, *Escherichia coli*. Each of these codes for a different O somatic type. There is similar specific variation in the antigenic structure of the protein components of bacterial flagellae and also in the carbohydrate components of bacterial capsules, all of which contribute to the more specific and detailed identification of bacterial strains. Since most of these bacterial cell components are antigenic to mammals, the antibodies produced as a result of infection may often be used diagnostically, such as in the diagnosis of syphilis or typhoid, and, equally, antibodies produced in laboratory animals may be used as a means of identifying bacterial isolates by serotyping.

The importance of these antigens in the classification of bacteria varies from genus to genus. Thus in *Esch. coli* the O somatic antigens from the bacterial cell wall enable the microbiologist to recognise those serotypes especially associated with infection of the urinary tract (O6, O8, O18,

Table 4.3 Kingdom Procaryotae division II. The bacteria.

| Major group | Taxas with medically important members | | |
	Family	Genus	Species examples
1. Spirochaetes	Spirochaetaceae. Helically coiled unicellular bacteria, motile but non-flagellate	*Borrelia* *Treponema* *Leptospira*	*Borr. recurrentis* *Tr. pallidum* *Lept. interrogans*
2. Spiral and curved bacteria	Spirellaceae. Rigid, helically curved rods with polar flagellae	*Spirellum* *Campylobacter*	*Sp. minor* *Camp. fetus*
3. Gram-negative aerobic rods	Pseudomonadaceae. Straight or curved rods; flagellate strict aerobes; oxidase positive	*Pseudomonas*	*Ps. aeruginosa*
4. Gram-negative facultatively anerobic rods	Enterobacteriaceae. Motile or non-motile; ferment carbohydrate oxidase negative	*Escherichia* *Salmonella* *Shigella* *Klebsiella* *Enterobacter* *Proteus*	*Esch. coli* *S. typhi* *Sh. dysenteriae* *Kl. pneumoniae* *Enter. cloacae* *Pr. mirabilis*
	Vibrionaceae. Usually motile; ferment carbohydrates; oxidase positive	*Vibrio*	*V. cholerae*
	Genera of uncertain affiliation. Motile or non-motile; ferment carbohydrates, oxidase positive or negative	*Haemophilus* *Pasteurella*	*H. influenzae* *Past. multocida*
5. Gram-negative anaerobic bacteria	Bacteroidaceae. Uniform or pleomorphic rods, motile or non-motile; strict anaerobes	*Bacteroides* *Fusobacterium*	*Bact. fragilis* *Fus. nucleatum*
6. Gram-negative aerobic cocci and coccobacilli	Neisseriaceae. Cocci in pairs or masses, or plump rods in short chains; non-flagellate; most are oxidase positive	*Neisseria* *Branhamella* *Moraxella*	*N. gonorrhoeae* *Bran. catarrhalis* (formerly *N. catarrhalis*) *Mor. lacunata*
7. Gram-positive Cocci	Micrococcaceae. Cocci in clusters; aerobic or facultatively anaerobic	*Streptococcaceae*	*Staph. aureus*
	Streptococcaceae. Cocci in pairs, chains or tetrads; faculative anaerobes	*Streptococcus*	*Strep. pyogenes*
	Peptococcaceae. Cocci in pairs, masses or chains, strict anaerobes; nutritionally exacting	*Peptococcus* *Peptostreptococcus*	*Pep. aerogenes* *Peptostr. anaerobius*

Table 4.3 Cont'd

| Major group | Taxas with medically important members | | Species examples |
	Family	Genus	
8. Endospore-forming rods	Bacillaceae. Mainly Gram positive. Motile or non-motile	*Bacillus* *Clostridium*	*B. anthracis* *C. tetani*
9. Gram-positive non-sporing rods	Lactobacillaceae. Rods single or in chains; usually non-motile; nutritionally exacting	*Lactobacillus*	*L. acidophilus* *L. casei*
	Genera of uncertain affiliation. Aerobic; Listeria, motile; Erysipelothrix, non-motile	*Listeria* *Erysipelothrix*	*L. monocytogenes* *E. rhusopathiae*
10. Actinomycetes	Coryneform group of bacteria. Gram-positive mainly non-motile; essentially aerobic	*Corynebacterium*	*C. diphtheriae*
	Propionibacterium. Gram positive; essentially aerobic	*Propionibacterium*	*P. acnes*
	Actinomycetaceae. Gram positive; non-acid fast; non-motile; no spores; essentially anaerobic	*Actinomyces*	*A. isreali*
	Mycobacteriaceae. Acid-fast rods; aerobic	*Mycobacterium*	*M. tuberculosis*
	Nocardiaceae. Gram positive; branched filaments; aerobic	*Nocardia*	*N. asteroides*
11. Rickettsias. Small Gram-negative rod-shaped organisms; mainly intracellular parasites	Rickettsiaceae. Transmitted by arthropods	*Rickettsia* *Coxiella*	*R. prowazekii* *C. burnetii*
	Chlamydiaceae. Multiply in living cells; non-motile	*Chlamydia*	*C. trachomatis* *C. psittaci*
12. Mycoplasmas. Gram-negative pleomorphic organisms with a single, triple-layer membrane but no cell wall; will grow on cell-free media	Mycoplasmataceae. Require sterol for growth	*Mycoplasma*	*M. hominis*
	Require cholesterol for growth	*Ureaplasma*	*U. ureolyticum*
	Acholeplasmataceae. Do not require sterol for growth	*Acholeplasma*	*A. laidlawii*

O75), those strains responsible for infantile gastroenteritis (O111, O127, etc), and those that are more frequently associated with neonatal meningitis (O6 and O18). By contrast, the lipopolysaccharide antigens from bacteria in the genus *Salmonella* are used to identify individual species of the genus. This forms the basis of the Kauffmann–White classification scheme. Thus *Salmonella paratyphi* A contains the O2 antigen and *S. paratyphi* B and *S. typhimurium* have the O4 antigen. Strains of salmonella are also typed according to their H, flagellar, antigens. Thus the speciation of the salmonellae is very precise and depends very largely on recognising the antigenic components of bacteria.

Not all bacterial antigens are specific, for example the O1 and O12 antigens in salmonella are widely distributed amongst a variety of strains. Similarly the K1 antigen of *Esch. coli* is also found in some strains of *Klebsiella* and other enteric Gram-negative rods.

Capsular antigens are also of considerable importance diagnostically. For example, the capsular antigens of *Neisseria meningitidis* and *Haemophilus influenzae* and the β-haemolytic streptococci are all used for the positive identification of bacterial isolates. The immunogenicity of bacterial antigens varies considerably. For example, it is more difficult to produce antibodies to *N. meningitidis* type b than to types a or c, and this contributes to the problems associated with producing a vaccine against the type b meningococcus. Similarly, patients frequently fail to produce specific antibody following infection with the β-haemolytic streptococci but instead produce a group streptococcal antibody. This is detected in the antistreptolysin O test. Finally, not all antibodies produced as a consequence of bacterial infection are protective, even though they may be of value diagnostically.

Most of the toxins produced by bacteria are also antigenic and, as a result, toxigenic strains of *Corynebacterium diphtheriae*, *Clostridium tetani* and *Cl. perfringens* (*welchii*) can be distinguished from non-pathogenic, non-toxigenic strains by simple serological tests. It is of interest that the toxigenic potential of *C. diphtheriae* is solely dependent on infection of the bacteria by a specific virus (bacteriophage) and that loss of this virus renders strains of the organism non-toxigenic.

Not only may different serotypes of bacteria be responsible for different types of infection, but differences may also be seen in geographical location. For example, the predominant strain of *N. meningitidis* in Europe is type b, whereas in the Middle East types a and c predominate. Similarly, *S. paratyphi* B is the cause of most paratyphoid fever in Great Britain while in other parts of the world *S. paratyphi* A or C may be the dominant isolate.

In addition to the antigenic cross reactions which occur amongst the Enterobacteriaceae such as the presence of the Vi antigen in bacteria other than *S. typhi* and the K1 antigen in various coliforms, there have also been reported some quite bizarre cross reactions. Possibly the most useful of these was the demonstration that certain strains of the genus *Proteus* (notably X19, X2 and XK) have antigens in common with strains of *Rickettsia* responsible for typhus infection. This observation resulted in the diagnostic test for typhus fever (Weil–Felix reaction), which enables serum samples from patients with typhus to be tested safely in the laboratory without recourse to cultures of the causative organism.

Epidemiological typing

In addition to serotyping, bacteria can be typed in a variety of other ways, usually for epidemiological purposes. The organisms under test are subjected to a range of antibiotics at carefully controlled concentrations (antibiogram) or to a range of other inhibitory substances (resistogram) and the pattern of sensitivity and resistance recorded. Identical strains, isolated from a single outbreak of infection, will have identical sensitivity patterns. Unless the bacteria under test have an unusual characteristic, these tend to be rather crude typing systems.

Of far greater value, especially with isolates of *Staphylococcus aureus* or *Pseudomonas aeruginosa*, is the system of phage (bacteriophage) typing. This consists of testing a group of bacterial isolates that are closely connected in time and space, such as might be isolated from an outbreak of staphylococcal or pseudomonas infection in a single ward over a period of 1 or 2 months, to the action of a range of phages which have been isolated, usually from bacteria of the same species. Strains of staphylococci and pseudomonas vary widely in their susceptibility to the action of phages. Only isolates derived from a common source are likely to have the same phage-susceptibility pattern. This therefore provides a very satisfactory means of typing bacteria in cases of suspected cross-infection. Although phage typing may be used for Gram-positive or Gram-negative bacteria, there are relatively few species in which the system is of real value. In the streptococci, for example, phage typing does not play a major role. This is because *Streptococcus pyogenes* and *Strep. pneumoniae*, both organisms associated with outbreaks of infection, can be reliably typed using specific antigenic components in the cell. In contrast, there is considerable need for an efficient phage typing system for *Staphylococcus epidermidis* to match that available for *Staph. aureus*. While these organisms are susceptible to the action of phages there is not at present a satisfactory typing system which can be used to determine the origin of the large number of coagulase-negative staphylococci (*Staph. epidermidis*) responsible for hospital infections, for example those occurring in many neonatal intensive care units.

Modes of action of antibiotics

The unique structural and chemical composition of bacteria provide the means whereby a variety of agents have been designed which are highly active against bacteria, fungi, protozoa, chlamydia, etc., but have little or no serious effect on the mammalian host. The β-lactam antibiotics (penicillins, cephalosporins, monobactams) all act on penicillin-binding proteins located in the bacterial cell wall at, or close to, the site of integration of NAM–NAG complexes. Since the reactions involved are unique to bacteria, it is not surprising that these groups of antibiotics show no direct toxicity to the mammalian host.

By contrast, because of the similarity between biological membranes, antibiotics such as polymyxin, which act on bacterial cell membranes show a high degree of toxicity towards the membranes of the host. The 70S ribosomal structure of bacteria is distinct from the 80S configuration found in mammals and as a result the antibiotics acting on bacterial protein synthesis, notably the aminoglycosides, chloramphenicol and the macrolides, do not as a rule have the same effect on mammalian protein synthesis. Nevertheless, many of these agents have toxic manifestations not associated with protein synthesis.

There has always been considerable concern about antibiotics which are active against the nucleic acid pathways of bacteria because of the similarities between bacterial and mammalian nucleic acid synthesis, and the processes involved in their replication. This concern has largely been directed towards their potential teratogenic effect. While such effects have been demonstrated in animals fed with very large concentrations of these antibiotics for considerable periods of time, there are no confirmed reports of teratogenicity arising from the routine use of antibiotics, such as metronidazole, when they have been used on women found subsequently to be pregnant.

Bacteria are unable to absorb preformed folic acid and therefore this has to be metabolized via *p*-amino benzoic acid and tetrahydrofolate. The sulphonamides and trimethoprim interfere with these intermediate steps in the synthesis of folic acid. Like the penicillins, because they act on a unique feature of the bacterial cell they are not directly toxic. However, the sulphonamides interfere with other mammalian metabolic processes, notably those associated with bilirubin, and exert toxic manifestations in this way.

The cell membranes of many fungal species contain sterols and the specific antifungal activity of the polyene antibiotics resides in the fact that they are only active on membranes containing sterol. The agents are, however, toxic in themselves such that nystatin cannot be used parenterally and amphotericin B can only be used with great care. The new imidazole antifungal drugs (econazole, myconazole) have high antifungal activity in vitro but have proved to be less effective in vivo.

Features of some important bacteria

1. The Gram-positive cocci.

a. Staphylococci. Staphylococcus aureus (pyogenes) is the major pathogen in the genus *Staphylococcus*.

It is characterised by golden-yellow colonies and the production of the enzyme coagulase as well as certain toxins. *Staphylococcus aureus* is an important pathogen causing wound infection and abscesses. It can be phage typed and the type strains divided into three groups: group I contains many hospital epidemic strains; group II strains are associated with impetigo and pemphigus neonatorum; group III contains many antibiotic-resistant strains and those producing enterotoxin. *Staphylococcus epidermidis* forms white colonies on agar and does not produce coagulase. The organism is pathogenic only under certain circumstances and infection is largely confined to patients who are immunocompromised. The majority of hospital isolates of *Staph. aureus* produce pencillinase (β-lactamase), which renders them resistant to penicillin and ampicillin. These organisms are sensitive to flucloxacillin, the cephalosporins and fusidic acid. Antibiotic resistance is a common feature of *Staph. aureus* and many hospitals currently have problems with methicillin-resistant strains (MRSA).

b. Streptococci. Streptococci are most conveniently divided according to their effect on red blood cells into β, α (green) and γ (non-haemolytic) strains. β-Haemolytic streptococci and some α-haemolytic streptococci can also be classified according to the Lancefield grouping system into groups A to O. The major human pathogens belong to Lancefield groups A, B, C and G. Group A streptococci (*Strep. pyogenes*) can be typed into more than 60 subtypes according to the M, T or R surface protein antigens. The Lancefield group A streptococcus is the major pathogen in this group and in the past was a major source of puerperal sepsis. Group B (*Strep. agalactiae* (GBS)) is an important cause of neonatal and puerperal infection.

The α-haemolytic streptococci include *Strep. pneumoniae*; the enterococci (faecal streptococci), many of which belong to Lancefield group D; the viridans streptococci of the respiratory tract and a group of low-grade pathogens, including *Strep. milleri*, an organism responsible for abscess formation. This group contains the organisms most frequently associated with endocarditis, particularly the viridans streptococci.

2. The Gram-positive bacilli.

a. *The genus* Corynebacterium. This group of bacteria includes *Corynebacterium diphtheriae* and many commensal bacteria (diphtheroids or coryneforms). These organisms show characteristic Chinese lettering or pallisading in stained smears, which occurs as a consequence of their longitudinal division. *Corynebacterium diphtheriae* is divided into three colonial biotypes, gravis, intermedius and mitis. Only toxin-producing strains of *C. diphtheriae* are significant pathogens. Toxin production is mediated by a bacteriophage. Toxigenic strains are recognised by the Elek test.

b. *The genus* Listeria. This group of bacteria also contains a single major pathogen, *Listeria monocytogenes*, a motile organism distributed widely in nature and responsible for serious infection in the newborn and the aged. *Listeria monocytogenes* is one of the eight species in this genus. While other species are occasionally isolated from human infections *L. monocytogenes* is the predominant human pathogen. Virulence factors associated with *L. monocytogenes* include the ability to survive within macrophages and the production of at least two haemolysins. The organism also produces lipolysin and cytotoxic substances such as hydrogen peroxide. Antibodies to flagellar and somatic antigens can be used to divide *L. monocytogenes* into 13 serovars, although only two are likely to cause human infections. The organism has been isolated from vegetables, the guts of wild birds and numerous species of mammal, including domestic cattle. Up to 70% of the human population can carry the organism in their gut at any one time. Outbreaks and sporadic cases of listeriosis have been associated with the ingestion of a variety of foods, including milk, cheese, meat, diary products and salads. The organism can frequently be isolated from cooked chilled food sold in supermarkets and in up to 60% of raw chicken pieces. Although the minimum dose of *L. monocytogenes* is unknown, it is considered that the levels isolated from many of these foods are dangerous since the food is subsequently cooked little if at all. Nosocomial cross-infection is a common feature of hospitalized cases of listeriosis. Among the factors that enable *L. monocytogenes* to survive and multiply in food are:

1. Resistance to alkaline conditions
2. The ability to grow under microaerophilic and anaerobic conditions

3. The ability to grow in certain foods in which the salt concentration may be as high as 10%
4. The ability to survive in concentrations of sodium nitrite that are permissible as food preservatives.

The range of illness caused by *L. monocytogenes* extends from asymptomatic infection to life-threatening conditions such as meningitis and septicaemia. Symptomatic infection is normally associated with persons whose immune response is impaired because of age (neonates and the elderly), in pregnancy and those treated with immunosuppressive drugs.

About one-third of all reported cases of *L. monocytogenes* infections are associated with pregnancy (maternal, fetal, neonatal). The fetus is usually affected. The condition may cause intrauterine death (20% of cases) or be apparent at or soon after delivery. Amongst infants infected, three-quarters die in utero or present with early-onset neonatal infection. The remaining one-quarter present as intermediate- or late-onset neonatal infections. Listeriosis occurs throughout pregnancy and should not be regarded as a disease exclusively of the third trimester. In one-third of mothers whose infants suffer intrauterine death or early neonatal sepsis, a pyrexial illness has not been reported. Serious infection of the central nervous system rarely occurs in pregnant women but it is reported in up to 60% of cases not associated with pregnancy; the reasons for this are not known. Recurrent listeriosis in the same woman during different pregnancies has been reported but is extremely rare. Listeriosis has not been implicated as a cause of recurrent human abortion.

c. *The genus* Clostridium. Organisms in this genus are characteristically anaerobic spore bearers. The major pathogens include *Cl. perfringens* (formerly *Cl. welchii*), *Cl. tetani* and *Cl. oedematiens*. Strains of *Cl. perfringens* may be distinguished according to the toxins (A–E) they produce. Classical gas gangrene and septic abortion are associated with type A strains. Food poisoning is due to a subgroup of type A, other human and animal infections are due to types B to E. The exotoxin produced by *Cl. tetani* contains a powerful neurotoxic component (tetanospasmin) and a tetanolysin which lyses red cells. *Cl tetani* may be harboured in the gut and is prevalent in well-manured soil. The germination of spores depends on a low oxygen tension in traumatised tissue. Neonatal tetanus and puerperal tetanus are frequently encountered in developing countries. The third pathogen in this genus, *Cl. botulinum*, produces an extremely potent toxin. This organism produces an intoxication not an infection. In adults this is consequent upon the ingestion of preformed toxin, which affects the cholinergic system blocking the release of acetylcholine at the presynaptic level. Neonatal botulism may arise as the result of the bacteria growing in the gut and liberating toxin as a consequence.

3. The Gram-negative cocci — the genus Neisseria. The major pathogens in this group are *Neisseria meningitidis* and *N. gonorrhoeae*. A third species, *N. catarrhalis*, has recently been reclassified as *Branhamella catarrhalis* and is implicated in low-grade infection. All these organisms have a characteristic bean-shaped diplococcal morphology. *Neisseria gonorrhoeae* is characteristically found inside polymorphonuclear leucocytes in the inflammatory exudate causing gonorrhoea or gonococcal ophthalmia. *Neisseria meningitidis* is spread from the nasopharynx of healthy carriers and is frequently associated with outbreaks of meningitis in military recruits, schools, etc. *Neisseria gonorrhoeae* cannot be isolated from patients who do not have gonorrhoea.

4. Enteric Gram-negative rods. This group includes several families of bacteria (the Enterobacteriaceae, the Pseudomonadaceae) and many genera (for example, *Escherichia*, *Salmonella*, *Klebsiella*, *Proteus*). The enteric Gram-negative rods are a mixed group of bacteria with many common features.

All of them may be isolated from the gut. They are divided initially into lactose-fermenting bacteria, such as the genera *Escherichia* and *Klebsiella*, and non-lactose-fermenting groups, such as the genera *Salmonella* and *Shigella*. The bacteria are identified by complex biochemical and serological techniques. The endotoxins of Gram-negative bacteria are complex lipopolysaccharides derived from bacterial cells. Multiple drug resistance and the transfer of drug resistance from one organism to another is a common feature of this group of bacteria. The salmonellae cause enteric fever, septicaemia and food poisoning. The shigellae are responsible for bacillary dysentery. *Escherichia coli* is renowned for its role in urinary tract infections and as a cause of neonatal meningitis. Many varieties of enteric Gram-negative rods may be isolated from the hospital environment where they are often associated with outbreaks of nosocomial infection.

5. Anaerobic Gram-negative bacteria. These are non-sporing bacilli or coccobacilli with strictly anaerobic growth requirements. The major genera in this group are *Bacteroides*, *Fusobacteria* and, more recently, *Mobiluncus*. These organisms form part of the normal flora of man, being harboured in the mouth, gut and vagina, and are responsible, with other anaerobes, for abscess formation, wound infections and, possibly, vaginosis. The group is classified on morphological, cultural and biochemical characteristics.

Mobiluncus species. These are microaerophilic motile curved rods first described in the early 1980s. They are present in large numbers in anaerobic (or bacterial) vaginosis. Two species have been distinguished by cell morphology, *Mob. curtisi* (short curved rods; Gram variable) and *Mob. mulieris* (long curved rods; Gram negative). Their role in the pathogenesis of vaginosis has not

been established. The term vaginosis is used to indicate one of the characteristic features of this non-specific infection, that is, that there is no inflammation of the vaginal mucosa and no inflammatory exudate (pus cells, etc., in the discharge). There is a foul-smelling (fishy) discharge that may be distressing to the patient but no pain or irritation. The pH of the vaginal secretions is above 5.0 and the addition of a drop of potassium hydroxide to the secretions on a glass slide releases a strong fishy smell due to amines. The bacteria associated with vaginosis are *Gardnerella vaginalis*, bacteriodes species of the melaninogenicus–oralis group as well as *mobiluncus*. A characteristic feature of non-specific vaginosis is the presence of 'clue cells' in the Gram film of vaginal swabs. These are vaginal epithelial cells coated with Gram-variable bacilli.

Mycoplasmas

These are a range of microorganisms which bridge the gap between bacteria and viruses. The major distinguishing features of these organisms are shown in Table 4.4. The mycoplasmas are an exception to the rule that bacterial cells are encased in rigid cell walls. Their cells are essentially

Table 4.4 Distinctive features of the major microbial groups

	Bacteria	Mycoplasmas	Rickettsiae	Chlamydia	Viruses
Growth on inanimate culture media	+	+	−	−	−
Multiplication by binary fission	+	+	+	+	−
DNA or RNA	Both	Both	Both	Both	Either but not both
Presence of ribosomes	+	+	+	+	−
Energy-producing enzymes	+	+	+	+	−
Sensitivity to antibiotics	+	+	+	+	−
Sensitivity to interferon	−	−	−	+	+
Rigid cell wall	+	−	+	−	−

protoplasts, that is, a bacterium with a thin elastic semipermeable cytoplasmic membrane but without a rigid peptidoglycan (NAM–NAG) cell wall. Mycoplasmas are smaller than other bacteria (~ 0.25 μm diameter), they grow and reproduce like bacteria but their lack of a cell wall means that they are of variable shape and can survive only under isotonic conditions. They have much in common with the mutant forms of normal bacteria known as L-forms and, in lacking a cell wall, are, by definition, resistant to antibiotics of the penicillin and cephalosporin groups.

Rickettsiae, *Coxiella burnetii* and chlamydiae

These organisms should be regarded as bacteria because they contain both ribonucleic acid (RNA) and DNA and have muramic acid in their outer coats. They reproduce by binary fission and are susceptible to the action of antibacterial drugs that have no effect on viruses. On the other hand, with diameters of only 0.2–0.5 μm they are nearer in size to viruses than to the bacteria, and they are also, with only one known exception, unable to reproduce except inside the cells of the host organisms. Rickettsiae and coxiella are pleomorphic, forming cocci, bacilli or filaments. By contrast, chlamydiae are spherical and have an unusual type of predominantly intracellular developmental cycle. The infective forms (elementary bodies) are about 0.3 μm in diameter. They are phagocytosed by host cells and develop within them into larger forms (reticulate bodies) up to 2 μm in diameter. More reticulate bodies are formed by binary fission during the next 20 hours or so but by about 40 hours these have become reorganised into large numbers of elementary bodies. Rupture of the host cells at 48–72 hours after infection releases the elementary bodies, which can then infect new host cells. Intracellular clusters of chlamydiae can be seen as basophilic inclusion bodies in Giemsa-stained smears. By contrast the inclusion bodies formed by viruses are acidophilic.

Viruses

With the possible exception of some of the pox-viruses, all human viruses are too small to be seen with the ordinary light microscope, unless they form inclusion bodies. Inclusion bodies may occur in the cytoplasm of the host cell, e.g. those of pox-virus infections, or within its nucleus, for example those associated with infection due to herpes simplex and the adenoviruses. Most inclusion bodies contain active viruses and are intracellular 'colonies'. Viruses have no metabolism of their own and cannot reproduce independently of the host cell. It is therefore arguable whether they should be described as living organisms. For this reason, viruses which are able to invade host cells and replicate are described as active rather than alive, and those which have lost the ability to reproduce are described as inactivated rather than dead. The virus particle is called a virion, not a cell. At its simplest, as in the virus of poliomyelitis, this particle is only 25–30 nm in diameter and consists only of a nucleic acid core (the genome), packed within a protein coat (the capsid), which protects the genome during transmission between host cells. At the other extreme the virions of poxviruses measure approximately 200×300 nm and are chemically and structurally considerably more complex, though they are still developments of the same basic plan.

The nucleic acid found in a virus is either RNA or DNA but never both, in contrast to bacteria and other cellular organisms. Viruses are divided according to whether they contain RNA, e.g. the entero-, rota- and retroviruses or DNA, e.g. the herpes-, pox- and parvoviruses. Viruses increase in number not by fission but by replication inside bacterial, plant or animal host cells which they have converted into virus production units. A variety of classification systems have been devised for viruses; examples from a system which is widely accepted are shown in Tables 4.5 and 4.6. The characteristics used in delineating the main groups within this system include:

1. Particle size. The size of virus particles is now determined by electron microscopy by comparison with particles of known size.

2. Nature of the nucleic acid in the genome.

3. Symmetry of the capsid. This is determined by the shapes and mutual attractions of the units within the capsid. These units are called capsomeres. The capsid may be an icosahedron

Table 4.5   Basic features of some DNA-containing viruses

Group	Examples	Important characteristics	Pathogenic qualities
Poxvirus	Variola Vaccinia *Molluscum contagiosum*	Large brick-shaped particle 230–300 × 200–250 nm visible by light microscopy. Resists drying. If dry, survives 10 mins at 100°C. Grows in chick embryo. Produces haemagglutinins	Smallpox, vaccinia, molluscum contagiosum, cowpox, milker's nodes. Localised skin lesions and generalised rashes
Herpesvirus	Herpes simplex virus Varicella zoster virus Epstein–Barr virus Cytomegalovirus	Enveloped icosahedral nucleocapsid — 62 capsomeres. Grows in nucleus. Ether sensitive. Labile at room temperature. No haemagglutinin	Vesicular skin lesions. Prolonged latency and repeated recrudescences. Stomatitis. Encephalitis. Chickenpox and shingles
Adenovirus	Many serotypes causing human infection	Naked icosahedron has 240 hexamers and 12 pentamers with fibres and knobs attached. Multiplies in nucleus. Ether resistant. Serotypes distinguished by neutralisation. One CF group. Some types produce haemagglutinins	Latent infections of lymphoid tissue. Bronchiectasis. Feverish pharyngitis, mild respiratory disease, pneumonia, conjuctivits and keratitis
Papovavirus	Human warts	Icosahedral. Multiply in nucleus. Slow growth cycle. Ether stable. Resists 56–65°C. Produces haemagglutinins	Human warts and oncogenic viruses of animals
Parvovirus	Minute viruses of man and animals	Very small, 18–22 nm in diameter. Ether resistant	Fifth disease (erythema infectiosum; aplastic crises if marrow under stress)

— a hollow, nearly spherical structure with 20 identical triangular faces. These viruses are said to show 'cubic symmetry', and their classification is based upon the number of capsomeres. In other groups the capsomeres form a spherical arrangement producing a hollow cylinder; these are said to show 'helical symmetry'. Some viruses have a more elaborate structure and are described as complex; for example, the brick-shaped poxviruses and the tadpole-like viruses which attack bacteria (bacteriophages).

4. Presence of an envelope. In some virus groups the nucleocapsid, i.e. the nucleic core plus the capsid, is surrounded by a loose membranous envelope consisting of lipids, proteins and carbohydrates derived from the host cell membrane as the virus is liberated from the cell, e.g. the myxoviruses. Enveloped viruses may be described as ether sensitive or resistant dependent upon whether or not they are inactivated by treatment with ether. This suggests that in sensitive viruses the lipid components of the envelope are necessary for viral activity. Closely associated with the envelopes of the myxoviruses are numerous projections associated with their haemagglutination activity. Viruses that do not have envelopes are described as naked.

Bacteriophages

Bacteriophages are a mixed group of viruses. They are found in many bacterial species but show a

Table 4.6   Basic features of some RNA-containing viruses

Group	Representative viruses	Important characteristics	Pathogenic qualities
Orthomyxovirus	Influenza viruses A, B, and C	Spherical or filamentous, RNA helix of 8 nm diameter. Enveloped by a lipoprotein membrane including haemagglutinin or neuraminidase subunits. Marked antigenic variation. Matures at cell membrane. Ether sensitive	Epidemic and endemic influenzae, pneumonia, bronchitis
Paramyxovirus	Parainfluenza viruses Measles	Small, naked icosahedra, but larger RNA helix 18 nm in diameter	Acute respiratory infections, colds, croup, measles, mumps
Togavirus	Yellow fever and dengue viruses	Icosahedra enveloped by a lipid-containing envelope which contains a protein haemagglutinin. Arthopod vectors. Antigen-sharing in several groups	Meningoencephalitis, lymphadenopathy, bleeding and purpuric rashes, yellow fever
Picornavirus	Enterovirus groups: contains three polio, >24 ECHO and >30 Coxsackie viruses, rhinoviruses, foot-and-mouth disease viruses. Rotaviruses	Small naked isosahedra, cubical symmetry, ether and acid resistant. Rhinoviruses are acid labile at pH 5.3. Stable at atmospheric temperatures for several weeks	Neuronal damage and paralyses (mainly polio 1 and 3 viruses), aseptic meningitis, epidemic myalgia (Bornholm), herpangina myocarditis and pericarditis, common colds, foot and mouth disease
Coronavirus	Human and animal viruses	Elliptical or spherical with club-shaped surface projections about 20 nm long. Ether sensitive	Colds and acute respiratory infections
Retrovirus	Oncoviruses: HTLV-I,II. Lentiviruses: HIV-I,II	Small spherical enveloped virus with single-stranded RNA genome. Unique form of RNA replication in which viral RNA-transcribed DNA is integrated into the host cell genome	Multiple immunological defects. Viruses have specific trophism for T4 (helper) cells

high degree of host specificity so that any one phage is usually limited not only to a single bacterial species but to certain strains within that species. This specificity is of practical value in subdivision of bacterial species for epidemiological purposes by phage typing. Bacteriophages differ in size and form but as a group they have the greatest structural complexity of any viruses. The nucleic acid is DNA in most of those that have been studied. The best known group of phages are the T-phages of *Escherichia coli*. These are tadpole shaped with a head containing the DNA core surrounded by a protein coat that corresponds to the capsid. From the head emerges a thin hollow tubular tail with an end-plate and terminal fibres by which the virus becomes attached and absorbed to the cell wall of its bacterial host. Once attached and absorbed the phage digests a small area of bacterial cell wall, the tail then contracts, injecting the viral DNA into the bacterial cell.

Cytomegalovirus

Cytomegalovirus (CMV) is one of the human herpesviruses. These are characterised by their ability to lie latent in the body following primary infection only to be reactivated periodically and to produce recurrent infection. CMV is an ubiquitous virus that infects most people during their lifetime. The acquisition rate varies inversely with socioeconomic status, being highest among people in developing countries and lowest among those of high socioeconomic status in industrialised countries. CMV infection in adults is almost always symptomless. About 40% of women in Great Britain do not have antibody to CMV and are therefore susceptible. Approximately 1% of susceptible women will have a primary infection during pregnancy and in 20–50% of cases the virus will be transmitted to the fetus or newborn infant. CMV infection of susceptible pregnant women may result from kissing or sexual contact, from their young children or, rarely, from blood transfusion. More than 90% of primary CMV infections are asymptomatic. Both primary and recurrent maternal CMV infection can lead to transmission of the virus to the fetus. This occurs in about 40% of pregnancies complicated by primary CMV infection. The virus may reach the fetus by the haematogenous route, by vertical transmission or, following delivery, through an infected birth canal. Transmission may occur at all stages of pregnancy but the risk of severe congenital infection is probably higher when maternal infection is acquired during the first 20 weeks. The consequences of intrauterine infection with CMV range from fetal loss to congenital malformation and symptomatic or asyptomatic infection. In Great Britain, 0.3–0.4% of infants are congenitally infected with CMV and a fifth of infected infants are damaged. Even among infants who appear normal at birth the consequences of congenital CMV infection may become manifest later in life. Delivery through an infected birth canal results in CMV acquisition in about half the patients, but excretion of the virus by these infants is not apparent before 4–12 weeks of age. Infants with symptomatic CMV infection are usually born of women who had a primary infection during pregnancy. Recurrent infection in the mother only rarely results in symptomatic congenital infection. Maternal immunity to CMV does not prevent the vertical transmission of the virus but does reduce the risk of fetal damage from such infection. Routine screening of women during pregnancy for evidence of primary or recent CMV infection would not be helpful Even when infection is known to have occurred, termination of the pregnancy is not a realistic or sensible option. At the present time, vaccination also offers no help in preventing congenital infection.

Rubella

It is 50 years since Gregg first described the association between maternal rubella infection in pregnancy and the occurrence of congenital effects in the offspring. However in spite of the availability of safe and effective vaccines a significant proportion of women of childbearing age continues to be susceptible and, in consequence, congenital infection is still reported. The virus of rubella, is purely a parasite of man with no arthropod or other vector. It is a separate genus Rubivirus within the family Togaviridae. The disease is generally mild and unimportant in children and non-pregnant adults, but when contracted by a pregnant woman it can have serious effects on the fetus, especially when infection occurs during the first trimester. Infection in the mother may lead to fetal loss or to birth of an infant with varying degrees of abnormality. In Great Britain, approximately 10% of women of childbearing age are susceptible despite the availability of an effective vaccine. In the absence of a protective level of antibody in the maternal serum, the virus can reach the placenta and may infect the baby. The chances of this happening and the extent of any associated fetal damage depend on the stage of pregnancy. Infections occurring after the 20th week of pregnancy rarely result in congenital defects. Infection during the first 20 weeks of pregnancy may result in a variety of defects, not all of which are apparent at birth. Amongst those appearing later in life are nerve deafness, mental retardation, seizures and choroidoretinitis. Infected babies may be profuse excretors of virus during the early months of life and constitute a potential hazard to other nonimmune pregnant mothers and their fetuses. Approximately a third of infants born with congenital rubella die within a few months. Prenatal screening would reassure the majority of women that they were protected from rubella and identify those who should be immunised before conception; however, in the majority of cases, women are only tested when they come to the antenatal clinic. As a result, those who are susceptible cannot be vaccinated until after delivery. The policy in Great Britain is to immunise schoolgirls and non-pregnant fertile women with a live attenuated rubella vaccine. Pregnancy should be avoided for 3 months following vaccination. However, congenital abnormalities have not been reported in cases where the mother was inadvertently vaccinated immediately prior to, or early in, pregnancy. In Great Britain, susceptibility to rubella is significantly higher among Asian antenatal patients (6%) than amongst non-Asians (2%) and the incidence of notified congenital rubella is 2.3 times higher among Asians compared with the non-Asian population.

Hepatitis

The alphabet of viral hepatitis includes a range of very different and unrelated human pathogens.

The hepatitis A virus, enterovirus type 72, is a small RNA virus similar to the picornavirus family. It is the cause of infectious or epidemic hepatitis, which is transmitted by the faecal–oral route.

The hepatitis B virus is a double-stranded DNA virus, which replicates by reverse transcription. The disease, which is epidemic in the human population and hyperepidemic in many parts of the world, is spread parenterally. Persistent infection — chronic carriage — is estimated to affect more than 300 million people.

The hepatitis C virus has been identified recently as a single-stranded enveloped RNA virus which is unrelated to hepatitis A. About 80% of patients worldwide with blood-borne non-A/non-B hepatitis have antibody to hepatitis C although the frequency of antibodies in donor blood is low. Infection is spread parenterally. In common with hepatitis B there are chronic sequelae of hepatitis C

infection which include chronic active hepatitis, cirrhosis and primary liver cancer.

The hepatitis D virus, the δ agent, is an unusual virus in having a single-stranded circular RNA genome. It requires a 'helper' function provided by the hepatitis B virus. It is transmitted with the hepatitis B virus and is an important cause of acute and severe chronic liver damage in many parts of the world.

Enterically transmitted non-A/non-B hepatitis (hepatitis E) occurs in both epidemic and sporadic forms and is generally associated with drinking water which has become contaminated with sewage. Person-to-person spread may also occur. Large epidemics have been reported from the Indian subcontinent, parts of the Soviet Union and the Far East. Outbreaks have also been reported from Africa and Mexico. The infection mainly affects young and middle-aged adults and, in pregnant women, is associated with a very high mortality, up to 40%. The epidemiological features of the infection resemble those of hepatitis A, although the agents are not serologically related, and patients who have recovered from, and are immune to, hepatitis A are susceptible to infection with hepatitis E. The biophysical properties of hepatitis E demonstrated so far suggest that it is similar to the calciviruses, such as the Norwalk virus, which are usually associated with severe diarrhoea.

Retroviruses

The discovery in 1977 of an epidemic form of agressive adult T cell leukaemia (ATL) heralded a host of dramatic events which have had profound implications throughout medicine. The clinical description of ATL was closely followed by isolation of the causal agent, human T cell leukaemia/lymphoma virus (HTLV-I), and the demonstration of specific antibody in infected patients. The implications of the discovery of HTLV-I were overshadowed by the subsequent development of the acquired immune deficiency syndrome (AIDS) epidemic and the necessary work on the human immunodeficiency virus (HIV-1), previously classified as HTLV-III. HIV-I and HTLV-I are both retroviruses, although they are now classified into separate groups. The retroviruses are RNA viruses which induce DNA transcription from viral RNA so that DNA can be intregrated into the host cell genome. In their natural history and cellular effects the two viruses are totally distinct.

Detection of specific HIV antibody indicates exposure to the virus and, as infection is believed to persist, possibly for life, it is a marker of infection. Patients in the early stages of infection may be virus positive but antibody negative for an indeterminate period of time until seroconversion occurs. Infection with HIV is transmitted mainly by sexual intercourse and, in consequence, HIV infection is especially relevant to obstetric and perinatal practice. At present the majority of cases of heterosexual AIDS is confined to intravenous drug users. However, the number of heterosexual cases in the non-addict population is increasing; in the USA there was an increase of 135% between 1985 and 1986.

While the HIV virus is transmitted more effectively from male to female than vice versa, there is no doubt that infection can be transmitted from women to men. The fetus can often be infected antenatally, during delivery and by breast feeding.

Fungi

These are generally larger than bacteria and are commonly multicellular. Fungal cell walls do not contain peptidoglycan (NAM–NAG) but owe their rigidity to fibrils of chitin embedded in a matrix of protein and mannan or glucan. Inside the cell wall lies a sterol-containing cytoplasmic membrane, which is the target for the polyene antifungal agents such as nystatin and amphotericin B.

Most fungi that infect man grow in a wide range of temperatures, although the optimal temperature for the majority is between 25 and 30°C. The dermatophytes responsible for superficial infections, such as ringworm, grow best between 28 and 30°C, while organisms such as *Candida albicans* or *Aspergillus fumigatus*, which are responsible for systemic infections, grow best at 37°C. Fungi are predominantly aerobic but many yeasts can produce alcohol by fermentation as an end product

of anaerobic metabolism. Virtually all fungi have the potential to reproduce by a process of mitosis, forming asexual spores. These may be conidia, produced in large numbers by filamentous fungi, such as aspergillus or the dermatophytes, or chlamydospores produced in small numbers, for survival in extreme conditions, by fungi such as *C. albicans*. The majority of fungi pathogenic in man were thought to lack a sexual phase in their life cycle and were therefore classified as the 'fungi imperfecti'. A sexual phase has now been demonstrated in the laboratory for many of these pathogenic fungi; however, it is convenient in the medical context to leave them under a single grouping of the 'fungi imperfecti'.

Pathogenic fungi

There are four main groups of pathogenic fungi: moulds (filamentous fungi), true yeasts, yeast-like fungi and dimorphic fungi.

Filamentous fungi. These grow as long filaments called hyphae, and the branched hyphae intertwine to form a 'mycelium'. Reproduction is by spores, including sexual spores, which are characteristic and are important in identification. The fungi all grow on Sabouraud's medium and often appear as powdery colonies due to the presence of abundant spores. The majority of fungi in this group come under the general heading of the dermatophytes, that is, the fungi responsible for superficial skin, nail and hair infections, and belong to the genera *Trichophyton*, *Microsporum* and *Epidermophyton*.

True yeasts. These are unicellular, round or oval fungi. Reproduction is by budding from the parent cell. Cultures in vitro characteristically show creamy colonies. The major pathogen in this group is *Cryptococcus neoformans*, which is characterised by a large polysaccharide capsule. Encapsulated yeasts in biological fluids are diagnostic of cryptococcal infection.

Yeast-like fungi. These organisms appear like yeasts as round or oval cells and reproduce by budding, but they also form long-branching filaments known as 'pseudohyphae'. *Candida* is the characteristic genus in this group with *C. albicans* being the major pathogen. Chlamydospores distinguish *C. albicans* from other members of the genus.

Dimorphic fungi. These grow as yeast forms in the body and at 37°C on culture media, but grow in a mycelial form in the environment or on culture media at 22°C. Several members of this group of fungi grow intracellularly in reticuloendothelial cells in infected patients, for example *Histoplasma capsulatum*.

Protozoa

These are unicellular organisms which are much larger than bacteria, and show clear differentiation of their protoplasm into nucleus and cytoplasm. They are eukaryotes. Their reproductive mechanisms vary from simple binary fission with nuclear replication by mitosis to complex life cycles involving sexual and asexual phases and the formation of cysts.

Parasitic protozoa are a small proportion of the whole subkingdom of protozoa but representatives of one group or another infect most vertebrate and invertebrate animals. Parasitic protozoa can multiply either sexually or asexually, or both; replication occurs in the host. In particular, their capacity for very rapid asexual reproduction accounts in a large part for their ability to reproduce clinically overwhelming infections. The protozoa of medical importance are placed in three phyla, Sarcomastigophora, Ampicomplexa and Ciliophora. A list of the medically important species is given in Table 4.7. The two protozoa of obstetric importance are *Trichomonas vaginalis* and *Toxoplasma gondii*.

Table 4.7 Some protozoan infections of man

Region	Protozoan
Intestinal	*Entamoeba* ssp. *Giardia intestinalis* *Cryptosporidium* ssp.
Blood	*Plasmodium* ssp. (malaria)
Blood and tissues	*Trypanosoma* ssp.
Tissues	*Toxoplasma gondii*
Lung	*Pneumocystis carinii*
Genital	*Trichomonas vaginalis*

Trichomonas vaginalis is common throughout the world and, in the developed world, is probably the commonest protozoan pathogen. It is transmitted by sexual intercourse and causes vaginitis in women and non-specific (non-gonococcal) urethritis in men. There are reported to be between 1.5 and 2 million cases annually in Great Britain. The parasite is oval or pear shaped with an undulating membrane along one side and four anterior flagellae. It measures 15 μm long by 7 μm wide. No cyst stage is known, and the parasite probably multiplies by simple binary fission. Transmission is direct and occurs during sexual contact; no non-human hosts are known. Infection of the vagina is usually accompanied by a purulent frothy discharge and by changes in the surface epithelium and submucosa of the vagina and cervix. Parasites are usually found on the mucosal surface and in fluid exudate but they do not invade. The severity of infection in women ranges from asymptomatic carriage to severe vaginitis. In contrast, the infection in men is generally mild or asymptomatic and often self-limiting. The treatment of choice is metronidazole. Successful treatment depends on tracing and treating all sexual contacts of a case.

Toxoplasma gondii is an intracellular protozoan with a worldwide distribution, causing infection in man and a wide range of animals. The asexual phase of the organism (trophozoite) is able to develop in the tissues of a wide variety of vertebrate hosts, including man, but the definitive host is the cat family, not only the domestic cat but also wild cats in which the sexual cycle occurs in the intestine after a prolonged latent period. Human infection rates may be as high as 90% in some populations. Infection is most often acquired by ingesting trophozoites in undercooked meat, though it may follow ingestion of oocysts resulting from the sexual cycle in the intestine of a cat and which are then excreted in its faeces. Thus the danger to women during childbearing years is from cat litter trays and from gardening, where the soil is likely to have been contaminated by cat excreta. After ingestion, the parasites are distributed to many organs and tissues via the blood stream and invade nucleated cells in all parts of the body and fetus. They multiply within the host cells, disrupting and finally destroying them. Focal areas of necrosis occur in many organs, particularly the muscles, brain and eye and contain infective cysts. Infection in man is usually subclinical but may produce a glandular fever-like syndrome or choroidoretinitis. Transplacental infection may occur during an acute infection in the mother, which may not be diagnosed but may result in serious disease in the fetus. Congenital toxoplasmosis is reported to complicate about 0.5% of pregnancies in Great Britain, but is known to be significantly under-reported. Infection results from maternal infection acquired during pregnancy with transplacental transmission to the fetus. Infection early in pregnancy may result in a stillbirth, or the birth of a live baby with disseminated infection that may result in choroidoretinitis, microcephaly or hydrocephalus, intracranial calcification, hepatosplenomegaly and thrombocytopenia. Maternal infection during the third trimester can also be transmitted to the fetus, but at this stage of development it usually causes no damage. Maternal infection is commonly subclinical and goes unnoticed unless serological screening is carried out. A rise in the mother's toxoplasma antibody titre during pregnancy or the finding that she has immunoglobulin IgM antibodies, indicating recent infection, raises the question whether to treat the infection, given that treatment does not guarantee the infant will be unaffected, or to terminate the pregnancy even though it is not certain that the fetus has been damaged. As with congenital syphilis the sooner after fetal infection the treatment is started the better the prognosis for the fetus. Spiramycin is the drug of choice for treatment of the mother and her fetus. An infant with congenital infection is treated with alternate courses of spiramycin and sulphadiazine plus pyrimethamine plus folinic acid for the 1st year, with prednisolone added if there is choroidoretinitis.

Helminths (worms)

The helminth parasites of man belong to three zoologically distinct groups: trematodes (flukes, cestodes), tapeworms and nematodes (roundworms). None of the infections with helminths have special significance during pregnancy.

IMMUNOLOGY

Introduction

Ever since Medawar and his colleagues discovered the laws of transplantation immunology in the late 1940s, the survival of the fetal allograft in a potentially hostile environment has puzzled and perplexed immunologists. Medawar crystallised the paradox in these words: 'The immunological problem of pregnancy may be formulated thus: How does the pregnant mother contrive to nourish within itself, for many months or weeks, a fetus that is an antigenically foreign body?'

Many have speculated on the wide-ranging benefits that might accrue from the unravelling of the mechanisms by which the fetus eludes the maternal immune system: rational strategies might evolve for the treatment of diseases of pregnancy thought to have an immunological basis (e.g. recurrent spontaneous abortion, pre-eclampsia and intrauterine growth retardation); organ transplantation programmes might benefit by emulating nature's strategies in creating a perfect allograft; clues might emerge as to how tumours escape immunosurveillance, and new treatments might therefore be developed. Although a great deal has been learnt over the past two decades, the paradox remains unresolved. Indeed, it has become apparent that the fetus is not a conventional allograft. To understand the current concepts of the maternofetal relationship a basic knowledge of immunology is essential.

The immune system

The basic function of the immune system is to combat the numerous pathogens present in the environment. It is customary to divide the immune system into two functional units, namely the *innate* system, and the *adaptive* system. The important elements of the two systems are given in Table 4.8. Although innate immunity acts mainly as a first line of defence, and adaptive immunity as a secondary line, in fact there is a great deal of interaction between the two systems: macrophages, which are conventionally assigned to the innate system, play a central role in processing and presenting antigens to T cells, which are assigned to the adaptive system.

Table 4.8 Elements of innate and adaptive immunity

	Innate immunity	Adaptive immunity
Cellular elements	Phagocytes, natural killer (NK) cells	T cells, B cells, Null cells
Soluble elements	Complement, lysozyme, acute-phase proteins	Antibody, cytokines
Other characteristics	No memory	Demonstrates memory
Previous exposure	Response not affected by previous exposure	Response quicker and more vigorous with previous exposure

The innate immune system

The essential cellular elements of innate immunity are the phagocytes and natural killer (NK) cells, while the soluble elements are complement, acute-phase proteins and interferon. The skin provides an extensive barrier against potential pathogens. Thus, most pathogens enter the body via the epithelial surface of the nasopharynx, gut, lungs and genitourinary tract. The distribution of elements of the innate immune system is designed to minimise this.

Phagocytes

Although there are several different types of phagocytes, all are derived from bone marrow stem cells. They are given different names depending on their location: blood phagocytes include the neutrophil polymorph and the monocyte; microglial cells are found in the brain; the Kupffer cells line the sinusoids of the liver; synovial A cells line the synovial cavity; alveolar macrophages are found in the lungs and mesangial phagocytes are found in the kidney. The phagocytes are thus strategically placed to encounter and combat pathogens, which they engulf, internalise, destroy and sometimes *process* before *presenting* to cells of the adaptive immune system.

Natural killer (NK) cells

These are leucocytes which recognise cell surface changes on cancerous or virus-infected cells, and which have the capacity to engage and kill these cells. The activity of NK cells is enhanced by interferons, which are produced by virus-infected cells (see below).

Soluble factors

Complement is a system of up to 20 proteins whose activity is analogous to the blood-clotting system: the activation of the first component triggers a *cascade* reaction. Complement can be activated by antigen-antibody interactions (the *classical* pathway) or by the surface molecules of a number of microorganisms (the *alternative* pathway); thus, complement activity can occur as part of the innate or adaptive immunity. The products of complement activation have various functions: some adhere to pathogens and promote phagocytosis (opsonisation); some attract phagocytes to the site of the reaction (chemotaxis); other components have an intrinsic ability to lyse the cell membranes of many bacterial species.

Interferons are produced by virus-infected cells. They promote the activity of NK cells, and also render hitherto uninfected cells resistant to virus infection. They are produced early in infection and are thus the first line of resistance against many viruses.

Acute-phase proteins (e.g. C-reactive protein) are serum proteins whose concentration rises by up to 190-fold during infection. Their function is primarily to coat pathogens and promote their phagocytosis (opsonisation).

The events occurring in the acute inflammatory reaction typify the cellular and humoral interactions in the innate immune system.

The acquired immune system

There are four fundamental features of adaptive immunity, namely:

1. Memory
2. Specificity
3. Diversity
2. Tolerance of self.

Memory

This is demonstrated by the fact that we rarely suffer twice from certain infections (e.g. chicken pox): the first contact with an infectious agent imparts memory, so that subsequent infection is repelled. This introduces the concept of primary and secondary immune responses: the primary response occurs on first contact with a pathogen, is slower and less vigorous; the secondary response, due to memory, is characterised by a more rapid and vigorous response. This is also the rationale behind vaccination: a relatively harmless form of a pathogen (e.g. a killed virus) is used to invoke a primary response and imprint memory: any subsequent contact with the virulent pathogen results in a secondary response which is early and more vigorous.

Specificity

Contact with one pathogen does not confer protection against other pathogens: the immune system differentiates specifically between two organisms.

Diversity

The environment is full of millions of potential pathogens, yet the immune system demonstrates a remarkable capacity to mount a response to most of them. This diversity of the immune response is an essential feature if the body is to successfully combat infection. The basis of this diversity is dealt with in the section on the genetics of the immune response.

Tolerance to self

The immune system must not only distinguish between two pathogens but must also distinguish between self and non-self. Occasionally the system breaks down and autoimmunity develops. The tolerance to self-antigens is established in early life before the maturation of the immune system: those circulating body components which reach the developing lymphoid system in the perinatal period induce a permanent self-tolerance, so that when immune maturity is established there is an inability to respond to self components.

Organisation of the lymphoid system

The lymphoid system is the collective term for cells, tissues and organs involved in the immune response. All the leucocytes are derived from bone marrow stem cells: B lymphocytes in the mammalian fetus are initially generated in the liver, and mature in the bone marrow, while T lymphocytes mature in the thymus — the bone marrow and thymus are thus primary lymphoid organs. The secondary lymphoid organs, which include the spleen, lymphoid tissue of mucosal surfaces (e.g. tonsils, Peyer's patches) and lymph nodes, contain mature T and B cells and accessory-cells. Circulation or traffic of lymphocytes throughout the lymphoid organs, and through blood, is not an entirely random process, but can be greatly influenced by the presence of antigen; for example, when antigen first arrives at the lymph node of a primed individual there is an immediate shut-down of lymphocyte traffic through the node.

The lymphatic system communicates with the blood circulation: most of the lymphatic vessels from the trunk and lower limbs ultimately drain into the right thoracic duct, which returns the lymph to the circulation. Thus the traffic of lymphocytes and antigen-presenting cells through the blood stream and lymphatic system facilitates the contact of lymphocytes with antigen.

Cellular elements of adaptive immunity

T cells

T cells are lymphocytes which, having originated from bone marrow stem cells, develop and differentiate in the thymus before seeding the secondary, peripheral lymphoid tissue. Events in the thymus are not completely understood, but they are undoubtedly crucial to normal immune function: it is thought, for instance, that it is in the thymus that T cells which have the potential to recognise self-antigens are selected out and die (clonal deletion); and rearrangement of the genes encoding the T cell receptor is thought to occur during this maturation phase. Three main types of T cell can be distinguished according to function and surface proteins: T helper (T_h) and suppressor (T_s) and cytotoxic (T_c) cells. T_h cells are characterised by the surface marker cell differentiation antigen 4 (CD4). They cooperate with B cells in the production of antibodies against protein antigens (T-dependent antigens); interact with macrophages and other cells by secreting cytokines, and also promote the development of T_c

cells. T_c and T_s cells both express the surface molecule CD8, and as yet are morphologically indistinguishable. There are, however, thought to be two distinct populations on the basis of functional differences. T_c cells destroy virally infected or mutant cells, while T_c cells regulate/suppress immune responses. T cells recognise antigen only if the latter is presented in association with molecules encoded by the major histocompatibility complex (MHC).

B cells

These lymphocytes originate from stem cells in the bone marrow and develop and differentiate there. They are responsible for antibody production. They can recognise antigen directly by their surface receptors — membrane-bound immunoglobulins (Ig) which are identical to the antibody produced by that B cell. Other B cell surface molecules include MHC class II molecules, complement receptors, Fc receptors, and receptors for B cell growth and differentiation factors. To produce an antibody response to most protein antigens, B cells require both the antigen and help from antigen-specific T_h cells. Antigens which necessitate such help are called T dependent. Carbohydrate and other non-protein antigens (e.g. components of bacterial cell walls) are T independent: antibody responses by B cells do not require T cell help.

   B cells activated by antigen proliferate and differentiate into either memory cells or plasma cells. The latter are end-stage cells which produce antibody.

Null cells

These are lymphocytes which express neither T nor B cell surface markers, but express a mixture of lymphocyte and macrophage surface markers. Some of these cells possess receptors for the Fc portion of IgG: they can thus recognise target cells coated with specific antibody, and they bind via the Fc receptor and kill the target cell, hence these cells have been designated killer (K) cells. These are thought to be distinct from a further subclass of null cells which kill virally infected cells or cells

with tumour antigens, but do not act via Fc receptors, the NK cells referred to above.

Antigen-presenting cells (APCs)

APCs take up antigen, and process and modify it into an immunogenic form, before presenting it in association with MHC molecules to T lymphocytes. Many types of cells subserve the function of antigen presentation: they include macrophages, dendritic cells, Langerhans cells of the skin — even B cells themselves can present antigen to T_h cells.

   The function of antigen presentation thus illustrates the intimacy of the interaction between cells conventionally regarded as part of innate immunity and those of acquired immunity: the division of the two systems is thus artificial, but is convenient for descriptive purposes.

Humoral elements of adaptive immunity

Immunoglobulins, complement and cytokines are the three principal humoral elements of adaptive immunity.

Immunoglobulins (Igs)

Igs are produced by B cells, and can be divided into five classes on the basis of chemical, physical and biological characteristics. Each class is designated by a single capital letter after the abbreviation Ig, thus: IgG, IgM, IgA, IgD and IgE. There are, in addition, subclasses for some of them — IgG has four subclasses. The characteristics of the five Ig classes are listed in Table 4.9. All Igs are structurally similar: each one is constructed from a basic unit consisting of two identical heavy (H) polypeptide chains and two identical light (L) chains bound together by disulphide bridges. Each chain is composed of constant and variable regions. The variable region of one L chain and one H chain form an antigen-binding site. The constant regions of the Ig molecule are involved in interactions between antibody and receptors (Fc receptors) on the body's cells. Thus, antibody can act as a bifunctional adaptor, cross-

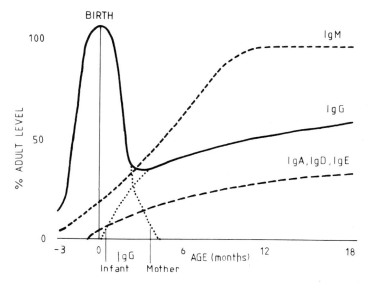

Fig. 4.7 Fate of maternal and neonatal Ig in the baby following birth. Note that the infant's IgG does not reach a large proportion of adult values until the maternal IgG is metabolised. When these curves cross, the baby is most susceptible to many infections. (Reproduced with permission from Roitt, *Essential Immunology* and Blackwell Scientific Publications.)

a wide range of pathogens before its own immune system is mature (Fig. 4.7). Occasionally, maternal IgG may be harmful to the fetus, e.g. Rhesus ISO immunisation or maternal immune thrombocytopenic purpura. It is unclear whether there is any significant non-pathological exchange of cellular elements.

A great deal has been learnt in recent years, but we are no nearer the truth. An understanding of the mechanism of fetal survival might allow the development of rational strategies for combating pregnancy disorders that may have an immunological basis, including RSA, pre-eclampsia and intrauterine growth retardation.

Immunopathology

In certain circumstances the regulatory mechanisms of the immune system breakdown: the ability to tolerate self-antigens may be lost and autoimmunity develops; or the immune responses become excessive and cause gross tissue damage (hypersensitivity). Autoimmune diseases form a wide spectrum and may involve humoral or cellular elements of the immune response or both, and the responses may be organ specific or non-organ specific. Hashimoto's thyroiditis is a typical example of an organ-specific disease, while systemic lupus erythematosus (SLE) is a typical example of a multisystem autoimmune disease where autoantibodies are formed against several body constituents, including DNA, cell surface antigens and basement membrane. SLE in particular is associated with increased reproductive wastage, e.g. recurrent miscarriage.

Four main types of hypersensitivity reactions are recognised, and these are described in Fig. 4.8. A type V reaction has been proposed for the immunostimulation responses caused by some non-complement-fixing antibodies (e.g. thyroid stimulating Igs), but this category is not associated with immunological damage. It is important to realise that the four types of reactions are not mutually exclusive and that they may coexist.

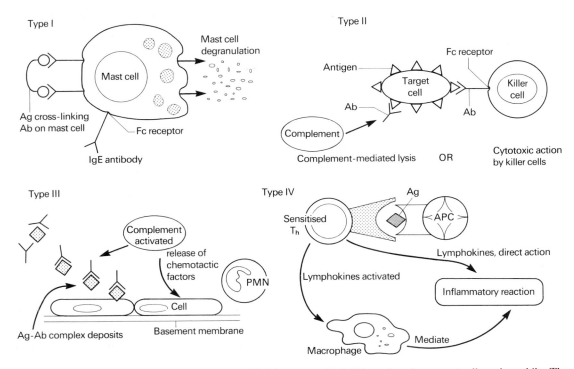

Fig. 4.8 Hypersensitivity reactions. **Type I**   Antigen (Ag) interacts with IgE bound to tissue mast cells or basophils. The cross-linking of IgE by Ag results in membrane destabilisation and release of vasoactive mediators such as histamine. Typical examples of type I reactions are asthma, rhinitis and conjunctivitis. Susceptible individuals are thought to have a genetic defect in Ag processing, which results in synthesis of IgE rather than IgG in response to certain allergens, e.g. grass-pollen, house dust, etc. **Type II**   Autoimmune haemolytic anaemias (including rhesus disease) and glomerulonephritis are typical examples of this reaction. Antibody (Ab), usually IgM or IgG, interacts with Ag on cells (erythrocytes or basement membranes) and activate complement and accessory cells to produce extensive tissue damage. **Type III**   Here Ab and Ag interact to form immune complexes in the circulation or in tissues: they may activate complement and accessory cells and thus damage tissue. Clinical examples include serum sickness, systemic lupus erythematosus and extrinsic allergic alveolitis. **Type IV**   These reactions are initiated by delayed hypersensitivity T cells (Td) which react with Ag and release lymphokines that execute their function either directly or through recruitment of macrophages, which release vasoactive amines.

5. Biochemistry

PROTEINS, PEPTIDES AND AMINO ACIDS

Introduction

Each of the many cell types in the body makes a unique set of proteins. There is considerable variation in the types of protein made by each cell type and a particular cell only synthesises a fraction of the total human protein repertoire. For example, despite the large amount of albumin present in blood plasma, it is only the hepatocytes in the liver that synthesise albumin; no other cell type does so in the adult. This is despite the fact that every cell contains within its nucleus a copy of the gene for albumin along with a copy of every other human gene. This concept is referred to as 'totipotency'; every cell has a copy of every gene even though only a fraction are expressed. During development and differentiation, the deoxyribonucleic acid (DNA) within each cell type comes under a regulatory mechanism such that some genes are expressed and others are completely repressed. In the case of some proteins, expression does not occur all the time but does so in response to a specific signal such as a hormone. The control of protein expression is aberrant in many tumours and inappropriate proteins are produced.

The proteins synthesised by a cell play a number of different roles. Some proteins have a structural role. This can be intracellular and there are proteins that provide the structural basis for the membrane around the cell and the membranes around the nucleus, mitochondria and the other discrete subcellular organelles. Figure 5.1 is a diagrammatic representation of a cell; each of the subcellular organelles contains structural proteins. Other proteins are secreted by a cell and are then used to support an extracellular structure. An example here is collagen. There are a number of forms of collagen which are encoded by discrete genes. The different collagens play specific roles; for example, collagen type I is the form found in bone, collagen type II is found in cartilage and collagen type IV is found in the basement membranes of epithelia. Collagen type III is found in the tissues of the fetus but this is replaced by type I following birth. Adults have little type III although it does reappear during the wound response. Collagen type I is a major component of bones, skin and a number of other tissues and this single protein comprises more than 50% of the total protein in the body.

Another role of proteins is enzymic function. The human genome encodes many hundreds of proteins which act as enzymes for specific reactions; these include synthetic reactions, degradative reactions, energy-producing reactions and

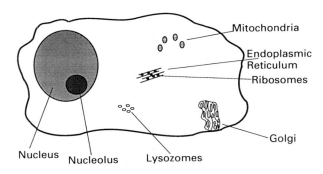

Organelle	Function
Nucleus	Contains chromosomal material and apparatus for cell division
Nucleolus	RNA and ribosome production
Lysozomes	Degradation of macromolecules
Golgi apparatus	Modification of proteins and their secretion and re-cycling
Endoplasmic reticulum	Membrane system for protein synthesis
Ribosomes	Catalyse peptide bond formation in protein synthesis
Mitochondria	Contain many enzymes involved in metabolism and energy production

Fig. 5.1 Structure of a cell.

energy-storing reactions. Very few biochemical reactions occur in the absence of enzymes and thus this catalysis is essential for life.

Some proteins are synthesized and then secreted to carry out a particular function that is non-structural. Hormones and neurotransmitters fall into this category as do the large number of proteins found in plasma that play a role in transport. One of the functions of albumin is to transport free fatty acids, and the plasma protein transferrin carries iron from the gut to tissues. In blood there are different classes of lipoproteins that carry lipids in circulation; chylomicrons carry triglycerides from the gut to adipose tissue and the liver. Low-density lipoproteins carry much of the cholesterol that is required by tissues; some of the cholesterol comes from dietary sources but most has been synthesized in the liver.

Some proteins in plasma play a hormone binding role. Other major constituents of plasma are the immunoglobulins (antibodies) and complement proteins that are part of the immune system.

Amino acids

There are 20 amino acids used in the synthesis of proteins. The generalized structure of an amino acid is shown in Figure 5.2, and Figure 5.3 shows the chemical structure of the amino acids used by man along with the two notations that are used to denote them. One is a three-letter code but, as there are so many protein sequences now available, a one-letter code has now become the preferred notation.

Man is able to synthesise some amino acids but not others. Those that can be synthesised are referred to as the non-essential amino acids and comprise the following:

Alanine   Glutamine
Aspartic acid   Glycine
Asparagine   Proline
Cysteine   Serine
Glutamic acid   Tyrosine.

The essential amino acids are:

Arginine
Histidine   Phenylalanine
Isoleucine   Threonine
Leucine   Tryptophan
Lysine   Valine.
Methionine

The situation is slightly more complex than this since man can synthesise cysteine if there is sufficient methionine present; similarly, tyrosine can be synthesised if there is sufficient phenylalanine present. Also histidine and arginine are not strictly essential but are required for normal growth.

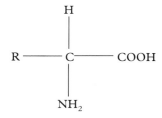

Fig. 5.2 General structure of an amino acid. R is an organic group (see Fig. 5.3)

AMINO ACID	STRUCTURE	SYMBOL
	Basic amino acids	
Arginine	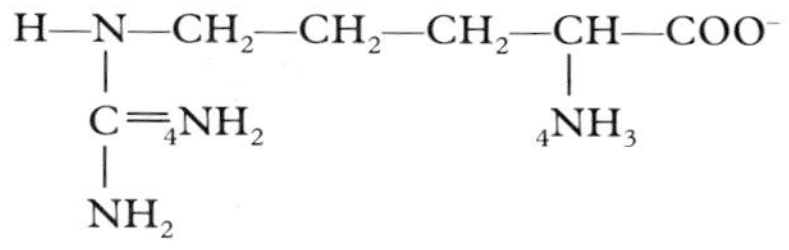 $H-N-CH_2-CH_2-CH_2-CH-COO^-$ $\quad\quad\mid\quad\quad\quad\quad\quad\quad\quad\quad\quad\mid$ $\quad\quad C=_+NH_2\quad\quad\quad\quad\quad _+NH_3$ $\quad\quad\mid$ $\quad\quad NH_2$	Arg (R)
Lysine	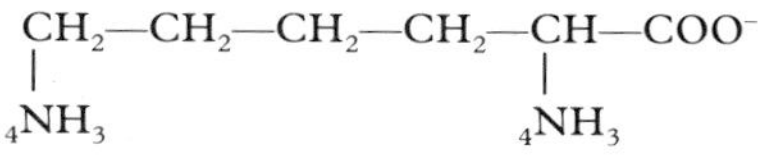 $CH_2-CH_2-CH_2-CH_2-CH-COO^-$ $\mid\quad\quad\quad\quad\quad\quad\quad\quad\quad\quad\mid$ $_+NH_3\quad\quad\quad\quad\quad\quad\quad _+NH_3$	Lys (K)
Histidine	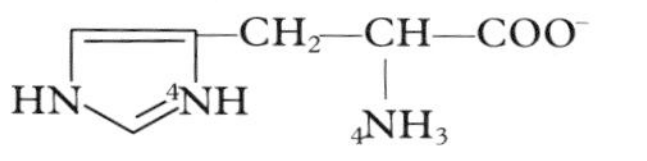 $-CH_2-CH-COO^-$ $HN\diagdown _+NH\quad\quad _+NH_3$	His (H)
	Acidic amino acids	
Aspartic acid	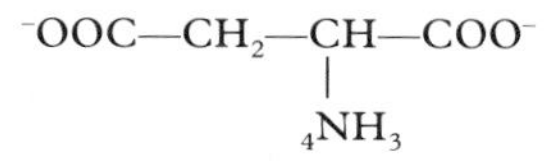 $^-OOC-CH_2-CH-COO^-$ $\quad\quad\quad\quad\quad\mid$ $\quad\quad\quad\quad _+NH_3$	Asp (D)
Glutamic acid	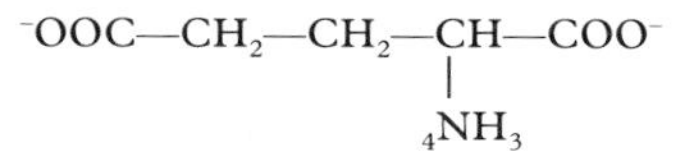 $^-OOC-CH_2-CH_2-CH-COO^-$ $\quad\quad\quad\quad\quad\quad\quad\mid$ $\quad\quad\quad\quad\quad\quad _+NH_3$	Glu (E)
Asparagine	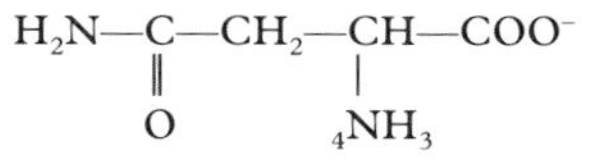 $H_2N-C-CH_2-CH-COO^-$ $\quad\quad\parallel\quad\quad\quad\mid$ $\quad\quad O\quad\quad _+NH_3$	Asn (N)
Glutamine	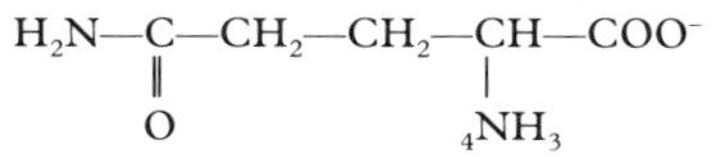 $H_2N-C-CH_2-CH_2-CH-COO^-$ $\quad\quad\parallel\quad\quad\quad\quad\quad\mid$ $\quad\quad O\quad\quad\quad\quad _+NH_3$	Gln (Q)
	Aromatic amino acids	
Phenylalanine	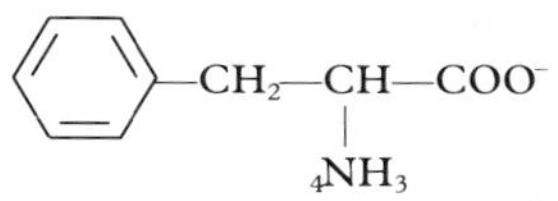 $-CH_2-CH-COO^-$ $\quad\quad\quad\quad\mid$ $\quad\quad\quad _+NH_3$	Phe (F)

Fig. 5.3   The structures of the amino acids.

AMINO ACID	STRUCTURE	SYMBOL
Aromatic amino acids		
Tyrosine	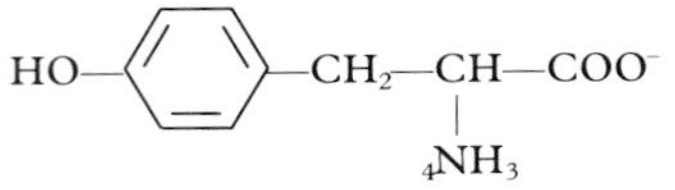 HO—⟨benzene ring⟩—CH_2—CH—COO^- with $_4NH_3$ below CH	Tyr (Y)
Tryptophan	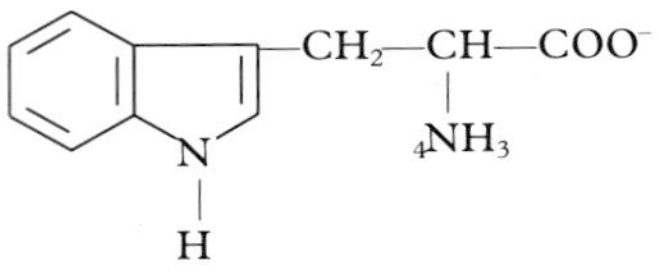 ⟨indole ring with N—H⟩—CH_2—CH—COO^- with $_4NH_3$ below CH	Trp (W)
Amino acids with aliphatic chains		
Glycine	H—CH—COO^- with $_4NH_3$ below CH	Gly (G)
Alanine	CH_3—CH—COO^- with $_4NH_3$ below CH	Ala (A)
Valine	H_3C and H_3C joined to CH—CH—COO^- with $_4NH_3$ below	Val (V)
Leucine	H_3C and H_3C joined to CH—CH_2—CH—COO^- with $_4NH_3$ below	Leu (L)
Isoleucine	CH_3—CH_2 and CH_3 joined to CH—CH—COO^- with $_4NH_3$ below	Iso (I)

Fig. 5.3   (Cont'd)

sugar chains remain intact, the protein continues to circulate in plasma. When the sugar chains become cleaved or modified then the proteins are removed from circulation and degraded. The liver has a most efficient mechanism for detecting altered circulating proteins. There are in the newly formed proteins no terminal galactose residues; there is a sialic acid residue after the galactose. If the galactosyl groups are revealed following damage to the protein it is immediately removed from circulation by hepatocytes which contain at their surface a receptor for the terminal galactose.

METABOLISM

Overall energy metabolism

Every cell has to maintain an adequate supply of energy. There are several sources of energy and each is metabolised to produce adenosine triphosphate (ATP). The ATP is essential for cellular processes such as protein synthesis, transport and the maintenance of ionic gradients across the plasma membrane. Carbohydrate and fatty acids are the normal energy sources but under certain circumstances amino acids can also be used. Which particular energy source is used depends upon a number of parameters such as dietary status, circadian rhythm, etc. In this section the individual metabolic pathways will be described followed by the controls that operate and the interrelationships between the pathways.

The metabolism of carbohydrates (sugars), fats (fatty acids) and amino acids begins with pathways that are specific for each energy source. The produces from these pathways then feed into common pathways. The overall interaction of the pathways is shown in Figure 5.6.

Sugars, fatty acids and amino acids are metabolised to produce acetate in the form of acetyl-coenzyme A (acetyl-CoA). The acetyl group has to be covalently linked to CoA for stabilisation.

The acetyl-CoA then enters the tricarboxylic acid (TCA) cycle, which is also known as the citric

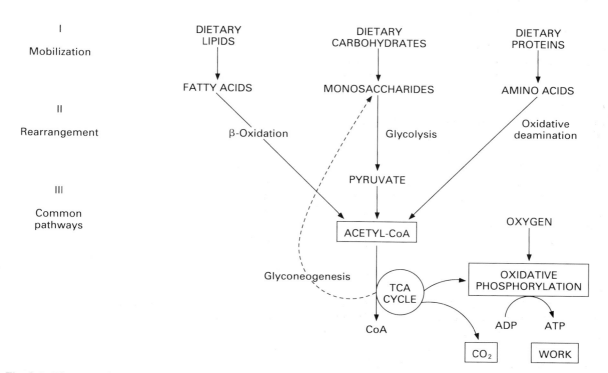

Fig. 5.6 The processing of dietary constituents.

acid cycle or the Krebs cycle, after the biochemist who was involved in its discovery. The TCA cycle results in the complete degradation of acetyl groups. The products are carbon dioxide and hydrogen in the form of nicotinamide adenine dinucleotide (NADH); the role of this cofactor will be described later. The NADH feeds into the respiratory chain inside the mitochondrion and the energy of the NADH is used to drive oxidative phosphorlyation to produce ATP from adenosine diphosphate (ADP). This reaction within the respiratory chain requires molecular oxygen, hence the name 'respiratory chain'.

Molecules such as glucose and fatty acids are sources of energy because there is an intrinsic energy within the bonds of the molecule and this energy is released when the molecule is broken into smaller parts. What nature has done is to evolve a mechanism by which this energy can be harnessed to produce ATP which acts in turn as the energy source to drive most biological reactions. Looking at the sequence of events for a molecule of glucose, the glycolytic pathway converts glucose to three acetate groups:

$$C_6H_{12}O_6 \rightarrow 3 \ C_2H_4O_2$$

The three molecules of acetate enter the TCA cycle in the form of acetyl-CoA and are converted to six molecules of carbon dioxide and 24 atoms of hydrogen in the form of NADH:

$$(3 \ C_2H_4O_2) + (6 \ H_2O) \rightarrow 6 \ CO_2 + 24 \ H$$

The carbon dioxide diffuses out of the cell and is expired by the lungs. The NADH enters the respiratory chain in the mitochondrion and, with the consumption of oxygen, is converted to water:

$$24 \ H + 6 \ O_2 \rightarrow 12 \ H_2O$$

This part of the reaction brings about the conversion of ADP to ATP.

The overall reaction has been

$$C_6H_{12}O_6 \rightarrow 6 \ CO_2 + 6 \ H_2O$$

i.e. the complete oxidation of a molecule of glucose to carbon dioxide and water. Nature has evolved an efficient sequence of reactions and most of the energy within the glucose molecule is utilised in the production of ATP from ADP. A single molecule of glucose can result in the formation of 38 ATP molecules. The chemical combustion of glucose in the presence of excess oxygen would yield 686 000 cal per mol. Each time an ADP molecule is converted to one of ATP, 7300 cal are required. Thus, since there is a net profit of about 36 molecules of ATP, this indicates that the process is approximately 40% efficient. The remaining energy is released as heat.

Glycolysis

The enzymes of the glycolytic pathway are found in the cytoplasm of the cell. The pathway converts a molecule of glucose that contains six carbon atoms to two molecules of pyruvic acid, each containing three carbon atoms. The pathway for glycolysis is shown in Figure 5.7 and it can be seen that in the first few steps the glucose becomes doubly phosphorylated; this consumes ATP and is thus energy dependent. Glucose is converted to glucose-6-phosphate, which is in turn isomerised to fructose-6-phosphate. (Here, isomerization is the rotation of two bonds around a carbon atom.) The fructose-6-phosphate is then phosphorylated to fructose-1,6-diphosphate and this is then hydrolysed to produce one molecule of 3-phosphoglyceraldehyde and one of dihydroxyacetone phosphate.

The next step is the conversion of the dihydroxyacetone phosphate into 3-phosphoglyceraldehyde. Thus, two molecules of 3-phosphoglyceraldehyde have been generated from one molecule of glucose. These two molecules are then converted to pyruvic acid via the intermediate stages 1,3-diphosphoglyceric acid, 3-phosphoglyceraldehyde and phosphoenolpyruvic acid. The two steps involving the metabolism of 1,3-diphosphoglyceric acid and phosphoenolpyruvic acid are worthy of note. In both cases the phosphate group that is transferred is of a 'high-energy' type. (This means that the phosphate bonding has high internal energy.) These groups are transferred to ADP to generate ATP.

Although more ATP is formed during glycolysis than ATP expended, there is only a net production of two molecules of ATP. Unlike the respiratory chain which is where the bulk of cellular ATP is

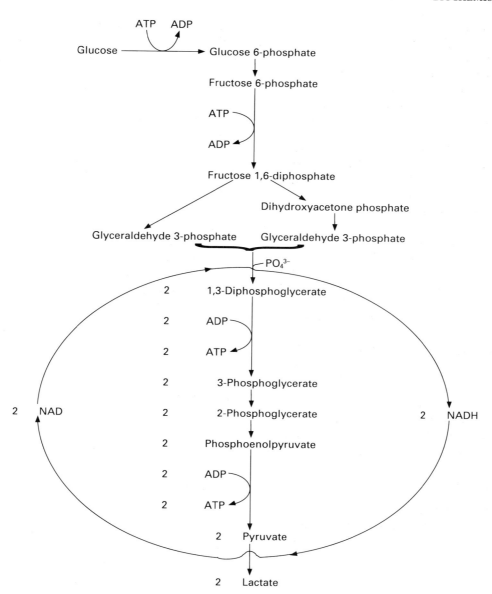

Fig. 5.7 Glycolysis, a metabolic rearrangement in which hexose sugars are converted to pyruvate or lactate. The major attack is the cleavage of fructose 1,6-diphosphate to two trioses. Note that two molecules of ATP are used up in the phosphorylation reactions in the first half of glycolysis, while two pairs of ATP molecules are produced in the second half, for an overall gain of two ATP molecules. The two NAD molecules reduced in oxidative phosphorylation of glyceraldehyde-3-phosphate are used in the anaerobic reduction of pyruvate to lactate.

produced, the glycolytic pathway does not require oxygen. Thus, for short periods of time the cell can survive without consuming oxygen by generating ATP via glycolysis.

Citric acid cycle

The enzymes that carry out the citric acid cycle are located inside the mitochondria. Pyruvate ions diffuse into the mitochondrion and become covalently attached to CoA, which acts as a carrier. Nicotinamide adenine dinucleotide (NAD⁺) plays a role in these reactions and it is necessary to know some molecular details.

Hydrogen can exist in a molecular form in which two atoms are bonded together. Although this molecular hydrogen (H_2) is highly reactive, under some conditions it is quite stable. Hydrogen never exists in an atomic state under normal conditions. Hydrogen is the simplest element and in theory consists of a nucleus with one proton and a single electron orbiting this nucleus. The reason molecular hydrogen can exist is that there are two electrons surrounding the two nuclei, which is a more stable electronic structure. When hydrogen is part of a more complex molecule, ionization can occur and the proton of hydrogen can leave the original molecule and bind to water. If this happens to an appreciable extent then the resulting solution is an acid because free protons or, rather, hydrated protons are what constitutes an acid.

NAD⁺ contains a positive charge because it is protonated, i.e. the nucleus of a hydrogen atom is part of the NAD molecule while the electron from the hydrogen has gone somewhere else. During the citric acid cycle it will be seen below that a number of metabolic steps involve NAD⁺ and as part of the enzymic reaction a hydrogen atom is transferred to NAD⁺ and a proton is released. The reaction can be viewed as

$$NAD^+ + H \rightarrow NADH + H^+$$

NADH can be viewed as a molecule containing high intrinsic energy. The NADH feeds into the respiratory chain and in the presence of oxygen will provide the energy for production of most of the ATP that is produced by any cell.

Figure 5.8 shows how the cycle operates and which are the steps that produce NADH; the structures of the substrates are shown separately for clarity.

The pyruvate is supplied into the cycle in the form of acetyl CoA, but should be viewed as a two-carbon moiety which is combined with oxaloacetate (four-carbon structure) to yield the six-carbon citric acid. After a rearrangement to isocitric acid, α-ketoglutaric acid is produced with the formation of carbon dioxide and NADH. The

next step also generates a molecule of carbon dioxide and of NADH when succinic acid is formed. There is then a series of rearrangements to fumaric and then to malic acid. In the final part of the citric acid cycle a further molecule of NADH is produced as malic acid is converted to oxaloacetate. Thus the starting substrate has been regenerated and another molecule of pyruvate (acetyl-CoA) can now react to initiate another round of the cycle.

Respiratory chain

The respiratory chain, otherwise known as the electron transport chain, resides in the mitochondria. A single molecule of NADH has sufficient energy to generate three ATP molecules from ADP. The function of the chain can therefore be considered to be a mechanism by which this energy is drawn off in a controlled fashion. The chain consists of a series of electron carriers which can accept and then donate electrons while the resulting production of energy is used to stimulate the formation of ATP via oxidative phosphorylation. Figure 5.9 shows an outline of the respiratory chain and the points where energy is produced for ATP production. There is a linear change in the redox potential of the carriers in the chain.

Fatty acid oxidation

Many tissues produce most of their energy by the oxidation of fatty acids. Tissues such as the heart and other muscles only derive limited energy from glucose and rely on circulating free fatty acids. Parts of the kidney are completely unable to utilise glucose or other carbohydrates as energy sources and therefore depend upon a source of fatty acids.

Triacylglycerols (triglycerides) are stored in adipose tissue and, in response to one of a variety of signals, a lipase enzyme becomes activated that cleaves the three fatty acids from the glycerol. The free fatty acids then travel to other tissues bound to albumin; fatty acids are insoluble in water and therefore have to be transported by albumin. The glycerol that is formed as a result of triglyceride hydrolysis does not travel to other tissues. It is either used to resynthesise new

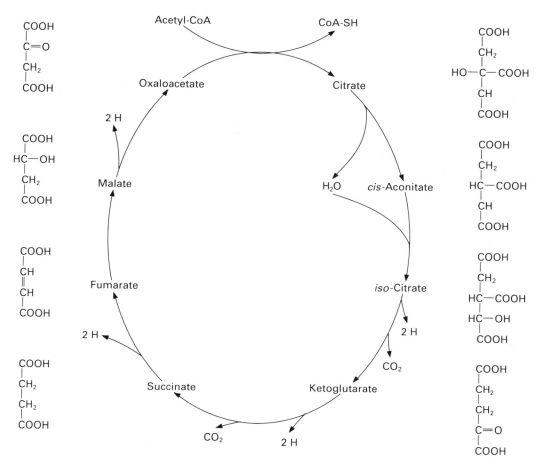

Fig. 5.8 The tricarboxylic acid cycle. For each turn of the cycle, at four points, two hydrogen atoms become available. At two points carbon dioxide is released: this accounts for the complete combustion of the acetyl group of acetyl-CoA, while acetoacetate is again ready to accept another molecule of acetyl-CoA.

triglycerides or, alternatively, it is phosphorylated to 3-phosphoglycerate which is a component of the glycolytic pathway.

Once a free fatty acid has reached the cell in which it is going to be used, it is subjected to a pathway called β-oxidation. Figure 5.10 shows the sequence of reactions involved. The fatty acid is activated by combination with CoA. There are then four enzymic steps in which the fatty acyl-CoA is reduced, hydrolysed, reduced again and finally hydrolysed to yield a molecule of acetyl-CoA and a molecule of acyl-CoA where the acyl group is now two carbon atoms shorter than the original. The acetyl-CoA feeds into the citric acid

cycle and the acyl-CoA goes through the process repeatedly until it is completely degraded. Thus, a molecule of palmitic acid which has 18 carbon atoms will be degraded to nine molecules of acetyl-CoA which will be further metabolised to produce ATP.

The metabolism described above refers to saturated fatty acids only, i.e. those with no unsaturated double bonds. There are three polyunsaturated fatty acids which are essential for health. Linoleic acid has 18 carbon atoms and two double bonds while linolenic acid has 18 carbon atoms and three double bonds. Arachidonic acid is 20 carbon atoms long with four double bonds.

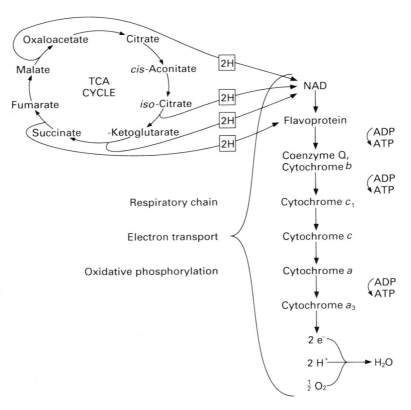

Fig. 5.9 The relationship between the tricarbocylic acid cycle and electron-transport and oxidative phosphorylation. Three pairs of hydrogen atoms form to reduce NAD, the fourth reduces a flavoprotein. Each pair of hydrogens ultimately reduces one atom of oxygen, and in the process three molecules of ATP are produced. Each turn of the cycle thus yields 12 ATP molecules. Respiratory oxygen is linked via the respiratory chain and the tricarboxylic acid cycle to the combustion of acetyl-CoA and the production of the carbon dioxide that is breathed out.

Although all three are required by cells, since man can synthesise linolenic and arachidonic acids from linoleic acid an adequate dietary supply of linoleic acid is sufficient. There are a number of biochemical pathways that require the essential unsaturated fatty acids and the production of leukotrienes and prostaglandins have been especially well studied.

Regulation of metabolic pathways

In an adult there is turnover within tissues and so the diet has to provide the nutrients for replacement as well as energy utilisation. The nutritional requirement includes amino acids, vitamins, salts and trace elements. There are considerable differences in the rates at which tissues turn over. Thus a tissue such as bone has a very slow rate of turnover and the macromolecules in the matrix

will be degraded and renewed with half-times measured in weeks if not months. At the other end of the range, the surface of the gut has a high rate of turnover and renewal. Like most epithelia, there is a constant movement and desquamation of cells. This must be balanced by replacement within the germinal layers.

An individual exists in different metabolic states throughout the day and, while at one point in time, energy may be derived from carbohydrate, at another ATP might be produced exclusively from oxidation of fatty acids. Following a meal, the body is in an absorptive state and there will be high levels of free glucose, triglycerides and amino acids in the blood stream. The tissues will use some of these components but most will be stored. The liver becomes active and will take up glucose and convert some to the storage polymer glycogen.

Carbon Atoms

Fig. 5.10 β-Oxidation of even-numbered long-chain fatty acids. Reaction I, the initial attack on the α- and β-carbon atoms, with removal of a hydrogen atom from each and the formation of a double bond between them, is catalysed by fatty acyl-CoA dehydrogenases with an electron-transferring flavoprotein as cofactor. Next (reaction II) comes hydration of this double bond, followed by reaction III, oxidation of the secondary alcoholic group to a keto group on the β-carbon atom, catalysed by a β-hydroxy fatty acyl-CoA dehydrogenase. The final step (reaction IV) is cleavage with CoA, catalysed by β-thiolase, to give acetyl-CoA. The resulting fatty acyl-CoA is in the same form as the starting material, and can undergo reaction I again, but is two carbon atoms shorter. Ultimately the fatty acid is completely disassembled to two-carbon acetyl-CoA units.

Some glucose can be converted to triglyceride.

Triglyceride travels in the circulation in the form of chylomicrons, which are aggregates of lipid and a small amount of protein. Some of the triglyceride in chylomicrons is taken up directly into adipose tissue while some is taken up in the liver where the triglycerides are used to make other species of lipoprotein. Very low-density lipoprotein and low-density lipoprotein contain different proportions of triglyceride, phospholipid, cholesterol and protein. Both forms of lipoprotein are secreted from the liver and then circulate to all the tissues where they supply lipids.

As all the circulating products from digestion are taken up into cells, the body turns to a postabsorptive state. Most tissues cannot store adequate amounts of carbohydrate and lipid for their energetic needs and so during the postabsorptive state the liver and adipose tissue release glucose and triglyceride for use by other tissues. It is often not appreciated that the glycogen in the liver is only able to provide glucose for a matter of an hour or two and (apart from the brain) most tissues use fat in the form of free fatty acids as their energy source for most of the day. The liver can also produce ketone bodies such as β-hydroxybutyrate and acetoacetic acid. Ketone bodies can be used as an energy source by a number of tissues and even the central nervous system after an adaptation period can metabolise ketone bodies to provide ATP.

There are very effective control processes that ensure adequate levels of ATP and that the ATP is derived from the most suitable energy source. In general, a cell will not be deriving ATP from carbohydrate and lipid at the same time.

Most of the regulation of and between the metabolic pathways occurs via a mechanism known as allosteric control. Some key enzymes in each pathway have, in addition to the binding sites for substrate, sites at which other components of the metabolic pathways can bind. When these other components bind to the enzyme its activity is altered. For example, the enzyme phosphofructokinase is part of the glycolytic pathway and is very sensitive to cellular concentrations of ATP, ADP and AMP. When concentrations of ATP are high then the activity of the enzyme is down-regulated since glycolysis should be slowed down in order to conserve carbohydrate stores. Phosphofructokinase is also regulated by the concentration of citrate and this provides a mechanism for regulation between different metabolic pathways. If there are high concentrations of acetyl-CoA which have been derived from fatty acid oxidation then this will result in high levels of citrate formation. High concentrations of citrate down-regulate phosphofructokinase and thus the use of fat for energy production will have a conserving effect on carbohydrate stores.

It is now known that many metabolic enzymes can be regulated. In addition to allosteric control, the concentrations of cofactors will also regulate enzyme activity. The status of the respiratory chain will influence NAD/NADH ratios. Since the sum of NAD and NADH concentrations is held fairly constant, if there are high levels of NADH then there will be insufficient substrate for several enzymes in the citric acid cycle and it will consequently be down-regulated.

An example of a control that operates in a metabolic cycle, which is important in the neonate, follows. The enzyme ATP-citrate lyase hydrolyses citrate and reverses the first step of the citric acid cycle. Although energy is consumed in this reaction the step is important for the neonate since it ensures levels of acetyl-CoA are maintained. During growth, cellular proliferation requires adequate lipid for membrane biosynthesis. ATP-citrate lyase ensures that, at a time in development when dietary lipid can be low, fatty acids are not used too extensively as an energy source. This maintains adequate supplies for growth.

CATABOLISM

All the red cells, white cells and platelets in circulation originate in the bone marrow. The stem cells within the marrow divide and differentiate to form the different cellular elements of blood. The process is regulated by a series of peptide growth factors. Erythropoietin, for example, is the peptide that promotes the formation of erythrocytes; it is synthesised and secreted by the juxtaglomerular apparatus of the kidney and it circulates to the bone marrow where it promotes proliferation.

Erythrocytes have a half-life of about 125 days before they are removed from circulation by the spleen. In order for constant replacement of these lost cells to occur the bone marrow is very active in erythropoiesis. As well as cellular proliferation, there has to be synthesis of haemoglobin. This oxygen-binding molecule is composed of two pairs of globin chains and a haem ring. The haem ring is synthesised in the mitrochondria and needs a sufficient supply of iron, which can frequently become the rate-limiting step. The uptake of iron across the gut is not an efficient process and even in the presence of sufficient dietary iron, the plasma concentration can become limiting.

Unless there is sufficient iron available the production of the globin peptide chains is redundant. For this reason there is a sophisticated control mechanism that operates. Only in the presence of sufficient haem does the synthesis of globin chains proceed. Protein synthesis involves a number of elongation factors whose activity is controlled by phosphorylation and dephosphorylation, and the enzymes responsible are regulated by haem levels.

When erythrocytes are degraded in the spleen (or indeed at the site of a wound response following tissue trauma), the haemogloblin is catabolised. The globin chains are degraded to amino acids which are reutilised. Haem cannot be reused and is catabolised in a number of enzyme steps, which finally produce bilirubin. This all occurs at the site of erythrocyte breakdown. The bilirubin is then transferred to the liver; because it is highly insoluble it travels to the liver bound to albumin. After diffusion into the hepatocytes, bilirubin is solubilised and detoxified by the coupling of two glucuronic acid residues. The conjugated bilirubin is then excreted into the bile.

Urea cycle

In the developed world, most individuals have a diet that is far in excess of requirement. Thus an individual consumes an amount of protein, which when hydrolysed to amino acids is considerably more than will be required for normal cellular turnover. Like most chemicals with free amino groups, these amino acids will become toxic if allowed to accumulate. There is an efficient detoxification mechanism which results in more than 95% of the nitrogen being excreted via the urine in the form of urea.

Figure 5.11 shows a sequence of metabolic reactions which constitute the urea cycle. The detoxification of amino acids begins before the urea cycle when a transaminase enzyme results in the transfer of the amino group from the acid onto α-ketoglutaric acid. The product, glutamic acid, is itself one of the amino acids but it is through this intermediate that all amino groups are metabolised. The glutamate is oxidatively deaminated to

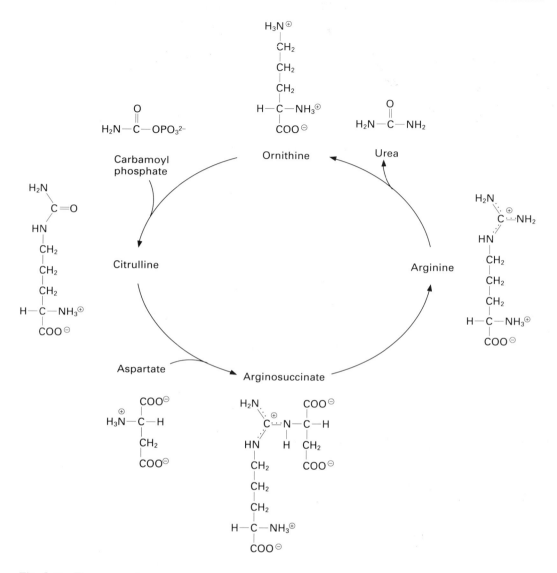

Fig. 5.11 The urea cycle.

produce ammonia, which immediately becomes an ammonium ion.

In a reaction requiring ATP, carbon dioxide and ammonium ions form carbamoyl phosphate and it is this that feeds into the urea cycle. The first step is the formation of citrulline from ornithine and carbamoyl phosphate. Then, in another ATP-dependent reaction a molecule of aspartic acid combines with citrulline to generate arginosuccinate. This is next hydrolysed to yield fumarate

and arginine and, in the final reaction, arginase releases urea from arginine, leaving ornithine. Thus the cycle is completed.

Most amino acid detoxification in man occurs in the liver, although small levels of the urea cycle enzymes are found in other tissues. The first few reactions occur in the mitochondria while the latter part of the cycle takes place in the cytoplasm. The urea diffuses out of the liver into systemic circulation. Like all small molecules urea is filtered through the glomerulus of the kidney but while nutrients such as glucose and amino acids are reabsorbed by the kidney tubules, urea is not and passes quantitatively into the urine. This excretory process is vital and, in chronic kidney failure, accumulation of urea can become a life-threatening process.

ENZYMES

Enzymes are proteins that act as catalysts. They bring about the enormous range of sophisticated chemical reactions that are necessary for life. In strict thermodynamic terms, it is incorrect to state that enzymes make reactions occur. Rather, an enzyme shifts the equilibrium of a reaction so that it is more favourable for it to proceed. This is accomplished by reducing the activation energy that is needed to promote the reaction. The catalysis occurs on a part of the enzyme called the active site.

The three-dimensional conformation of an enzyme is crucial to activity and the ability to act as a catalyst can be lost if the three-dimensional shape is altered. A change of shape and resulting loss of activity is referred to as denaturation and can be brought about in a number of ways. Heating an enzyme usually results in complete loss of activity. The three-dimensional structure of the protein is maintained in part by hydrogen bonds. These are fairly weak in nature and can be readily disrupted by heat. Most enzymes are destroyed at 50–60°C.

Organic solvents will usually destroy enzymic activity. The solvent disrupts the internal bonding of the protein, in particular the interactions of the hydrophobic amino acids. Even after removal of the solvent it is rare that the protein can refold in such a way as to regenerate enzyme activity.

Changes in pH will also affect enzyme activity. Because amino acids are zwitterions and partially charged, the local pH will influence the degree to which they are charged. Changes in pH can thus affect the charge of amino acid residues, which in turn affects the interactions between the amino acids and can result in denaturation. Some proteins are extremely sensitive and lose activity with small pH changes; others are less sensitive.

Enzyme kinetics

Enzymes are usually present at low concentrations inside the cell. The substrate binds to the enzyme and by reducing the activation energy for the reaction, the enzyme brings about a shift in equilibrium and this allows formation of product. If the reaction only involves a single substrate then this can be described by

$$\text{Enzyme + Substrate} \rightarrow \text{Enzyme/substrate complex} \rightarrow \text{Enzyme + Product}$$

The rate of reaction is dependent upon the concentrations of enzyme and substrate, but at high concentrations of substrate the enzyme will become saturated. At this point the rate of the reaction is maximal (and is depicted as V_{max}). In order to describe the activity of an enzyme the Michaelis constant (K_m) is used and this is the concentration of substrate at which the velocity of the reaction is half-maximal. K_m is a measure of how tightly a substrate binds to the enzyme. The lower the value of K_m, the more tightly the substrate can bind. Values for the Michaelis constant are commonly in the micromolar range.

Values for K_m and V_{max} can be calculated by measuring enzyme rates of reaction at a number of substrate concentrations and plotting the reciprocals of both parameters against one another. This is called a Lineweaver–Burk plot and normally produces a straight line.

Enzyme inhibitors can act in a competitive or non-competitive manner. In the case of competitive inhibitors, there is direct competition between the substrate and inhibitor for binding to the active site of the enzyme: K_m is increased but V_{max} is unaltered. In the case of a non-competitive inhibitor, K_m remains the same while V_{max} is reduced because the inhibitor binds at a location away from the active site but brings about a reduction in activity of the enzyme without affecting substrate binding. Figure 5.12 shows a Lineweaver–Burk plot for the two types of inhibitor.

Vitamins (see also pp. 190–2)

Many enzymes require a cofactor in order to operate. The cofactors are small in comparison to

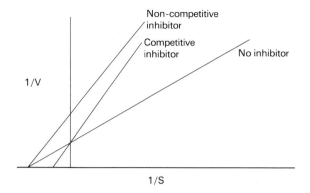

Fig. 5.12 Lineweaver–Burk plots for enzyme inhibitor. V is the reaction rate and S is the substrate concentration.

the enzyme but play an essential role in the binding and activation of the substrate. Most of the cofactors cannot be synthesised by man and the factor or its precursor have to be supplied in the diet. The dietary components are known as vitamins. To give an example, pyridoxine (also known as vitamin B_6) is a vital dietary requirement. Once it has been absorbed across the gut and transported to a tissue, it is converted enzymically inside the cell by enzymes to pyridoxal phosphate, which is then in turn used as a cofactor for transaminase enzymes.

Vitamins are classified as water or fat soluble and Table 5.1 shows the vitamins required by man and the enzymic pathways in which they are used. The water-soluble vitamins are the B series and vitamin C, which are all used in a large number of enzymic reactions that concern intermediary metabolism. The four fat-soluble vitamins, A, D, E and K, take part in diverse unrelated reactions ranging from formation of blood-clotting proteins (vitamin K) to formation of visual pigments (vitamin A).

The bacteria in the colon produce some of the vitamins required by man and this can act as a limited source. Some vitamins turn over fairly rapidly and so a deficiency state can arise soon after withdrawal. In the case of other vitamins, such as vitamin B_{12}, the body maintains significant reserves of material and man can survive for months without this particular vitamin in the diet.

Table 5.1 The vitamins

Water-soluble vitamins	
Vitamin	*Role*
Thiamine (vitamin B_1)	Oxidative decarboxylation
Riboflavin (vitamin B_2)	Oxidation/reduction enzymes
Pantothenic acid (vitamin B_5)	Coenzyme A formation
Niacin (nicotinic acid)	Oxidation/reduction enzymes
Pyridoxine (vitamin B_6)	Transaminase enzymes
Biotin	Carboxylation reactions
Cobalamin (vitamin B_{12})	Homocysteine and methyl-malonyl CoA reactions
Folic acid	'One-carbon' transfers
Ascorbic acid (vitamin C)	Hydroxylation of proteins — especially collagen

Fat-soluble vitamins	
Vitamin	*Role*
Vitamin A (retinol)	Formation of visual pigments
Vitamin D (calciferol)	Dihydroxy form essential for calcium homeostasis
Vitamin E (tocopherol)	Anti-oxidant significant in fertility
Vitamin K (menaquinone)	Modification of proteins — especially those in blood clotting

The role of enzymes in digestion
(see also pp. 188–9)

The diet contains proteins, fats and complex carbohydrates. None of these can be absorbed by the gastrointestinal tract and enzymic digestion has to occur in order to generate products that can be absorbed into the blood stream or lymphatic circulation.

Protein

Digestion of protein begins in the stomach. The 'chief' cells secrete pepsinogen. The parietal (oxyntic) cells secrete hydrochloric acid and the resulting low pH causes the hydrolysis of pepsinogen into pepsin, which is a proteolytic enzyme. Pepsin shows specificity and causes peptide bond hydrolysis only next to three particular amino acids, namely tryptophan, phenylalanine and tyrosine; these are all amino acids with aromatic side chains. Pepsin therefore generates peptide fragments from large proteins.

The pancreas synthesizes three protease enzymes in inactive precursor form. These are trypsinogen, procarboxypeptidase and chymotrypsinogen. These are secreted in inactive forms and released into the gut via the pancreatic duct. The mucosa of the proximal part of the small intestine secretes an enzyme called enterokinase which cleaves trypsinogen, converting it to trypsin. Trypsin in turn cleaves and activates procarboxypeptidase and chymotrypsinogen. In all these cases the release of a small peptide fragment generates active enzyme.

Chymotrypsinogen is like pepsin and cleaves next to amino acids with aromatic side chains. Trypsin cleaves next to the basic amino acids lysine and arginine while carboxypeptidase cleaves sequential amino acids starting at the carboxyl terminus. The action of these enzymes is to convert proteins to either amino acids or very small peptides with two or three amino acids.

In the small intestine the single amino acids are transported by the enterocytes into systemic circulation. The microvilli of the intestinal mucosa contain peptidases that cleave the di- and tripeptides into single amino acids which are then also transported into the blood stream. The small intestine is highly efficient and most of the amino acids are absorbed across the wall of the duodenum and jejunum.

Carbohydrate

Most of the carbohydrate in the diet is starch, which is a large polymer of glucose. The diet will also contain some sucrose and lactose, which are both disaccharides. Sucrose is composed of glucose and fructose while lactose is composed of glucose and galactose.

The salivary glands and the pancreas both secrete amylases which break down starch into the disaccharides maltose and isomaltose. These two carbohydrates, along with lactose and sucrose, are then taken up by a similar mechanism. The mucosal villi contain the four enzymes maltase, isomaltase, lactase and sucrase and these break down the relevant disaccharide into monosaccharides which are transported into the blood stream. The transport of glucose and galactose is an active process and ATP is required; the transport of fructose is passive.

Glucose is the most utilised carbohydrate energy source. Most cells take up glucose from circulation and the insulin released from the pancreas following a meal stimulates this process. The glucose can be used immediately for energy production or it can be stored in the form of glycogen which is a branched polymer of glucose. When the cell requires to use the glucose stored as glycogen then the enzyme phosphorylase is activated by the cyclic adenosine monophosphate (cAMP) pathway (see Fig. 5.13) and glucose-6-phosphate is produced. When glucose is transported into the cell it is also phosphorylated by the enzyme hexokinase or glucokinase. In either case it is glucose-6-phosphate that enters the metabolic pathway.

Fat

The predominant dietary fat is triglyceride, i.e. three fatty acids esterified to a single molecule of glycerol. It is not until the small intestine that digestion of fat begins. The first stage is the emulsification of the fats with the bile salts. The liver synthesises bile salts and acids but they are stored in the gall bladder. In response to cholecystokinin, bile is ejected into the small intestine and causes dispersal of dietary fat into small droplets. This has the effect of increasing the surface area, thereby increasing the rate of action of the lipase enzymes secreted by the pancreas. The products are fatty acids and monoacylglycerol and these diffuse into the epithelial cells lining the gastrointestinal tract. Inside the cell, the monoacyl glycerols are broken down to fatty acid and glycerol. The epithelial cells then resynthesise triglycerides and then, along with a small amount of phospholipid, cholesterol and specific protein are assembled into chylomicron particles, which diffuse into the lacteals of the lymphatic system. The process of fat digestion in the healthy individual is also very efficient and is completed in the duodenum and jejunum.

The chylomicrons diffuse into the lymphatic lacteals and then travel along the lymphatic vessels. Ultimately they enter the blood stream

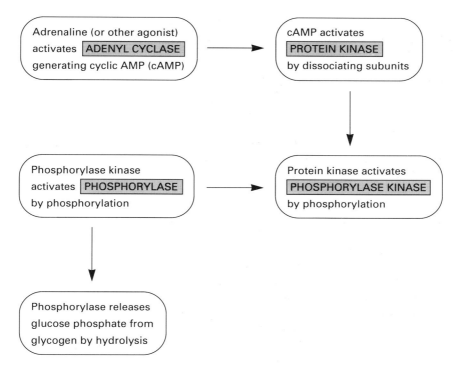

Fig. 5.13 Activation of phosphorylase by the cyclic AMP-dependent pathway.

when the lymph in the thoracic duct flows into the left subclavian vein. The triglycerides in the chylomicrons are taken up and stored by adipose tissue. When there is demand then this fat can be used by a number of organs and tissues. Free fatty acids are transported to the site of utilisation. Lipases within the adipose tissue will hydrolyse the triglycerides and the resulting fatty acids diffuse out of the adipocytes and become bound to albumin in the blood stream.

6. Physiology

BIOPHYSICAL DEFINITIONS

1 mol of an element or compound is the atomic weight or molecular weight, respectively, in grams. Thus 1 mol of sodium is 23 g (at. wt Na = 23) and 1 mol of sodium chloride is 58.5 g (at. wt Cl = 35.5; 35.5 + 23 = 58.5). A normal (molar) solution contains 1 mol per litre of solution. Therefore a normal solution of sodium chloride contains 58.5 g and is about a 6% solution. Note that this is very different from a physiological 'normal' solution of sodium chloride, where the concentration of sodium chloride (0.9%) is adjusted so that the sodium has the same concentration as the total number of cations in plasma (154 mmol/l). The concentrations of

biological substances are usually much weaker than molar. The conventional nomenclature for decreasing molar concentrations is given below. The same prefixes may be used for different units of measurement.

1 millimole (mmol)	=	1×10^{-3} mol
1 micromole (μmol)	=	1×10^{-6} mol
1 nanomole (nmol)	=	1×10^{-9} mol
1 picomole (pmol)	=	1×10^{-12} mol
1 femtomole (fmol)	=	1×10^{-15} mol
1 attomole (amol)	=	1×10^{-18} mol

1 equivalent = 1 mol divided by the valency. Thus 1 Eq of sodium (valency 1) = 23 g, and 1 mol of sodium = 1 Eq or 1 mmol = 1 mEq.

However, 1 Eq of calcium (valency 2, mol. wt 40) = 20 g. 1 mol of calcium = 2 Eq, and 1 mmol Ca^{2+} = 2 mEq Ca^{2+}.

Measurements in medicine are wherever possible being made in SI (Systeme Internationale) units. Under this system the concentration of biological materials is expressed in the appropriate molar units (often mmol) per litre.

The units used in the measurement of osmotic pressure are considered below.

THE DISTRIBUTION OF WATER AND ELECTROLYTES

A normal 70 kg man is composed of 60% water, 18% protein, 15% fat and 7% minerals. Obese individuals have relatively more fat and less water. Of the 60% (42 litres) of water, 28 litres (40% of body weight) are intracellular; the remaining 14 litres of extracellular water are made up of 10.5 litres of interstitial fluid (extracellular and extravascular) and 3.5 litres of blood plasma. The total blood volume (red cells and plasma) is 8% of total body weight, or about 5.6 litres.

Total body water can be measured by giving a patient deuterium oxide (D_2O), 'heavy water', and measuring how much it is diluted. Extracellular fluid volume can be measured with inulin by the same principle. Intracellular fluid volume = total body water (D_2O space) less extracellular fluid volume (inulin space). Intravascular fluid volume can be measured with Evans blue dye. Total blood volume can be calculated knowing intravascular fluid volume and the haematocrit. Interstitial fluid volume = extracellular fluid volume (inulin space) less intravascular fluid volume.

The distribution of electrolytes and protein in intracellular fluid, interstitial fluid and plasma is given in Figure 6.1. Note that for reasons of comparability, concentrations are expressed in milliequivalents per litre of water, not millimoles per litre of plasma.

The major difference between plasma and interstitial fluid is that interstitial fluid has relatively little protein. As a consequence, the concentration of sodium in the interstitial fluid is less and so is the overall osmotic pressure (see below). There are further major differences between intracellular fluid and extracellular fluid. Sodium is the major extracellular cation, whereas potassium and, to a lesser extent, magnesium, are the predominant intracellular cations. Chloride and also bicarbonate

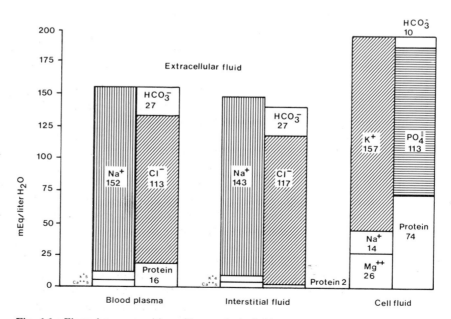

Fig. 6.1 Electrolyte composition of human body fluids.

are the major extracellular anions; protein and phosphate are the predominant intracellular anions.

Anion gap

In considering the composition of plasma for clinical purposes, account is often taken of the 'anion gap'. This is calculated by considering sodium the principle cation, 136 mEq/l, and subtracting from it the concentrations of the principal anions, chloride, 100 mEq/l and bicarbonate, 24 mEq/l. This leaves a positive balance of 12 mEq/l. The normal range is 8-16 mEq/l. The gap is considered to exist because of the occurrence of unmeasured anions, such as protein or lactate, which would balance the number of cations. An increase in the anion gap suggests that there are more unmeasured anions present than usual. This occurs in such situations as lactic acidosis, or diabetic keto-acidosis, where the lactate and acetoacetate are balancing the excess sodium ions. A more complete explanation of the anion gap would be to consider both the unmeasured cations as well as the unmeasured anions as in Table 6.1. Situations where the anion gap is increased include keto-acidosis, lactic acidosis, and hyperosmolar acidosis; poisoning with salicylate, methanol, ethylene glycol and paraldehyde and also hypo-albuminaemia. A decreased anion gap occurs in bromide poisoning and in myeloma.

Table 6.1 Anion gap (mEq/l)

Cation		Anion	
Na^+	136	Cl^-	100
		HCO_3^-	24
	136		124
		Gap	12
	136		136

The gap consists of unmeasured cations and anions:

K^+	4.5	Protein$^-$	15
Ca^{2+}	5	PO_4^{3-}	2
Mg^{2+}	1.5	SO_4^{2-}	1
		Organic acids	5
	11		23
	147		147

TRANSPORT MECHANISMS

These mechanisms account for the movement of substances within cells and across cell membranes. The transport mechanisms to be considered include diffusion, solvent drag, filtration, osmosis, non-ionic diffusion, carrier-mediated transport and phagocytosis. Not all of these mechanisms will be considered in detail.

Diffusion is the process whereby a gas or substance in solution expands to fill the volume available to it. Relevant examples of gaseous diffusion are the equilibration of gases within the alveoli of the lung, and of liquid diffusion, the equilibration of substances within the fluid of the renal tubule. An element of diffusion may be involved in all transport across cell membranes because recent research suggests that there is a layer of unstirred water up to 400 μm thick adjacent to biological membranes in animals.

If there is a charged ion that cannot diffuse across a membrane which other charged ions can cross, the diffusible ions distribute themselves as in the following example:

In	Out
K_i^+	K_o^+
Cl_i^-	Cl_o^-
Protein$^-$	

$$\frac{[K_i^+]}{[K_o^+]} = \frac{[Cl_o^-]}{[Cl_i^-]}$$ Gibbs–Donnan equilibrium

The cell is permeable to K^+ and Cl^- but not to protein. Since K_i is about 157 mmol/l and K_o is 4 mmol/l, the Gibbs–Donnan equilibrium would predict that the ratio of chloride concentration outside the cell to that inside should be 157/4. In fact, there is almost no intracellular chloride so that the ratio in vivo is even greater than 40. This is because there are other factors than simple diffusion affecting both potassium and chloride concentrations.

Solvent drag is the process whereby bulk movement of solvent drags some molecules of solute with it. It is of little importance.

Filtration is the process whereby substances are forced through a membrane by hydrostatic pressure. The degree to which substances pass through the membrane depends on the size of the holes in the membrane. Small molecules pass through the holes; larger molecules do not. In the renal glomerulus the holes are large enough to allow all blood constituents to pass through the filtration membrane, apart from blood cells and the majority of plasma proteins.

Osmosis describes the movement of solvent from a region of low solute concentration, across a semipermeable membrane to one of high solute concentration. The process can be opposed by hydrostatic pressure; the pressure that will stop osmosis occurring is the osmotic pressure of the solution. This is given by the formula:

$$P = \frac{nRT}{V}$$

where, P = osmotic pressure, n = number of osmotically active particles, R = gas constant, T = absolute temperature, V = volume. For an ideal solution of a non-ionised substance n/V equals the concentration of the solute. 1 osmole (Osm) of a substance in an ideal solution is then defined such that:

$$1 \text{ Osm} = \frac{\text{Molecular weight in grams}}{\substack{\text{Number of osmotically} \\ \text{active particles in solution}}}$$

So for an ideal solution of glucose

$$1 \text{ Osm} = \frac{\text{Molecular weight}}{1} = \text{Molecular weight}$$
$$= 180 \text{ g.}$$

However, sodium chloride dissociates into two ions in solution. Therefore, for sodium chloride,

$$1 \text{ Osm} = \frac{\text{Mol. wt}}{2} = \frac{58.5}{2} = 29.2 \text{ g.}$$

Calcium chloride dissociates into three ions in solution. Therefore, for calcium chloride,

$$1 \text{ Osm} = \frac{\text{Mol. wt}}{3} = \frac{111}{3} = 37 \text{ g.}$$

However, the molecules or ions of all solutions aggregate to a certain degree so that interaction occurs between the ions or molecules, and they each do not behave as osmotically independent particles and they do not form ideal solutions. Freezing point depression by a solution is also caused by the number of osmotically active particles. The greater the concentration of osmotically active particles, the greater the freezing point depression. In an ideal solution, with no interaction, 1 mol of osmotically active particles per litre depresses the freezing point by 1.86°C. Therefore, an aqueous solution which depresses the freezing point by 1.86°C is defined as containing 1 Osm/l. One which depresses the freezing point by 1.86°C/1000, i.e. 0.00186°C contains 1 mOsm/l. Plasma (osmotic pressure 300 mOsm/l has a freezing point of $(0-0.00186 \times 300)°C = -0.56°C$.

Osmolarity defines osmotic pressure in terms of osmoles per litre of solution. Since volume changes at different temperatures, osmolality which defines osmotic pressure in terms of osmoles per kilogram of solution is preferred, though not always employed.

The major osmotic components of plasma are the cations sodium and potassium, and their accompanying anions, together with glucose and urea. The concentration of sodium is about 140 mmol/l. This, and the accompanying anions will therefore contribute 280 mOsm/l. The concentration of potassium is about 4 mmol/l, which, with its accompanying anions will give 8 mOsm/l. Glucose and urea contribute 5 mOsm/l each to a total of 300 mOsm/l in normal plasma. During pregnancy, this falls to at least 290 mOsm/l.

We are now in a position to consider some of the forces acting on water in the capillaries (see Fig. 6.2). There is a difference of 25 mmHg in osmotic pressure between the interstitial water and the intravascular water due to the plasma proteins (see above). This force will tend to drive water into the capillary. At the arteriolar end of the capillary, the hydrostatic pressure is 37 mmHg; the interstitial pressure is 1 mmHg. The nett force driving water *out* is therefore $37 - 1 - 25 = 11$ mmHg, and water tends to pass out of the arteriolar end of the capillary. At the venous end of the capillary, the pressure is only 17 mmHg. The nett force driving water *in* the capillary is therefore $25 + 1 - 17 = 9$ mmHg. Fluid therefore enters the capillary at the venous end. Factors which would decrease fluid reabsorption and cause clinical oedema are a reduction in plasma proteins, so that the osmotic gradient between the intra-

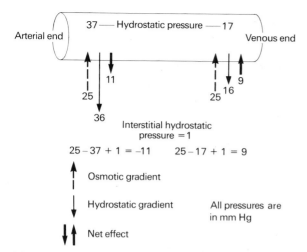

37 —— Hydrostatic pressure —— 17

Arterial end   Venous end

11

25   25   16   9

36

Interstitial hydrostatic
pressure = 1

$25 - 37 + 1 = -11$ $25 - 17 + 1 = 9$

Osmotic gradient

Hydrostatic gradient   All pressures are
in mm Hg

Net effect

Fig. 6.2 At the arterial end of the capillary the hydrostatic forces acting outwards are greater than the osmotic forces acting inwards. There is a nett movement out of the capillary. At the venous end of the capillary, the hydrostatic forces acting outwards are less than the osmotic forces acting inwards. There is a nett movement into the capillary.

vascular and interstitial fluids might be only 20, not 25, mmHg, or a rise in venous pressure so that the pressure at the venous end of the capillary might be 25 mmHg, rather than 17 mmHg.

Non-ionised diffusion is the process whereby there is preferential transport in a non-ionised form. Examples are transport of lipid-soluble drugs, e.g. propranolol across the lipids of the blood–brain barrier or the placenta.

Carrier-mediated transport, implies transport across a cell membrane, using a specific carrier. If the transport is down a concentration gradient from an area of high concentration to one of low concentration, this is known as facilitated transport, e.g. the uptake of glucose by the muscle cell, facilitated by the participation of insulin in the transport process. If the carrier-mediated transport is up a concentration gradient from an area of low concentration to one of high concentration, this is known as active transport, e.g. the removal of sodium from muscle cells by the sodium pump.

Phagocytosis and pinocytosis involve the incorporation of discrete bodies of solid and liquid substances respectively by cell wall growing out and around the particles so that the cell appears to swallow them. The reverse procedure is known as reverse pinocytosis.

ACID–BASE BALANCE

Normal acid–base balance

Acids and bases

A simple knowledge of chemistry allows some substances to be easily categorised as acids or bases. For example, hydrochloric acid is clearly an acid and sodium hydroxide is a base. But when describing acid-base balance in physiology, these terms are used rather more obscurely. For example, the chloride ion may be described as a base. A definition that is more applicable, is to define an acid as an ion or molecule which can liberate hydrogen ions. Since hydrogen ions are protons, acids may also be defined as proton donors. A base is then a substance which can accept hydrogen ions or a proton acceptor. If we consider the examples below, hydrochloric acid dissociates into hydrogen ions and chloride ions, and is therefore a proton donor (acid). If the chloride ion associates with hydrogen ions to form hydrochloric acid, the chloride ion is a proton acceptor (base). Ammonia is another proton acceptor when it forms the ammonium ion. Carbonic acid is an acid (hydrogen ion donor); bicarbonate is a base (hydrogen ion acceptor). The $H_2PO_4^-$ ion can be both an acid when it dissociates further to HPO_4^{2-} and a base when it associates to form H_3PO_4.

$$HCl \rightleftharpoons H^+ + Cl^-$$
$$NH_3 + H^+ \rightleftharpoons NH_4^+$$
$$H_2CO_3 \rightleftharpoons H^+ + HCO_3^-$$
$$H_3PO_4 \rightleftharpoons H_2PO_4^- + H^+$$
$$H_2PO_4^- \rightleftharpoons H_3PO_4^{2-} + H^+$$

pH

The pH is the negative $\log_{10}$ of the hydrogen ion concentration expressed in moles per litre. A negative logarithmic scale was used because the numbers are all less than 1, and because they vary over quite a wide range. Since the pH is the negative logarithm of the hydrogen ion concentration, low pH numbers, e.g. pH 6.2, indicate relatively high hydrogen ion concentrations, i.e. a relatively acidic solution. High pH numbers, e.g. pH 7.8, represent lower hydrogen ion concentrations, i.e. relatively alkaline solutions. The normal pH range in human tissues is 7.36–7.44. Although a neutral pH (hydrogen ion concentration equals hydroxyl ion concentration) at 20°C has the value 7.4, water dissociates more at physiological temperatures, and a neutral pH at 37°C has the value 6.8. Therefore, body fluids are mildly alkaline (higher the pH number, the lower hydrogen ion concentration).

A pH value of 7.4 represents a hydrogen ion concentration of 0.00004 mmol/l as we see in the following example:

$$
\begin{aligned}
pH &= 7.4 \\
[H^+] &= 10^{-7.4} \text{ mol/l} \\
&= 10^{-8} \times 10^{0.6} \text{ mol/l} \\
&= 0.00000001 \times 4 \text{ mol/l} \\
&= 0.00000004 \text{ mol/l} \\
&= 0.00004 \text{ mmol/l} \\
(1 \text{ mol/l} &= 1000 \text{ mmol/l}).
\end{aligned}
$$

Partial pressure of carbon dioxide (P_{CO_2})

In arterial blood, the normal value is 4.8–5.9 kilopascals (kPa) (36–44 mmHg). It is a fortunate coincidence that the figures expressing P_{CO_2} in mmHg are similar to those expressing the normal range for pH (7.36–7.44)

Henderson–Hasselbalch equation

This equation describes the relationship of hydrogen ion, bicarbonate and carbonic acid concentrations (equation (3)). It can be rewritten in terms of pH, bicarbonate and carbonic acid concentrations, as in equation (4), but carbonic acid concentrations are not usually measured. However, because of the presence of carbonic anhydrase in red cells, carbonic acid concentration is proportional to P_{CO_2} (equation (1)). Equation (4) can therefore be rewritten in terms of pH, bicarbonate and P_{CO_2} (equation (5)). All these data are usually available from blood gas analyses. If we know any two of these variables, the third can be calculated.

Carbonic anhydrase

$$CO_2 + H_2O \rightleftharpoons H_2CO_3 \tag{1}$$

$$H_2CO_3 \rightleftharpoons H^+ + HCO_3^- \tag{2}$$

By the Law of Mass Action

$$[H_2CO_3] = K [H^+] [HCO_3^-] \tag{2}$$

$$\therefore [H^+] = \frac{1}{K} \frac{[H_2CO_3]}{[HCO_3^-]} \cdot \tag{3}$$

By taking logarithms of the reciprocal:

$$pH = K' + \log \left(\frac{[HCO_3^-]}{[H_2CO_3]} \right).$$

K' is a constant (6.1):

$$pH = 6.1 + \log \left(\frac{[HCO_3^-]}{[H_2CO_3]} \right) \tag{4}$$

$$= 6.1 + \log \left(\frac{[HCO_3^-]}{P_aCO_2 \times 0.04} \right). \tag{5}\star$$

Control of pH

The Henderson–Hasselbalch equation, expressed in equation (5), indicates that the variables controlling pH are P_{CO_2} and bicarbonate concentration. Ultimately, P_{CO_2} is controlled by respiration. Short-term changes of pH may therefore be compensated for by changing the depth of respiration. Bicarbonate concentration can be altered by the kidneys, and this is the mechanism involved in the long-term control of pH. Further details of these mechanisms are given on pages 177 and 183.

Buffers

A buffer solution is one to which hydrogen or hydroxyl ions can be added with little change in the pH.

Consider a solution of sodium bicarbonate to which is added hydrochloric acid (Fig. 6.3). The hydrogen ions of the hydrochloric acid react with bicarbonate ions of the sodium bicarbonate to form carbonic acid. Carbonic acid does not dissociate so readily as hydrochloric acid. Therefore the hydrogen ions are buffered. Reading from right to

---

$\star$ For equation (5), because of the action of carbonic anhydrase, $[H_2CO_3]$ is proportional to P_aCO_2. For the given constants of equation (5), P_{CO_2} is expressed in mmHg.

left in Figure 6.3, we have a solution that starts as 100% bicarbonate ions, and becomes 100% carbonic acid, as hydrochloric acid is added. Initially, in the pH range 9–7, a very small change in bicarbonate concentration, requiring the addition of only a few hydrogen ions, is associated with a large change in pH. However, in the steep part of the curve, between pH 5 and 7, a considerable quantity of hydrogen ions can be added, as indicated by a marked fall in the proportion of bicarbonate remaining, with relatively little change in pH. It is in that pH range that the buffering ability of bicarbonate is greatest.

The pH at which 50% of the buffer is changed from its acidic to its basic form (or vice versa) is known as the pK. For bicarbonate the pK is 6.1, making bicarbonate rather poor as a buffer for body fluids, since the pK is considerably towards the acidic side of the physiological pH range (7.36–7.44). The buffer value of a buffer (millimoles of hydrogen ion per gram per pH unit) is the quantity of hydrogen ions which can be added to a buffer solution to change its pH by 1.0 pH unit from pK +0.5 to pK −0.5.

In blood, the most important buffers are proteins. These are able to absorb hydrogen ions onto free carboxyl radicals, as illustrated in Fig. 6.4. Of the proteins available, haemoglobin is more important than plasma protein, partly because its buffer value is greater than that of plasma

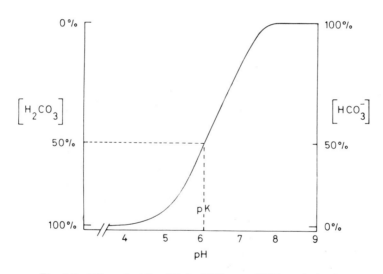

Fig. 6.3 Effect of adding H^+ (as HCl) to an HCO_3^- solution (as $NaHCO_3$). The pH changes from 9.0 when the solution is 100% HCO_3^- and 0% H_2CO_3 to less than 4 when the solution is 0% HCO_3^- and 100% H_2CO_3. At the pK valve when the HCO_3^- is 50% changed to H_2CO_3 the curve is steepest, indicating that there is relatively little change in the pH for a relatively large change in HCO_3^- in concentration. The pK is 6.1.

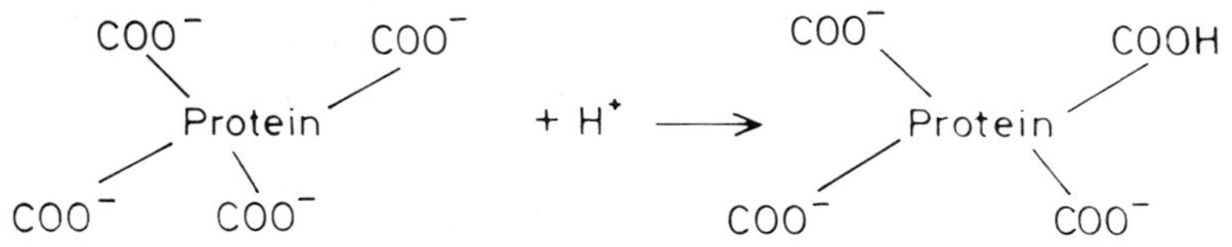

Fig. 6.4 The absorption of hydrogen ions onto free carboxyl radicals.

protein (0.18 mmol of hydrogen per gram of haemoglobin per pH unit, versus 0.11 mmol of hydrogen per gram of plasma protein per pH unit); but also because there is more haemoglobin than plasma protein (15 g haemoglobin per 100 ml versus 3.8 g of plasma protein per 100 ml). These two factors mean that haemoglobin has six times the buffering capacity of plasma protein. In addition, deoxygenated haemoglobin is a weaker acid and a more efficient buffer than oxygenated haemoglobin. This increases the buffering capacity of haemoglobin where it is more needed, after oxygen has been liberated in the peripheral tissues.

Buffer base and base excess

The buffer base is the total number of buffer anions (usually 45–50 mEq/l of blood) and consists of bicarbonate, phosphate and protein anions (haemoglobin and plasma protein).

Base excess is the difference between the actual buffer base and the normal value for a given haemoglobin and body temperature. It is negative in acidosis, and is then sometimes expressed as a positive base deficit, and positive in alkalosis. It gives an index of the severity of the abnormality of acid–base balance.

Standard bicarbonate

This is the carbon dioxide content of blood equilibrated at a P_{CO_2} of 40 mmHg and a temperature of 37°C when the haemoglobin is fully saturated with oxygen. In general it represents the non-respiratory part of acid–base derangement, and is low in metabolic acidosis and raised in metabolic alkalosis. The normal value for the standard bicarbonate is 27 mmol/l.

Abnormalities of acid–base balance

These are usually divided into acidosis (pH less than 7.36) and alkalosis (pH greater than 7.44). In addition, we consider respiratory acidosis and alkalosis where the primary abnormality is in respiration (carbon dioxide control) and metabolic acidosis and alkalosis, which are best defined as abnormalities that are not respiratory in origin. We will only consider initial, single abnormalities.

Table 6.2 Values of pH and P_{CO_2} characterising acidosis and alkalosis

	pH	P_{CO_2} kPa	P_{CO_2} mmHg
Normal	7.36–7.44	4.8–5.9	36–44
Respiratory acidosis	<7.36	>5.9	>44
Respiratory alkalosis	>7.44	<4.8	<36
Metabolic acidosis	<7.36	<5.9	<44
Metabolic alkalosis	>7.44	>4.8	>36

For these single uncomplicated abnormalities, respiratory and metabolic acidosis and alkalosis can be defined according to Table 6.2, which gives the values of pH and P_{CO_2} characterising each abnormality.

Respiratory acidosis

There is a low pH and a high P_{CO_2}. Here the basic abnormality is a failure of carbon dioxide excretion from the lungs. Carbon dioxide dissolves in the blood and in the presence of carbonic anhydrase, carbonic acid is formed which dissociates into hydrogen ions and bicarbonate (equations (1) and (2), p. 162). Respiratory acidosis may arise from abnormalities of respiration which may range from impaired respiratory control due to excessive sedation, to obstructive airways disease. In the long term, respiratory acidosis is compensated for by bicarbonate retention in the kidneys, which increases pH towards normal values.

Respiratory alkalosis

There is a high pH and a low P_{CO_2}. This is induced by hyperventilation, whatever the cause. Perhaps the commonest clinical presentation is anxiety, where the acute fall in hydrogen ion concentration due to blowing off carbon dioxide may be such as to cause paraesthesiae, or even tetany (*main d'accoucheur*). Tetany occurs because more plasma protein is ionised when the pH is high. This protein binds more calcium, lowering the ionised (metabolically effective) calcium level (see p. 195). However, respiratory alkalosis is also seen in the early stages of exercise, at altitude and in patients who have had a pulmonary embolus. In pregnancy, there is hyperventilation but the kidney excretes sufficient bicarbonate to compensate fully for the fall in carbon dioxide, and there is therefore no change in pH.

Metabolic acidosis

There is a low pH and the P_{CO_2} is not elevated. This may occur because of excessive acid production, impaired acid excretion, or excessive alkali loss. Examples of excess acid production are diabetic ketoacidosis and methanol poisoning, in which methanol is metabolised to formaldehyde, which subsequently forms formic acid.

Failure of acid excretion occurs in chronic renal failure, and, more specifically, in renal tubular acidosis, where the patients are not initially uraemic, but acid excretion by the kidney is impaired. Acetazolamide is a diuretic drug which inhibits ammonia formation within the kidney, and this too causes metabolic acidosis. Patients who have ureterosigmoid anastomoses develop such a severe metabolic acidosis that this has limited the application of this palliative operation. The metabolic acidosis arises partly because there is an element of chronic renal failure, due to previous hydronephrosis and chronic urinary tract infection; also, hydrogen ions secreted in the urine into the bowel are reabsorbed from the colon.

Excess alkali loss is seen in patients who have a pancreatic fistula or prolonged diarrhoea, since both the body fluids lost are alkaline.

Metabolic alkalosis

The pH is high and the P_{CO_2} is not reduced. This may occur, due to the loss of acidic fluid, because of prolonged vomiting. It also occurs in excessive alkali ingestion, seen in patients who take antacids for peptic ulceration. Metabolic alkalosis frequently accompanies hypokalemia.

THE CARDIOVASCULAR SYSTEM

In this section we describe the electrical activity of the heart, the conducting system, haemodynamic changes during the cardiac cycle, the electrocardiograph, control of blood pressure and changes in blood pressure and cardiac output during pregnancy.

The conducting system of the heart (see Fig. 6.5)

Specialised conducting tissue is necessary within the heart to ensure the orderly and synchronous contraction of atria followed by the ventricles. The electrical impulse starts at the sinoatrial (SA) node located in the right atrium at the entry of the superior vena cava. From there, the impulse spreads through the smooth muscle to the atrioventricular (AV) node, situated in the right atrium above the atrioventricular ring, near the interatrial septum. There is no specialised conducting tissue between the SA node and the AV node. However, specialised tissue, the bundle of His, is necessary to conduct the impulse from the AV node through the atrioventricular ring, which acts as an insulator, to the septum where the bundle divides into right and left branches, innervating the right and left ventricles respectively. The more distal fibres of the conducting system are known as the Purkinje system. The right bundle is a relatively narrow group of fibres. The left bundle is a much wider sheet of fibres; thus, right bundle branch block due to damage to the right bundle occurs relatively easily, and is not necessarily of pathological significance. Left bundle branch block

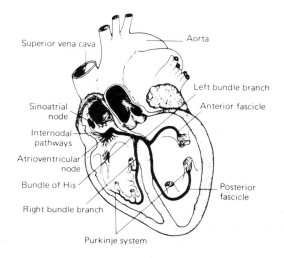

Fig. 6.5 The conducting system of the heart. Internodal pathways in the atria are not specialised conducting tissue in normal individuals. Aberrant pathways have been found in subjects susceptible to dysrhythmias. (Reproduced with permission from W. H. Ganong, *Review of Medical Physiology*, Lange Medical Publications.)

implies considerable additional damage to the underlying myocardium to interrupt such a wide sheet of fibres, and is always pathological. Some people have abnormal conducting tissue which bypasses the AV node. These patients are at risk from tachyarrhythmias, such as occur in the Wolff–Parkinson–White syndrome. Interruption of, or damage to, the conducting system is the main cause of the various degrees of heart block.

Factors affecting heart rate

The activity of the SA node is controlled neurogenically by the sympathetic and parasympathetic nervous systems, directed by the vasomotor and cardioinhibitory centres respectively (see below). At rest, the dominant tone is parasympathetic, mediated via the vagus nerve (a muscarinic effect; see Table 6.3).

In addition, the discharge rate from the SA node and therefore heart rate is increased by the direct actions of thyroxine and high temperature, by β-adrenergic activity, and by atropine which blocks dominant parasympathetic tone; it is decreased by hypothyroidism, hypothermia, and β-adrenergic blockade. SA node activity is also decreased in ischaemia, and, under these circumstances, other pacemakers (AV node, ventricles) can take over the pacemaker activity of the heart at a slower intrinsic rate.

The electrocardiogram

Figure 6.6 shows the normal electrocardiogram. The P wave represents atrial depolarisation, the QRS complex ventricular depolarisation, and the T wave represents ventricular repolarisation. Atrial repolarisation is not seen separately, since it occurs during the time of the QRS complex. Each small square of the electrocardiogram represents 0.04 seconds; each large square represents 0.2 seconds. In the vertical axis the electrocardiogram is calibrated so that 1 cm equals 1 mV. To determine the heart rate with the electrocardiogram running at conventional speed, divide 300 by N, where N is the number of large squares between successive R waves.

The PR interval should be between 0.1 seconds and 0.2 seconds. If it is greater than 0.2 seconds,

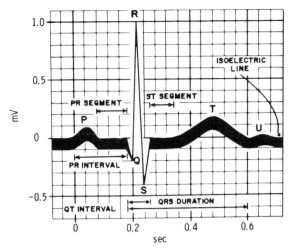

Fig. 6.6 The normal electrocardiogram. (Reproduced with permission from Ganong, W. H. *Review of Medical Physiology*, Lange Medical Publications.)

there is a delay in conduction from the atria to ventricles, i.e. heart block. If the PR interval is less than 0.1 seconds, conduction from the atria to the ventricles is abnormally rapid, implying aberrant conduction systems, as occurs in the Wolff–Parkinson–White syndrome.

The QT interval is between 0.3 and 0.4 seconds; it is much more dependent on heart rate than is the PR interval; it is increased in hypocalcaemia, hypokalaemia, rheumatic carditis and after medication with quinidine. It is decreased by hypercalcaemia, hyperkalaemia and digoxin.

Pressure and saturations in the cardiac chambers

Blood in the right side of the heart is relatively desaturated, so that the normal mixed venous oxygen saturation is about 60%. However, because the blood entering from the superior vena cava usually has a higher saturation than inferior vena caval blood, and because blood of a different saturation enters from the coronary sinus into the right atrium, a sample of true mixed venous blood can only be taken from the pulmonary artery. This problem is further accentuated by the streaming which occurs in the right atrium and right ventricle, so that proper mixing does not occur in these chambers. Blood in the left side of the heart is 96% saturated with oxygen, giving a P_{CO_2} of 90–100 mmHg (100 mmHg = 13.3 kPa). There is no difference in saturation between blood in the left atrium and blood in the left ventricle.

All pressures in the circulation should be measured relative to a fixed reference point, ideally the level of the right atrium. Using this reference point, the mean right atrial pressure is usually 1–7 mmHg (average 4 mmHg). This is determined indirectly when one assesses the jugular venous pressure, and, more directly, at measurement of central venous pressure. The pressure in the left atrium is about 10–15 mmHg, and this can be measured by determination of the wedged pulmonary artery pressure. At the bedside, a Swan–Ganz catheter with a balloon tip can be floated through the right heart from a peripheral vein, and become wedged in a distal pulmonary artery. Under these circumstances, the pressure in the tip of the catheter is approximately the same as the left atrial pressure. The same Swan–Ganz catheter is used for measuring cardiac output by indicator dilution, injecting a bolus of cold saline in the right atrium and measuring the area under the curve of the temperature trace recorded in the pulmonary artery. In the right ventricle, the pressure in systole should not exceed 35 mmHg, and at the end of diastole averages 4 mmHg. The pressure in the pulmonary artery should not exceed 35/15 mmHg. In the left ventricle, the systolic pressure depends on the systemic arterial pressure; a normal value would be about 140 mmHg. The left ventricular pressure at the end of diastole is 10 mmHg.

Haemodynamic events in the cardiac cycle and their clinical correlates (see Fig. 6.7)

This section only describes events in the left side of the heart. The events in the right side of the heart are similar. However, left atrial systole occurs after right atrial systole and left ventricular systole precedes right ventricular systole.

At the very beginning of ventricular systole, the mitral valve is open; the pressure in the left atrium is somewhat greater than that in the left ventricle. As ventricular systole continues, the pressure in the left ventricle exceeds that in the left atrium, thus closing the mitral valve. Shortly after, the

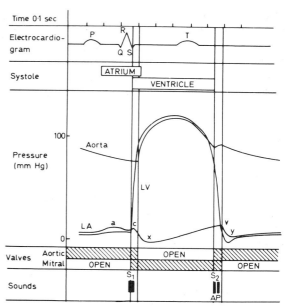

Fig. 6.7 Haemodynamic and electrocardiographic correlates of events in the cardiac cycle. (Reproduced with permission from Blackwell Scientific Publications and the editors of *Companion in Medical Studies.*)

pressure in the left ventricle exceeds that in the aorta, and this opens the aortic valve; ejection of blood then occurs from the left ventricle. As the ventricle starts relaxing, the pressure in the left ventricle falls below that in the aorta; initially, the aortic valve stays open because of the forward kinetic energy of the ejected blood. With a further fall in pressure in the left ventricle, the aortic valve then closes. As the pressure in the left ventricle continues to fall below and becomes lower than that in the left atrium, the mitral valve opens, and blood passes from the atrium to the ventricle.

In the period of rapid filling, early in diastole, blood falls from the atria to the ventricles. However, the remaining one-third of ventricular filling is caused by atrial systole, which, in turn, causes the *a* wave in the jugular venous pressure trace. The *c* wave coincides with the onset of ventricular systole, making the tricuspid valve bulge into the atrium and raising the pressure there. The *v* wave is due to the filling of the atrium while the tricuspid valve is shut, and the upward movement of the tricuspid valve at the end of ventricular systole.

During the early part of ventricular systole, both mitral and aortic valves are closed. The volume of blood within the ventricle must then remain the same. This is therefore known as the period of isovolumetric contraction. As the ventricle relaxes, there is a similar period when both aortic and mitral valves are closed, the period of iso-volumetric relaxation.

In those with normal hearts, valve closure is associated with heart sounds; but valve opening is not. The first sound is caused by mitral valve closure, and the second sound by aortic valve closure. Patients with abnormal valves may have an ejection click (aortic stenosis) at aortic valve opening or an opening snap (mitral stenosis) at mitral valve opening. The third heart sound occurs at the period of rapid ventricular filling; the fourth heart sound is related to atrial systole. The fourth heart sound is therefore absent in patients with atrial fibrillation. Heart sounds, other than the first and second, are usually considered pathological, although the third heart sound in particular is very commonly heard in pregnancy and in young people.

The electrical events of the electrocardiograph precede mechanical ones. Thus, the P wave representing atrial deplorisation occurs before the fourth heart sound, and the QRS complex representing ventricular depolarisation, occurs at the onset of ventricular systole. The T wave (ventricular repolarisation) is already occurring at the height of ventricular systole.

Alterations in heart rate are associated with changes in the length of diastole rather than the length of systole. This can be a problem in patients where filling of the ventricles is impaired, as in mitral stenosis; such patients are very intolerant of rapid heart rates.

Since right ventricular systole occurs a little later than left, the second sound is split, the second component being due to the closure of the pulmonary valve. During inspiration, the delay of ejection of blood from the right side of the heart is even greater, so that splitting of the second sound widens.

Control of stroke volume

Stroke volume and heart rate are the two factors that govern cardiac output. The resting cardiac output is about 4.5 l/min in females, 5.5 l/min in males. The difference is partly due to males being bigger. The cardiac index is the cardiac output divided by the calculated body surface area in square metres. It is normally about 3.2 l/min/m² and is less dependent on body size than is cardiac output. Heart rate changes have already been described on page 166. Starling's law of the heart states that the force of contraction is proportional to the initial muscle fibre length. The initial fibre length depends on the degree of stretch of the ventricular muscle, or the amount that the ventricle is dilated in diastole, i.e. the venous return. As end diastolic volume increases, the force of contraction increases until a maximum is reached and the heart starts to fail (see Fig. 6.8).

Factors affecting end diastolic volume (also called preload) are those factors that control effective blood volume, i.e. the total blood volume, the body position (pooling of blood in the lower limbs in the upright posture) and the pumping action of muscles in the leg which encourages the venous return. Venous tone also affects effective blood volume. The veins are the capacitance vessels of the circulation. If venous tone is increased, venous return is also increased. Intrathoracic pressure is

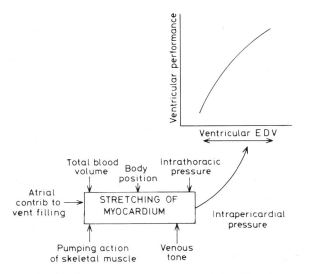

Fig. 6.8 Relation between ventricular end diastolic volume (EDV) and ventricular performance (Frank–Starling curve), with a summary of the major factors affecting EDV. Atrial contribution to vent filling = atrial contribution to ventricular filling. (Reproduced with permission from B. Ward et al., 1967, Mechanisms of contraction of the normal and failing heart, *New England Journal of Medicine*.)

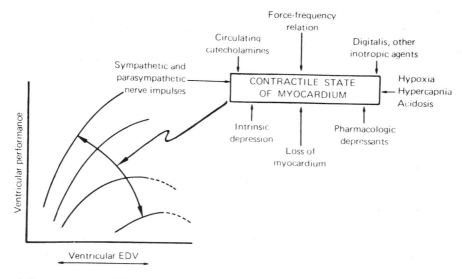

Fig. 6.9 Effect of changes in myocardial contractility on the Frank–Starling curve. The major factors influencing contractility are summarised on the right. EDV = end diastolic volume. (Reproduced with permission from B. Ward et al., 1967, *Mechanisms of contraction of the normal and failing heart*, *New England Journal of Medicine*.)

also important. If intrathoracic pressure is high, as in patients who are being artificially ventilated, blood does not return so effectively to the heart. When patients have a pericardial effusion, intra-pericardial pressure may be high, the heart cannot dilate and ventricular filling is impaired, so that cardiac output falls. Atrial systole, as described above, contributes one-third of ventricular filling.

Figure 6.8 shows one curve relating ventricular performance to end diastolic volume. However, one can also draw a series of such curves (Fig. 6.9) showing how ventricular performance may be increased without change in end diastolic volume. Such an increase moving from a lower to a higher curve represents an increase in contractility. This is seen in treatment with digoxin and other 'inotropic' agents such as aminophylline; with sympathetic nerve stimulation and with β adrenergic catecholamines, e.g. adrenaline and isoprenaline. The reverse is seen with drugs such as β adrenergic blocking agents (e.g. propranolol) and quinidine which are pharmacological depressants of myocardial activity, in hypoxia, hypercapnia and acidosis, in patients who have lost myocardial tissue as after a myocardial infarction and with increased systemic arterial pressure. Systemic arterial pressure is a major component of afterload, the resistance against which the heart must work

to pump out blood. (Cf. inotropic and chronotropic drugs. Chronotropic drugs such as atropine exert their effect by a change in heart rate.)

Changes in blood volume and cardiac output in pregnancy (see Fig. 6.10)

During pregnancy, plasma volume increases from the non-pregnant level of 2600 ml to about

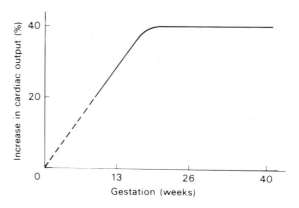

Fig. 6.10 Changes in cardiac output through pregnancy. Note that cardiac output is considerably increased by the end of the first trimester, and the increase is maintained until term. (Reproduced with permission from F. Hytten and G. Chamberlain, *Clinical Physiology in Obstetrics*, Blackwell Scientific Publications.)

3800 ml. This increase occurs early in pregnancy and there is not much further change after 32 weeks gestation. The increased plasma volume is related to the size of the fetus. The red cell mass also increases from a non-pregnant level of 1400 ml to 1650–1800 ml depending on whether iron supplementation has been given. The increase in red cell mass occurs steadily until term. However, since plasma volume increases proportionately more than red cell mass, the haematocrit and haemoglobin concentration fall during pregnancy. A haemoglobin level of 10.5 g/l would not be unusual in healthy pregnancy. Cardiac output also rises by about 40% from about 4.5 l/min to 6 l/min. This rise can be seen early in pregnancy, and cardiac output reaches a plateau at 24–30 weeks' gestation. The rise is maintained through labour, and declines to prepregnancy levels over a rather variable time course after delivery. If the patient is studied lying supine, the gravid uterus constricts the inferior vena cava, and decreases the venous return, thus falsely decreasing cardiac output. This is also the mechanism of hypotension seen in patients lying flat on their backs at the end of pregnancy (supine hypotensive syndrome) and may be a contributory factor to fetal distress in patients lying in this position during labour.

The vasodilator substance bradykinin is formed from protein precursors (kininogens) in the plasma and tissues under the influence of the kallikrein enzymes. Bradykinin is inactivated by angiotensin-converting enzyme (see p. 172).

Cardiac output increases by about 40%; but heart rate increases by only about 10% from 80 beats per minute to 90 beats per minute during pregnancy. Therefore, there must be an associated increase in stroke volume. The increase in cardiac output is more than is necessary to distribute the extra 30–50 ml of oxygen consumed per minute in pregnancy. Therefore, the arteriovenous oxygen gradient decreases in pregnancy.

Figure 6.11 indicates the distribution of the increase in cardiac output seen in pregnancy. At term, about 400 ml/min goes to the uterus, and about 300 ml/min extra goes to the kidneys. The increase in skin blood flow could be as much as 500 ml/min. The remaining 300 ml would be distributed amongst the gastrointestinal tract, breasts and the other extra metabolic needs of pregnancy,

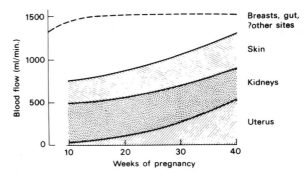

Fig. 6.11 Distribution of increased cardiac output during pregnancy. (Reproduced with permission from F. Hytten and G. Chamberlain, *Clinical Physiology in Obstetrics*, Blackwell Scientific Publications.)

such as respiratory muscle and cardiac muscle. Early in pregnancy, uterine blood flow has not increased, although cardiac output and renal blood flow have. There is therefore a disproportionately higher quantity of extra blood perfusing skin, breasts and other organs at this time.

Blood flow and pressure control

These are both general and local control mechanisms. The integration of changes in cardiac output and all the various control mechanisms for peripheral resistance is very complicated.

Blood pressure is proportional to cardiac output and peripheral resistance. Cardiac output is controlled by heart rate and stroke volume (see pp. 166, 168–9). Peripheral resistance is controlled neurogenically by the autonomic nervous system, and directly by substances that act on blood vessels: angiotensin II, serotonin, kinins, catecholamines secreted from the adrenal medulla, metabolites such as adenosine, potassium, H^+, P_{CO_2}, P_{O_2} and prostaglandins.

From the Poiseuille formula the flow (f) in a tube of radius (r) and length (L) is governed by the relation

$$f \propto \frac{Pr^4}{\eta L}$$

where P is the pressure gradient and η the viscosity of the fluid. Flow and peripheral resistance are therefore extremely sensitive to blood vessel radius. A 5% increase in vessel radius increases flow and decreases resistance by 21%. In blood, which is not a Newtonian fluid, viscosity rises markedly when the haematocrit rises above 45%. Such a marked increase in viscosity therefore causes a considerable reduction in blood flow.

The autonomic nervous system and blood pressure control

Receptors involved in blood pressure control in blood vessels and the heart are shown in Table 6.3. Both cholinergic and α and β-adrenergic receptors are involved. The major tonic effect is adrenergic vasoconstrictor, and vasodilatation is largely achieved by a reduction in vasoconstrictor tone rather than active vasodilatation.

The action of the autonomic system in controlling blood pressure is governed by the cardio-inhibitory and vasomotor centres. The cardio-inhibitory centre is the dorsal motor nucleus of the vagus nerve. Impulses pass from the cardio-inhibitory centre via the vagus nerve to the heart, causing bradycardia and decreasing contractility. These effects reduce cardiac output and therefore blood pressure. The input to the cardioinhibitory centre is from the baroreceptors (see below). An increase in baroreceptor firing rate stimulates the cardioinhibitory centre and so produces reflex slowing of the heart and a reduction in blood pressure. The cardioinhibitory centre also receives inputs from other centres, so that pain and emotion can both increase vagal tone. If the vagal stimulation caused by pain and/or emotion is severe enough, blood pressure is decreased to the point where cerebral perfusion is impaired and the subject faints.

Sympathetic output to the heart and blood vessels is controlled by the vasomotor centre. The input to the vasomotor centre is from the baroreceptors; a *fall* in baroreceptor activity is associated with increased output from the vasomotor centre, thus increasing blood pressure. The vasomotor centre also receives fibres from the aortic carotid body chemoreceptors so that a fall in the Po_2 or pH or a rise in the Pco_2 will stimulate the vasomotor centre and cause a rise in blood pressure. In addition, baroreceptors in the floor of the fourth ventricle, which are sensitive to cerebrospinal fluid (CSF) pressure innervate the vasomotor centre. These act so that a rise in CSF pressure causes an equal rise in blood pressure (Cushing reflex). Pain and emotion can also stimulate the vasomotor centre as well as the cardio-inhibitory centre. Therefore, these stimuli can cause a rise in blood pressure, as well as a fall in blood pressure.

The carotid sinus baroreceptor is located at the bifurcation of the internal carotid artery. Fibres of the glossopharyngeal nerve carry impulses at frequencies that, within certain limits, are proportional to the instantaneous pressure in the carotid artery. In experimental animals at pressures below 70 mmHg, the receptors do not fire at all. Between 70 and 150 mmHg the receptors fire with increasing frequency as the blood pressure rises. This frequency reaches a maximum at 150 mmHg. Therefore, the carotid sinus baro-

Table 6.3 Autonomic receptors affecting the heart and blood vessels

Location	Receptor	Comments
Heart muscle and conducting tissue	Cholinergic	↓ Heart rate ↓ Conduction velocity ↓ Contractility
	α-adrenergic	Nil
	β_2-adrenergic	↑ Heart rate ↑ Conduction velocity ↑ Contractility
Blood vessels	Cholinergic (vasodilator)	Muscle Coronary artery Salivary glands
	α-adrenergic (vasoconstrictor)	All tissues
	β_1-adrenergic (vasodilator)	Brain Skeletal muscle Intra-abdominal

receptors can modulate blood pressure between 70 and 150 mmHg, but not outside this range. In patients with hypertension, the baroreceptors adapt and shift upwards the pressures over which they respond.

Local control of blood flow

Metabolites that accumulate during anaerobic metabolism cause vasodilatation. This allows tissues to autoregulate their blood flow; vasodilatation allows an increased blood flow and decreases the tendency for anaerobic metabolism. The metabolites involved are hydrogen ions, potassium, lactate, adenosine (in heart but not skeletal muscle) and carbon dioxide. In addition, hypoxia itself causes vasodilatation.

Another form of autoregulation is the myogenic reflex. If the perfusion pressure in the arteriole decreases, thus tending to decrease local blood flow, the smooth muscle in the arteriole relaxes allowing vasodilatation and an increase in local blood flow. The converse occurs at high perfusion pressures: arteriolar smooth muscle then contracts, causing vasoconstriction, and a reduction in blood flow to offset the high perfusion pressure. Note that these changes induced by the myogenic reflex maintain local blood flow but will exacerbate changes in systemic blood pressure.

Other substances affecting the blood vessels locally are prostaglandins derived from fatty acids. Prostaglandin E and prostaglandin A cause a fall in blood pressure by reducing splanchnic vascular resistance. Prostaglandin F causes an increase in blood pressure due to vasoconstriction, although the site where this occurs is not known. Prostacyclin, the levels of which increase considerably in pregnancy and which is produced by blood vessels and the fetoplacental unit, causes a marked vasodilatation, which will cause a fall in blood pressure unless the cardiac output also increases. Thromboxane derived from platelets causes vasoconstriction.

Other locally active substances are the vasodilator endothelium-derived relaxing factor (EDRF), which has been shown to be nitric oxide locally made from L-arginine, and endothelin, a 21 amino acid peptide that is intensely vasoconstrictor. Another potent vasoconstrictor

agent is angiotensin II, produced under the influence of renin. Renin is an enzyme largely produced by the juxtaglomerular apparatus of the kidney, but also by the pregnant uterus, which splits angiotensin I, a decapeptide, from its substrate, one of the plasma proteins. Angiotensin I is then converted to angiotensin II in the lungs, by angiotensin-converting enzyme which removes a further two amino acid residues. The stimuli to renin secretion are β-adrenergic agonists, hyponatraemia, hypovolaemia, whether induced by bleeding or changes in posture, and pregnancy. A similar but smaller rise in renin levels is also seen in patients taking oestrogen-containing contraceptive pills. It is probable that angiotensin I has no physiological activity, but angiotensin II is intensely vasoconstrictive. In addition, angiotensin II also stimulates aldosterone production from the zona glomerulosa of the adrenal gland, and this will, in turn, cause a rise in blood volume, and blood pressure over the longer term, by sodium retention.

The action of angiotensin II can be inhibited by the competitive inhibitor saralasin. The angiotensin-converting enzyme is inhibited by the converting enzyme inhibitor captopril and other similar drugs.

Blood pressure changes in pregnancy

The marked rise in cardiac output which occurs in pregnancy does not cause a rise in blood pressure, unless a pathological process such as toxaemia of pregnancy occurs. Therefore, there must be a decrease in total peripheral resistance, and this vasodilatation accomodates the increased blood flow to the uterus, kidney, skin and other organs (Fig. 6.11).

The decreased peripheral vascular resistance does not always keep strictly in proportion with the increase in cardiac output and during the middle of pregnancy from, perhaps, 8 to 36 weeks, the systolic blood pressure may fall by up to 5 mmHg, and the diastolic blood pressure by up to 10 mmHg because the peripheral resistance falls by more than cardiac output rises (Fig. 6.12). Other factors affecting blood pressure are posture and uterine contractions, which act via the changes in cardiac output already described. Uterine con-

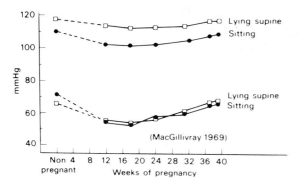

Fig. 6.12 Effect of pregnancy on systolic and diastolic blood pressure as found by MacGillivray. (Reproduced with permission from F. Hytten and G. Chamberlain, *Clinical Physiology in Obstetrics*, Blackwell Scientific Publications.)

tractions expel blood from the uterus, increase cardiac output and increase blood pressure. The supine position, by causing caval obstruction, decreases cardiac output and will decrease blood pressure.

RESPIRATION

The lungs

Respiration is the process whereby the body takes in oxygen and eliminates carbon dioxide. We need to consider the action of the lungs, and, in addition, transport of oxygen and carbon dioxide to peripheral tissues.

Gas composition

Table 6.4 shows the partial pressures of dry air, inspired air, alveolar air and expired air at body temperature and normal atmospheric pressure (760 mmHg or 101.1 kPa, where 100 mmHg = 13.3 kPa). Dry air consists of oxygen, nitrogen and a little carbon dioxide. We do not normally breathe completely dry air, and inspired air usually has some water vapour (partial pressure, 5.7 mmHg). Alveolar air is fully saturated with water (47 mmHg) and is in equilibrium with pulmonary venous blood. The small difference in the Po_2 between alveolar air (100 mmHg) and pulmonary venous blood (98 mmHg) shows the efficiency of gas exchange in the healthy lung. Expired air is a mixture of alveolar air and inspired air with regard to oxygen and carbon dioxide concentrations. As a result of this mixture, the partial pressure of nitrogen is less in expired air (570 mmHg) than in inspired air (596 mmHg). The total volume of alveolar air is about 2 litres; alveolar ventilation is about 350 ml for each breath. Alveolar ventilation is therefore a small proportion of total alveolar volume, and the alveolar gas remains relatively constant in composition.

Dead space

Although the alveolar ventilation is 350 ml per breath, the tidal volume is 500 ml per breath. The difference, 150 ml, is the anatomic dead space, the volume of air between the mouth or nose and the alveoli that does not participate in gas exchange. The anatomic dead space (millilitres) approximately equals body weight (pounds avoirdupois) (1 kg = 2.2 lb). In addition, on occasions, some alveoli, particularly in the upper part of the lungs, are well ventilated, but rather poorly perfused; whereas other alveoli in the dependent lower part of the lungs are well perfused, but poorly venti-

Table 6.4 Partial pressures of gases (mmHg)[a] in a resting, healthy man at sea level (barometric pressure = 760 mmHg)

	Dry air		Inspired air	Alveolar air	Expired air
Po_2	159.1	(21%)	158.0	100.0	116.0
Pco_2	0.3	(0.04%)	0.3	40.0	26.8
PH_2O	0.0	(0%)	5.7	47.0	47.0
PN_2[b]	600.6	(79%)	596.0	573.0	569.9
Total	760.0		760.0	760.0	759.7

[a] 1 kPa = 7.5 mmHg.
[b] Includes small amounts of rare gases.

lated. This mismatching of ventilation and perfusion represents a further source of wasted ventilation which, together with the anatomic dead space, makes up the total or physiological dead space. In healthy, supine individuals, the anatomic dead space nearly equals the physiological dead space. In patients who are sick with lung disease, or heart failure, the physiological dead space considerably exceeds the anatomic dead space.

Oxygen consumption

The normal oxygen consumption at rest is about 250 ml/min. The oxygen capacity of normal blood is about 20 ml per 100 ml (200 ml/l). Oxygen consumption of 250 ml/min at rest is achieved by delivering 1 litre of oxygen to peripheral tissues (cardiac output, 5 litres × 200 ml oxygen per litre = 1 litre), of which 25% is extracted and 75% is returned to the heart in venous blood. In extreme exertion, ventilation increases to about 150 l/min. This allows oxygen delivery of 3.2 l/min with a cardiac output of 16 l/min. (Cardiac output, 16 l/min × oxygen capacity, 200 ml/l = 3.2 l/min). Of this, 75% is extracted

and 25% is returned to the heart, giving an oxygen consumption of 2.4 ml/min, almost 10 times that at rest.

Lung volumes (see Fig. 6.13)

The total lung capacity is approximately 5 litres. Of this, 1.5 litres, the residual volume, remains at the end of forced expiration. The volume of gas, 3.5 litres, that can be inhaled from forced expiration to forced inspiration is the vital capacity. The normal tidal volume (500 ml) is a small proportion of the maximum 3.5 litres that is possible. The tidal volume is situated in the middle of the vital capacity, so that the inspiratory reserve volume is approximately 1.5 litres, as is the expiratory reserve volume.

Mechanics of ventilation

The chest cavity expands by the actions of the intrathoracic musculature, innervated from T1 to T11 and the diaphragm innervated by the phrenic nerve (C3–C5). Thus cord section below C5 allows

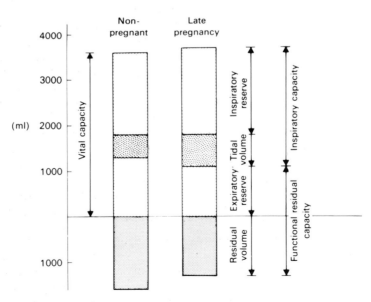

Fig. 6.13 Subdivisions of lung volume and their alterations in pregnancy. (Reproduced with permission from F. Hytten and G. Chamberlain, *Clinical Physiology in Obstetrics*, Blackwell Scientific Publications.)

spontaneous ventilation because of the phrenic nerve innervation. Phrenic nerve crush, as used to be performed for the treatment of tuberculosis, allows spontaneous ventilation because of the action of thoracic musculature. Damage to the spinal cord above the level of C3 needs permanent artificial ventilation, since both the phrenic nerve and thoracic innervation are inactivated.

At rest, the pressure in the potential space between the visceral pleura and the parietal pleura is −3 mmHg, i.e. 3 mmHg less than the atmospheric pressure. This pressure can be determined by connecting a balloon catheter with the balloon in the oesophagus at the level of the mediastinum to a pressure transducer. During quiet inspiration, the chest expands and the pressure in the intrapleural space decreases to −6 mmHg. This pressure gradient is sufficient to overcome the elastic recoil of the lung, which therefore expands following the chest wall. In forced inspiration, the pressure in the intrapleural space may fall to as low as −30 mmHg. Expiration is passive; the muscles of the diaphragm and chest wall relax, and the elastic recoil of the lung causes the lung and therefore the chest to contract. Forced expiration may be associated with muscular effort and a positive intrapleural pressure.

Resistance to air flow

The rapidity with which expiration occurs depends on the stiffness of the lungs and the resistance of the bronchi. This is measured clinically, by determining the forced expiratory volume in 1 second (FEV_1). Since this volume depends on the vital capacity it is easiest expressed as FEV_1/FVC. In normal individuals this ratio exceeds 75%. The ratio decreases in age but in asthma it may be as low as 25%, and the FEV_1, which in healthy individuals is about 3.0 litres, is less than 1 litre in patients with attacks of severe asthma. An alternative measurement of airway resistance is the peak flow rate, which should be greater than 600 l/min. Both peak flow rate and FEV_1/FVC depend on large airway calibre and the stiffness of the lung. To measure the stiffness of the lungs independently, it is necessary to use more complicated apparatus and to determine lung compliance.

Oxygen transfer

Oxygen is transferred across the 300 million alveoli which have a total surface area of about 70 m². Transfer occurs across the type 1 lining cells; apart from the epithelial cells, mast cells, plasma cells, macrophages and lymphocytes, the alveoli also contain type 2 granular pneumocytes, which make surfactant. The granules that these cells contain are thought to be packages of surfactant. Patients who are deficient in surfactant, such as premature infants or adults suffering from the adult respiratory distress syndrome, have type 2 pneumocytes which do not contain granules. Surfactant is necessary to lower the surface tension of alveoli and maintain patency of the alveoli. In the absence of surfactant, the surface tension of the fluid in the alveoli is so high that the alveoli collapse.

Effect of pregnancy

During pregnancy, ventilation is already increased during the first trimester. The total increase is about 40%. A similar, but smaller, effect is seen in patients taking contraceptive pills containing progestogens, and in the luteal phase of the menstrual cycle. It is therefore thought to be due to progesterone, which acts partly by stimulating the respiratory centre directly, and partly by increasing its sensitivity to carbon dioxide. Some patients are aware of the increase in ventilation and feel breathless; others are not. The increase in ventilation is achieved by increasing the tidal volume, rather than the respiratory rate. This is a more efficient way of increasing ventilation, since an increase in respiratory rate involves more work in shifting the dead space more frequently. The tidal volume therefore expands into the expiratory reserve volume and the inspiratory reserve volume (see Fig. 6.13). The consensus of opinion is that the vital capacity does not change. However, the residual volume decreases by about 200 ml, possibly due to the large intra-abdominal swelling. Therefore, the total lung capacity also decreases by about 200 ml. There is no change in FEV_1 or peak flow rate in pregnancy. The increase in ventilation is much greater than the increase in oxygen consumption, which is only about 50 ml extra at term. Of this 50 ml, 20 ml would be necessary for the fetus, 6 ml for the increase in cardiac output and 6 ml for the increase in renal work. This would leave a further 18 ml for the other increased metabolic activity in pregnancy.

The hyperventilation of pregnancy causes a fall in the P_{CO_2} from a normal value of about 40 mmHg to 31 mmHg. The bicarbonate level falls to maintain a normal pH, but because bicarbonate falls, sodium falls also. There is therefore a decrease in the total number of osmotically active ions and a fall in osmolarity of about 10 mmol/l. Such a fall in osmolarity would normally be associated with profound diuresis; so there must be an adaptation of the hypothalamic centres governing vasopressin secretion as well (see p. 184).

During pregnancy, bronchodilator stimuli are progesterone secretion (dilates smooth muscle) and prostaglandin E_2. Bronchoconstrictor influences are prostaglandin F_2, and the decrease in resting lung volume which decreases the overall space available for the airways to occupy. These factors balance each other out so that there is no overall change in airways resistance.

Control of respiration

Although several respiratory centres with different functions have been described in the midbrain on the basis of experiments performed in decerebrate or anaesthetised animals, it is not clear to what extent such localisation occurs in conscious man. It is therefore simpler to think of one diffuse medullary respiratory centre. The respiratory centre is responsible for controlling both the depth of respiration and its rhythmicity. Respiratory neurones are of two types, inspiratory and expiratory. When the inspiratory neurones are stimulated at the respiratory centre, the expiratory neurones are inhibited and vice versa. The respiratory centre receives input from higher voluntary centres and pain and emotion will also increase ventilation; but in most healthy patients, ventilation is automatic, and we do not need to be consciously aware of the need to breathe.

The most important input to the respiratory centre comes from chemoreceptors. There are two main groups of these: central chemoreceptors,

possibly on the surface of the upper medulla, but separate from the medullary respiratory centre, and peripheral chemoreceptors around the aortic arch and in the carotid body. The aortic arch chemoreceptors are innervated by the vagus nerve; the carotid body chemoreceptors by the glossopharyngeal nerve. The carotid body is highly specialised tissue, which has an exceedingly high blood flow rate. This makes it possible for the chemoreceptors in the carotid body to be sensitive to changes in the P_{O_2}, not to the oxygen content of blood. The carotid body chemoreceptors are the only chemoreceptors sensitive to changes in the P_{O_2}. Carotid and aortic body chemoreceptors are sensitive to changes in the P_{CO_2} and pH. The central chemoreceptors are probably only sensitive to changes in the pH, any effect of a change in the P_{CO_2} being mediated by the ensuing pH change. The chemoreceptors may also be stimulated by cyanide, lobeline, nicotine, nikethamide and doxapram. Of these respiratory stimulants, doxapram is now one of the most popular, since it does not have other stimulatory side-effects, in particular, the risk of causing convulsions in normal dosage.

The response to hypercapnia

If it were not for the activity of the chemoreceptors, a decrease in ventilation would be associated with a rise in the P_{CO_2} (curve A, Fig. 6.14) and

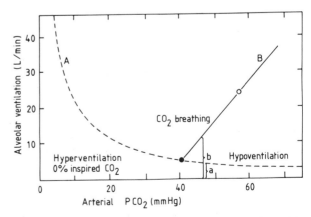

Fig. 6.14 Relations between alveolar ventilation and arterial (alveolar) P_{CO_2} at a constant rate of metabolic carbon dioxide production.

an increase in ventilation would be associated with a decrease in the P_{CO_2}. When the P_{CO_2} is less than 40 mmHg this does occur. However, the activity of the respiratory centre is such that any rise in the P_{CO_2} above 40 mmHg is associated with a marked increase in ventilation (curve B, Fig. 6.14). The ratio of ventilation observed (b, curve B) to ventilation expected (a, curve A) is the gain of the control system. In normal hyperoxic individuals, this varies between 2 and 5. It is decreased in age, and in trained athletes, and it increases in pregnancy to 8, thus increasing the sensitivity of the respiratory centre to carbon dioxide as indicated earlier. Hypoxia also increases respiratory centre sensitivity to carbon dioxide.

The response to hypoxia

This is more subtle than the response to the P_{CO_2} since the effect of hypoxia is modulated by the effects of ventilation on the P_{CO_2}, and by changes in the buffering ability of haemoglobin: any increased ventilation associated with hypoxia will also be associated with a decrease in the P_{CO_2}. A decrease in the P_{CO_2} will decrease respiratory drive (see Fig. 6.14) and this will therefore decrease the hyperventilation that would otherwise have been caused by falling P_{O_2}; also, a fall in the P_{O_2} is associated with increased quantities of deoxygenated haemoglobin. Deoxygenated haemoglobin is a better buffer than oxygenated haemoglobin, and therefore the patient becomes less acidotic. The stimulus to respiration caused by acidosis is therefore also reduced.

For these reasons, ventilation only shows marked increases when the P_aCO_2 falls below 60 mmHg (Fig. 6.15). A fall in oxygen saturation of haemoglobin 1% is associated with an increase in ventilation of 0.6 l/min. The response is blunted by chronic hypoxia, as occurs in patients living at altitude, with cyanotic congenital heart disease or by hypercapnia due to lung disease (Fig. 6.15).

The effect of changes in hydrogen ion concentration

A rise in hydrogen ion concentration causes an increase in respiration. This is due to peripheral

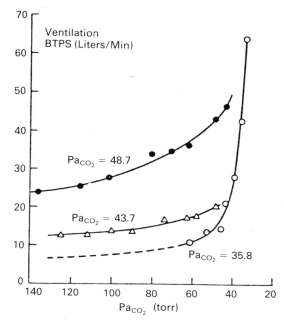

Fig. 6.15 Increase in ventilation due to hypoxia associated with low and high levels of carbon dioxide. (Reproduced with permission from Comroe, *Physiology of Respiration*, Chicago Year Books.)

and central stimulation of chemoreceptors. In metabolic acidosis, the increase in ventilation decreases P_{CO_2}, which, in turn, decreases the hydrogen ion concentration. In metabolic alkalosis, there is a decrease in ventilation which allows the P_{CO_2} to rise with a consequent compensatory increase in hydrogen ion concentration.

Other inputs to the respiratory centre are from proprioceptors in the chest wall. These sense respiratory movements, and an absence of respiratory movements causes stimulation of the respiratory centre. There are irritant receptors in the air passages (J receptors) and lungs which respond to foreign bodies and also stimulate respiration via the respiratory centre. These J receptors are possibly responsible for the increase in ventilation seen in patients with mild respiratory tract infections, where there is no alteration in blood gas composition.

It is not known to what extent the inflation and deflation receptors in the smooth muscle of the airways affect the control of normal respiration.

The baroreceptors have a trivial influence on respiration, in comparison to the profound effect that chemoreceptors have on the circulation. There are also receptors in the pulmonary arteries and coronary circulation, sensitive to veratrum alkaloids, stimulation of which causes decreased respiration and even apnoea. This is the Bezold–Jarrisch reflex.

Oxygen and carbon dioxide transport

The lungs maintain an alveolar P_{O_2} of 98 mmHg and a P_{CO_2} of 40 mmHg, but special transport mechanisms are needed to carry the oxygen absorbed at the lungs to the peripheral tissues and to transport carbon dioxide produced by the metabolism, from peripheral tissues to the lungs.

Oxygen transport

The haemoglobin molecule is specially adapted to transport oxygen. Each molecule has four iron atoms which can combine reversibly with four oxygen atoms. The haemoglobin molecule can alter its shape (quaternary structure) to favour uptake or unloading of oxygen.

However, throughout this combination, the iron remains in the ferrous state and the association of haemoglobin with oxygen is therefore referred to as oxygenation. If the iron is oxidised to the ferric form, methaemoglobin is formed, which does not act as an oxygen carrier.

Each gram of haemoglobin reacts with 1.34 ml of oxygen. Therefore, 100 ml of blood containing 15 g of haemoglobin can react with 19.5 ml of oxygen. In contrast, 100 ml of blood would only contain 0.3 ml of oxygen in solution at a P_{O_2} of 95 mmHg. Therefore, the presence of haemoglobin increases oxygen-carrying capacity 70-fold. Venous blood at a P_{CO_2} of 46 mmHg contains 3.0 ml of carbon dioxide in solution, and 49.7 ml of carbon dioxide as bicarbonate. The formation of bicarbonate (see below) therefore increases carbon dioxide transport 17-fold.

Figure 6.16 shows that the relationship between the P_{O_2} and oxygen saturation for haemoglobin is hyperbolic. The biggest change in saturation occurs between a P_{O_2} of 40 mmHg and of 70 mmHg, and of course this is the change be-

tween the P_{O_2} in peripheral tissues and the P_{O_2} in the lungs. There is little change in saturation as the P_{O_2} falls from 100 to 70 mmHg and, in this way, haemoglobin compensates for any minor falls in the P_{O_2} associated with lung disease or a decrease in inspiratory P_{O_2} which would occur at altitude. However, both acidosis and hyperthermia shift the haemoglobin dissociation curve to the right and decrease the affinity of haemoglobin for oxygen. A fall in the pH to 7.2 or an increase in temperature to 43°C will reduce the oxygen saturation to 90% at a P_{O_2} of 98 mmHg, and this can have a significant effect in patients who are ill with acidosis of any cause or high fever. The presence of methaemoglobin or of other abnormal haemoglobins such as haemoglobin S will also shift the dissociation curve to the right, decreasing affinity and decreasing the uptake of oxygen by haemoglobin.

The shape of the dissociation curve is also beneficial when haemoglobin unloads oxygen in peripheral tissues at a low P_{O_2}. Here acidosis (the Bohr effect) and hyperthermia, both of which will occur in metabolically active tissue, are an advantage. They decrease affinity and help haemoglobin to unload further oxygen. The formation of carbamino compounds by the combination of carbon dioxide and haemoglobin (see below) also shifts the curve to the right (Haldane effect) and assists unloading in metabolically active tissue. The position of the haemoglobin dissociation curve can be defined by the P_{50}, the P_{O_2} at which haemoglobin is 50% desaturated.

2,3-Diphosphoglycerate (2,3-DPG) is formed from 3-phosphoglyceraldehyde, a product of glycolysis via the Embden–Meyerhof pathway. It also affects haemoglobin dissociation in red cells and the presence of 2,3-DPG shifts the dissociation curve to the right. 2,3-DPG levels are decreased in acidosis and banked blood but increased by androgens, thyroxine, growth hormone, anaemia, exercise and hypoxic conditions (living at altitude and cardiopulmonary disease). Thus, banked blood does not give up its oxygen very easily but hypoxic individuals do unload oxygen easily even if their low haemoglobin affinity is less favourable for oxygen uptake.

The fetus clearly needs high-affinity blood since the P_{O_2} in the fetal umbilical vein is only about

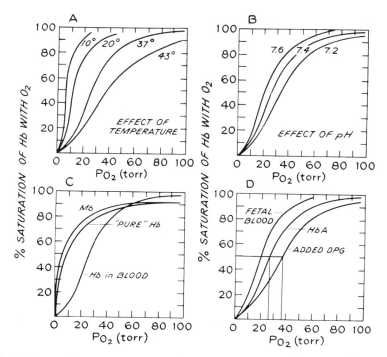

Fig. 6.16 Variations in the haemoglobin (Hb) oxygen dissociation curve. **A** effect of changes in temperature; **B** effect of changes in blood pH; **C** hyperbolic curve of 'purified' haemoglobin A (HbA) (dialysed to be salt free) is similar to curve of myoglobin (Mb); **D** the dissociation curve of fetal blood (but not pure HbF) is to the left of adult blood containing HbA; addition of diphosphoglycerate (DPG) shifts curve of blood with HbA to the right and increases P_{50} (decreases affinity of oxygen for Hb and facilitates unloading of oxygen in tissues). (Reproduced with permission from Comroe, *Physiology of Respiration*, Chicago Year Books.)

30 mmHg. Different mammalian species have different ways of increasing the affinity of fetal blood. In man, fetal haemoglobin has a low oxygen affinity and this is not the mechanism by which fetal red cells increase their affinity for oxygen. Instead, in human fetal red cells the fetal haemoglobin does not interact with 2,3-DPG, and it is this that accounts for the increased affinity of human fetal blood for oxygen.

Carbon monoxide

Carbon monoxide has 210 times the affinity for haemoglobin that oxygen does. Therefore, if the ratio of carbon monoxide to oxygen in inspired air is 1 to 210, equivalent to a 0.1% concentration of carbon monoxide in air, haemoglobin will be 50% oxygenated and 50% combined with carbon monoxide (n.b. the oxygen concentration is 21%).

This effect alone will reduce the oxygen capacity of haemoglobin by 50% and would be the same as giving the patient a haemoglobin concentration of 7.5 g per 100 ml. However, the presence of carboxyhaemoglobin also shifts the haemoglobin dissociation curve of oxygen to the left (increased affinity) so that even the oxygen that is combined with haemoglobin is not liberated in peripheral tissues, and this accounts for the profound tissue hypoxia that occurs in carbon monoxide poisoning. It also explains why such patients are not cyanosed, because the oxygen remains combined with haemoglobin. Cyanosis is not seen until the concentration of deoxygenated haemoglobin in the blood is at least 5 g per 100 ml. The cherry-pink colour that these patients do have is due to the presence of carboxyhaemoglobin.

The amount of carboxyhaemoglobin associated with smoking (5–8% carboxyhaemoglobin) is sufficient to shift the tissue P_{O_2} from 45 to 40 mmHg. This may account for the deleterious effect of smoking on ischaemic heart disease, and also for the intrauterine growth retardation seen in the fetuses of women who smoke in pregnancy.

Carbon dioxide transport

Carbon dioxide is transported in the plasma, partly in solution, partly by hydration to form carbonic acid (equation 1) and partly by the formation of carbamino compounds with the N-terminal end of plasma proteins (equation 2). Hydration is very slow because there is no carbonic anhydrase in the plasma. Hydrogen ions are formed from both reactions, and these are buffered by plasma proteins.

$$\text{Carbonic anhydrase (red cells only)}$$
$$CO_2 + H_2O \rightleftharpoons H_2CO_3 \rightleftharpoons H^+ + HCO_3^- \quad (1)$$

$$\boxed{\text{Protein}} - NH_2 + CO_2 \longrightarrow \boxed{\text{Protein}} - N \begin{matrix} H \\ \backslash \\ COOH \end{matrix}$$

$$\rightleftharpoons \boxed{\text{Protein}} - N \begin{matrix} H \\ \backslash \\ COO^- \end{matrix} + H^+ \quad (2)$$

Carbon dioxide also enters the red cells and is again transported in solution, and by hydration. However, hydration occurs rapidly in red cells because of the presence of carbonic anhydrase; also, the products of the reaction are dealt with. The hydrogen ions are buffered by the relatively high levels of deoxygenated haemoglobin (see p. 164), and bicarbonate ions are able to diffuse out of the red cells, into the plasma which has a relatively lower bicarbonate concentration. To maintain electrical neutrality, the chloride ions diffuse back into the red cells and this process is known as the chloride shift. The process of hydration is associated with a net increase in the total number of ions which are osmotically active, and therefore water also enters the red cells, which swell. The biconcave disc shape of the red cells allows them to swell without bursting.

In addition, carbon dioxide reacts with haemoglobin to form carbamino compounds, as in equation (2). The carbamino compounds are fully ionised, giving a further source of hydrogen ions to be buffered by haemoglobin.

The net effect of these reactions is that two-thirds of carbon dioxide are transported in the plasma as bicarbonate, but that the majority of hydrogen ions produced are buffered in the red cells.

THE URINARY SYSTEM

Introduction

The function of the kidney is to contribute to the homeostasis of the internal environment; in particular, the kidney is concerned with salt and water balance and hence blood volume, long-term adjustments in acid–base balance, and the regulation of the blood level of certain ions, such as calcium and phosphate. The kidney is the main pathway for the elimination of nitrogenous waste products, such as urea and some drugs, such as salicylate. It also has a major endocrine role in vitamin D metabolism and the production of renin and erythropoietin. Certain cells in the kidneys secrete prostaglandins, which probably affect local blood flow and tubular function.

Microanatomy

The functional unit of the kidney is the nephron (45–65 mm long) (see Fig. 6.17). Each human kidney contains approximately 1 million nephrons. Blood is filtered at the glomerulus, which is the beginning of the nephron, and the filtrate is subsequently modified by reabsorption or secretion in its passage through the nephron. Urine is the result of all the modifications to the glomerular filtrate after it has left the nephron at the collecting duct, although some minor alterations in composition may occur in the bladder.

The glomerulus is an invagination at the closed end of the renal tubule (Bowman's capsule). Blood is brought to the glomerulus by the afferent arteriole which drains into a network of capillaries which fill the glomerulus. The glomerular filtrate has to cross two layers of cells, the capillary endothelium and the tubular epithelium separated by an amorphous basal lamina, to pass from the blood

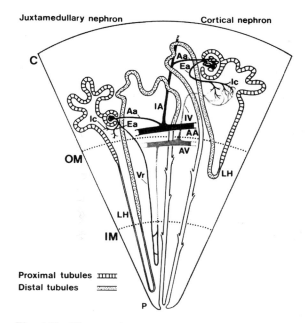

Fig. 6.17 Diagram of nephrons and their blood supply: AA, arcuate artery; AV, arcuate vein; Aa, afferent arteriole; Ea, efferent arteriole; IA, interlobular artery; IV, interlobular vein; Ic, intertubular capillaries; LH, loop of Henle; Vr, vasa recta; P, papilla; **C**, Cortex; **OM**, outer medulla; **IM**, inner medulla. (Reproduced with permission from *Companion to Medical Studies, Vol. 1*, 2nd edn, Blackwell Scientific Publications.)

Here the majority of the reabsorption of ions and water from the glomerular filtrate occurs. The proximal tubule leads to the loop of Henle, which is largely concerned with salt and water concentration. The loop of Henle then leads to the distal convoluted tubule, which, in turn, leads to the collecting duct. Between the ascending limb of the loop of Henle and the distal convoluted tubule is a portion of the tubule lined by specialised cells, the macula densa. This portion of the tubule is in close apposition to the efferent and afferent arterioles at the glomerulus, and this region is collectively known as the juxtaglomerular apparatus, which is the site of renin secretion. The loop of Henle differs between the tubules located in the cortex (cortical tubules, 85% of the total) and those located near the medulla (juxtamedullary tubules, 15% of the total). The juxtamedullary tubules have much longer loops of Henle and also only they have a thick portion to the ascending limb of the loop of Henle. This thick portion is thought to be essential for the reabsorption of chloride, an essential part of the mechanism for concentrating urine (see below).

The efferent arteriole leaves the glomerulus to form the blood supply to the tubule. It supplies a network of peritubular capillaries, which then drain into the renal vein. The juxtamedullary nephrons have specialised efferent arterioles, the vasa recta, which supply the loop of Henle (see Fig. 6.17).

Clearance

Substances such as creatinine or urea which are excreted by the kidney have a lower concentration in the renal vein than the artery; they are therefore said to be cleared by the kidney. But, with few exceptions, most substances are not completely cleared by the kidney. The clearance of a substance such as creatinine is a theoretical concept. Clearance equals the volume of blood that would be totally cleared of creatinine in unit time. Thus, if the creatinine clearance is 120 ml/min and the serum creatinine is 70 μmol/l (0.8 mg per 100 ml), the kidney excretes $70 \times \frac{120}{1000} = 8.4\mu$mol/min (0.1 mg/min). If the renal blood flow is 1.2 l/min, this would reduce the creatinine level by

vessels to the tubule. It is this barrier that is deranged in those forms of kidney disease which affect the glomerulus, such as glomerulonephritis. The filtrate passes out of the glomerular capillaries and across the epithelium of the tubule through epithelial pores, which electron microscopy suggest are 25 nm in diameter, although functionally they appear to be 8 nm in diameter, since molecules larger than 8 nm are not filtered. Therefore, the glomerular filtrate contains no red cells (diameter, 7.5 μm) and essentially no protein. In addition, the protein around the capillary pores is negatively charged. Therefore, negatively charged substances, such as albumin, whose molecules are less than 8 nm in diameter may not pass through the capillaries to any extent. The capillaries of the glomerulus are a portal system since they drain from the afferent arteriole to the efferent arteriole.

The next portion of the tubule after the glomerulus is the proximal convoluted tubule.

$8.4 \times \dfrac{1000}{1200} = 7.0 \ \mu mol$. So a creatinine clearance of 120 ml/min will maintain a renal vein creatinine level of 70 μmol/l if the renal artery creatinine level is 77 μmol/l.

To calculate the clearance of a substance it is best to work from first principles. For example, let us assume we are told that:

Serum creatinine	$= 70 \ \mu mol/l$	(1)
Urine creatinine	$= 6 \ mmol/l$	
24-hour urine volume	$= 2 \ l/24$ hours.	

Then,

$$\begin{aligned}
\text{24-hour urine} \\
\text{creatinine excretion} &= 2 \times 6 \ mmol \\
&= 2 \times 6 \times 1000 \ \mu mol
\end{aligned}$$

$$\begin{aligned}
\text{Excretion of} \\
\text{creatinine} &= \dfrac{2 \times 6 \times 1000 \ \mu mol}{60 \times 24} \\
\text{in 1 minute} &= 8.3 \ \mu mol. \qquad (2)
\end{aligned}$$

From (1), 1 μmol of creatinine occupies $\dfrac{1000}{70} = 14.3$ ml.

From (2), with 8.3 μmol excreted per minute, creatinine clearance $= 8.3 \times 14.3 = 119$ ml/min.

Glomerular filtration rate (GFR)

The clearance of a substance that is neither reabsorbed from the renal tubule nor secreted into the tubule is equal to the GFR. The plasma constituent that most closely approaches this is creatinine, and the creatinine clearance is therefore the usual measurement for estimation of the GFR. The normal GFR (both kidneys together) is 120 ml/min. It is proportional to body surface area, but about 10% less in women than men, even after adjustment for body surface area. Creatinine may be both secreted to and reabsorbed from the renal tubule, but has the great advantage that it is endogenously produced and the blood levels do not fluctuate much. For accurate determination of the GFR the inulin clearance may be used but inulin has to be infused to maintain a steady plasma level. The clearance of radioactive vitamin B_{12} has also been used for measurement of the GFR, but obviously not in pregnancy.

Renal blood flow

This is normally about 1.2 l/min. It varies with body surface and sex in the same way as the GFR does. Since only the plasma is concerned in the excretion of most substances, the term renal plasma flow (RPF) is often used, rather than renal blood flow. If the haematocrit is 45% the RPF is 660 ml/min when the blood flow is 1.2 l/min: $660 = 1200 \left(\dfrac{100 - 45}{100} \right)$ ml/min.

Renal blood flow could be measured directly by placing flow meters on the renal arteries; but this would be a highly invasive procedure. In practice we measure the clearance of substances such as p-aminohippuric acid (PAH) or iodopyracet (Diodrast), which are not metabolised by the kidney, and are assumed to be almost totally excreted through the kidney. Thus the renal vein concentration of PAH is assumed to be zero. Under these circumstances, which implies secretion of PAH into the renal tubule, PAH clearance equals renal blood flow.

The renal blood vessels are innervated by the autonomic nervous system via the renal nerves. Stimulation of the renal nerves causes vasoconstriction and a decrease in renal blood flow. This occurs via the vasomotor centre in systemic hypotension and also in severe hypoxia. Renal blood flow is also decreased by the direct action of catecholamines and both neural and humoral mechanisms are likely to be involved in the reduction of renal blood flow associated with exercise.

The filtration fraction is the ratio of GFR to RPF. The normal filtration fraction is $\dfrac{120}{660} = 0.18$. As the RPF falls in hypotension, the filtration fraction increases thus maintaining the GFR.

Handling of individual substances

Glucose and amino acids

Glucose and amino acids are reabsorbed by active transport at the proximal tubule. If the filtered load of glucose is too great for the proximal tubule to be able to reabsorb all the filtered glucose, glucose is excreted in the urine. This occurs in patients with hyperglycaemia due to diabetes mellitus. Patients with aminoaciduria, as occurs in the Fanconi syndrome, have a congenital abnormality of the proximal tubules so that they cannot reabsorb amino acids efficiently.

Sodium and chloride

The reabsorption of sodium by the renal tubule is a major feat, which consumes considerable energy. The filtered load of sodium presented to the renal tubules is about 0.2 million mmol/day. The vast majority of this is reabsorbed, so that the total quantity of sodium excreted varies between 1 and 400 mmol/day, depending on the salt and water balance of the individual. The chief controlling mechanisms accounting for the variation in the sodium reabsorption are the levels of aldosterone and other mineralocorticoids, glomerular filtration rate, variations in intrarenal pressure, which affects filtration fraction, and concomitant changes in potassium and hydrogen ion excretions. In addition a peptide secreted by the heart, atrial natriuretic peptide, increases the excretion of sodium but the mechanism of action and precise function of this substance are unclear.

The majority of sodium is reabsorbed actively in the proximal tubule. In addition, sodium is reabsorbed actively in the distal convoluted tubule, collecting duct and bladder under the control of mineralocorticoids. Sodium is also reabsorbed passively in the thick, ascending loop of Henle in exchange for chloride ions, which are themselves actively reabsorbed. The anions involved in sodium reabsorption are chloride (80%) and bicarbonate (19%). The remaining 1% of sodium reabsorption is accounted for by exchange for potassium (0.5%) and hydrogen (0.5%) ions.

Chloride is usually reabsorbed passively, following sodium and potassium reabsorption in the proximal convoluted tubule. It is also actively reabsorbed in the thick, ascending loop of Henle. Chloride reabsorption is decreased when bicarbonate reabsorption is increased, so that the levels of chloride and bicarbonate vary reciprocally in the plasma. Before the measurement of bicarbonate became freely available it was realised that chloride levels are high in those situations where the bicarbonate level is low, e.g. metabolic acidosis, and

much knowledge of acid-base balance was inferred from estimation of the chloride concentration; this is no longer necessary.

Bicarbonate

Bicarbonate is partly reabsorbed passively following sodium reabsorption; it is also reabsorbed by buffering hydrogen ions. Within the renal tubule, hydrogen ions react with bicarbonate to form carbonic acid. The carbonic acid is broken down under the influence of carbonic anhydrase in the brush border of the cells of the proximal convoluted tubule to form carbon dioxide and water. Carbon dioxide is reabsorbed across the tubular cell, and in the proximal tubular cell reacts again with water to form carbonic acid, which subsequently dissociates; bicarbonate is therefore reabsorbed as carbon dioxide, rather than as bicarbonate ions. This mechanism occurs so long as the plasma bicarbonate concentration is less than 28 mmol/l. Once the bicarbonate concentration exceeds this level, bicarbonate appears in the urine, which becomes alkaline.

Potassium

Potassium is reabsorbed actively in the proximal convoluted tubule, in exchange for chloride ions. It is also secreted into the distal convoluted tubule, in exchange for sodium ions, and this is under the control of aldosterone and other mineralocorticoids. High concentrations of aldosterone cause an increase in sodium reabsorption and potassium secretion in the distal tubule. The kidney is not as efficient in conserving potassium, as it is in conserving sodium. In hypokalaemia, the obligate excretion of potassium is about 10 mmol/day, whereas in hypovolaemia the kidney can reduce sodium excretion to 1 mmol/day.

Hydrogen ions

Hydrogen ions are actively excreted in the proximal and distal tubules in exchange for sodium. In the tubule the hydrogen ions are buffered by bicarbonate, phosphate and ammonia, which keeps the pH of the tubular fluid greater than 4.5, the minimum for hydrogen ion secretion.

Ammonia is produced locally in the kidney tubules by deamination of amino acids, and is secreted into the tubular fluid at the proximal and distal tubules, and collecting duct.

Water

Of the 170 litres of water that are filtered per day, all but 1.5 litres are reabsorbed under normal circumstances. However, in extreme hydration the total amount of water excreted may be as high as 50% of the glomerular filtration rate. This control of water reabsorption depends on the level of antidiuretic hormone, the glomerular filtration rate and the solute load. The bulk of water reabsorption occurs passively in the proximal tubule, where sodium and chloride are reabsorbed, and water is absorbed isotonically. Concentration of the urine occurs because of the high osmotic pressure achieved by reabsorption of chloride followed by sodium in the thick, ascending limb of the loop of Henle in the medulla of the kidney. As the filtrate passes down the collecting duct it becomes exposed to this high osmotic pressure and water is reabsorbed. The permeability of the collecting duct is altered by the level of antidiuretic hormone. High levels of antidiuretic hormone increase the permeability of the cells of the collecting duct, therefore allowing more water to be reabsorbed from tubular fluid, and a lower volume of concentrated urine to be finally secreted. Low levels of antidiuretic hormone decrease permeability of the cells of the collecting duct, so that large quantities of dilute urine are excreted.

Antidiuretic hormone is secreted from the posterior pituitary gland, under the influence of the hypothalamus. Its secretion is increased by stress, hypovolaemia, and increase in plasma osmolarity, adrenaline and certain drugs such as morphine. Its secretion is decreased by an increase in circulating blood volume, a fall in plasma osmolarity and by alcohol.

Urea

Urea accumulates in high concentration in the renal medulla. The kidney tubular cells are freely permeable to urea; when urine flows are low, urea can easily leave the kidney tubules and only 10–20% of the filtered urea is excreted. At high urine flow rates, 50–70% of filtered urea is excreted.

Additional functions

Non-excretory functions of the kidney include renin formation (see above and p. 172), erythropoietin formation and the metabolism of vitamin D. Erythropoietin is a circulating glycoprotein with molecular weight of about 23 000. It is thought to be formed by the action of another substance, renal erythropoietic factor, which acts on a plasma globulin produced in the liver. Erythropoietin is necessary for the production of red blood cells and acts to stimulate the formation of proerythroblasts from stem cells. The site of renal erythropoietic factor production in the kidney is not known; the kidney is not the only source of erythropoietic factor in man, since some erythropoietin is present after bilateral nephrectomy. Reduced levels of erythropoietin are thought to be one of the main reasons why patients with uraemia are anaemic.

Vitamin D is either produced in the skin by the action of sunlight or ingested in the diet. In the liver it is converted to 25-dihydroxycholecalciferol. In the kidney this is converted to the active metabolite 1,25-dihydroxycholecalciferol. It is this hormone which increases calcium uptake from the gastrointestinal tract, and mobilises calcium from bone. Renal rickets is in part due to the failure of the kidney to produce normal quantities of 1,25-hydroxycholecalciferol in renal failure. Calcium handling by the kidney is described on page 196.

The effect of pregnancy

During pregnancy the kidneys increase by about 1 cm in length, due to an increase in cell size rather than in cell number. The ureters are also dilated, partly because of the smooth muscle relaxant properties of progesterone, and partly because of obstruction by the growing uterus.

The renal blood flow increases from about 1.2 l/min in the nonpregnant state to at least 1.5 l/min in pregnancy. This increase appears early, probably within the first trimester. The effect is very dependent on posture, particularly in late pregnancy, when the gravid uterus obstructs the venous return in patients who are supine and

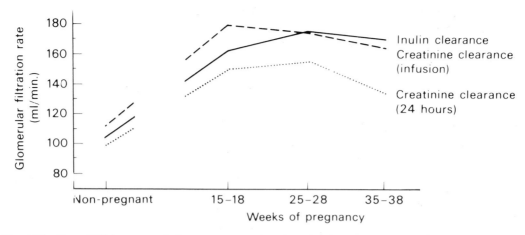

Fig. 6.18 Mean GFR in women during pregnancy and 8–12 weeks after delivery. (Reproduced with permission from F. Hytten and G. Chamberlain, *Clinical Physiology in Obstetrics*, Blackwell Scientific Publications.)

decreases cardiac output. However, in addition, renal blood flow is also decreased in patients in the erect posture, compared to those lying down, whether they are pregnant or not.

Associated with the rise in renal blood flow, there is an increase in glomerular filtration rate to 140–170 ml/min (Fig. 6.18). The increase in glomerular filtration rate causes a fall in the blood urea from 4.3 to 3.1 mmol/l and in the serum creatinine from 73 to 47 μmol/l. It is important for the clinician to be aware of these changes, since levels of urea and creatinine, which are normal in non-pregnant individuals, could represent quite severe renal disease in patients who are pregnant. The increased glomerular filtration rate increases the filtered load of glucose, and this is one reason why glycosuria is common in pregnancy, since the filtered load of glucose may be greater than the ability of the proximal tubule to reabsorb glucose. In addition, there is probably a specific abnormality induced in the renal tubule by pregnancy, so that the proximal tubules cannot reabsorb so much glucose in the pregnant state as they can in the non-pregnant state.

Physiology of micturition

The passive phase

The bladder fills with urine at approximately 1 ml/min. Folds of transitional cell epithelium be-

come flattened and the detrusor muscle fibres passively stretch with very little rise of intravesical pressure.

At the same time, the intraurethral pressure caused by the elastic tissue, the arteriovenous shunts and the tone of the smooth and striated muscle components is maintained at a higher level than the intravesical pressure.

Proprioceptive afferent impulses caused by the stretching of the detrusor fibres pass through the pelvic splanchnic nerves to the sacral roots of S2–S4. As urine volume increases, these impulses pass up the lateral spinothalamic tracts to the thalamus and thence to the cerebral cortex, thus bringing the sensation of bladder filling to a conscious level. The act of micturition is initially subconsciously and later consciously postponed by inhibitory impulses blocking the sacral reflex arc.

The active phase

At an appropriate time and place, a suitable posture is adopted through the organisation of the frontal lobes of the cerebral cortex and the anterior hypothalamus, and the following sequence of events take place in the act of micturition:

1. The muscles of the pelvic floor are voluntarily relaxed, causing a loss of the posterior urethrovesical angle and funnelling of the bladder neck.

2. At the same time, the voluntary fibres of the external sphincter are relaxed causing an overall fall of intraurethral pressure by at least 50%.

3. 5–15 seconds later, the inhibitory activity of the higher centres on the sacral reflex is lifted, allowing a rapid flow of efferent parasympathetic impulses, mainly from S3, to cause the detrusor to contract. As a result the intravesical pressure rises and can be augmented by the voluntary contraction of the diaphragm and the anterior abdominal wall musculature.

4. Urine flow commences when the intravesical pressure exceeds the intraurethral pressure. The urine flow may also further stimulate the sacral reflex by the conduction of afferent impulses from its lining to S2–S4.

5. At the end of micturition, the flow rate diminishes, the intravesical pressure falls and the striated musculature of the pelvic floor elevates the bladder neck; the external urethral sphincter interrupts the terminal flow in the region of the midurethra and obliterates the urethral lumen. The inhibitory influence of the higher centres is reestablished and the bladder becomes passive once more.

Urodynamic data in the normal adult female

a.	Residual urine	0–10 ml
b.	First sensation of bladder filling	Approx. 150–200 ml
c.	Voiding volume	Approx. 220–320 ml
d.	Voiding pressure	Approx. 45–70 cmH_2O
e.	Maximum urine flow rate	20–40 ml/s
f.	Bladder capacity	Approx. 600 ml
g.	Intravesical pressure rise (0–500 ml)	Approx. 0–10 cmH_2O. Detrusor contractions do not occur even with rapid filling or at full capacity
h.	Maximal urethral pressure in the absence of micturition	Approx. 50–100 cmH_2O, but varies with age and child bearing.

THE GASTROINTESTINAL TRACT

Mechanics

Mastication

This is accomplished by voluntary muscles innervated by the motor branch of the fifth cranial nerve.

Swallowing

There are two stages to this process:

1. Voluntary stage — food in the form of a bolus is pressed by the tongue upwards and backwards against the soft palate.

2. Involuntary stage — passage of food initially through the pharynx (1–2 seconds) and then by peristalsis down the oesophagus (4–8 seconds) to the stomach. The process is controlled by the deglutition centre in medulla and lower pons.

Gastro-oesophageal sphincter

There is tonic contraction of the circular muscle of the lower end of the oesophagus 2–5 cm above the gastro-oesophageal junction at all times other than when swallowing, eructating or vomiting. In addition, angulation at the lower end of the oesophagus by the diaphragm is increased on raising the intra-gastric or intra-abdominal pressure, so creating a shutter-valve effect.

In pregnancy, gastric relaxation and delayed emptying may predispose to incompetence of the cardia and so reflux of gastric acid.

Stomach

Storage of food in quantities up to nearly 1 litre is possible. Mixing of food into chyme occurs by a combination of constrictor waves and peristalsis. Emptying is promoted by:

1. Increased gastric volume causing antral peristalsis.

2. Release of gastrin by food (especially meat) causing acid secretion. This in turn stimulates the pyloric pump while at the same time relaxing the pylorus.

Emptying is inhibited by:

1. Enterogastric reflex from the duodenum to pylorus when there is excess of chyle, acid, hyper- or hypotonic fluids, or excess of protein breakdown products.

2. A possible hormonal reflex from the duodenum to pylorus — especially when chyle contains excess of fats.

During pregnancy, gastric emptying is either unchanged or slowed. Foodstuffs of high osmolarity (e.g. glucose) are especially liable to delay emptying.

Gall bladder

This structure stores and concentrates bile. Emptying is brought about by fat in the small intestine causing cholecystokinin–pancreozymin to be released from the mucosa. Cholecystokinin stimulates the gall bladder to contract and the sphincter of Oddi to relax.

Small intestine

Distension is the main stimulus to peristalsis, by autonomic fibres to the myenteric plexus (see Fig. 6.19). The parasympathetic fibres stimulate movement; the sympathetic fibres inhibit movement.

Ileocaecal sphincter and valve

The sphincter mechanism here allows about 750 ml of chyle a day into the caecum.

Both ileal peristalsis and gastrin release relax the ileal sphincter whilst increased caecal pressure and irritation of the caecum constrict it.

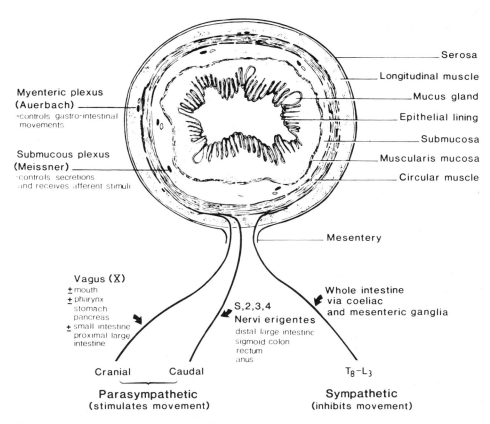

Fig. 6.19 Schematic transverse section of the gut showing nerve supply.

Colon

In the ascending colon the haustrations propel semisolid food by combined contractions of circular and longitudinal muscle. In the transverse and sigmoid colon, mass movement drives solid faeces towards the rectum.

Defaecation

Faeces entering the rectum stimulate reflex parasympathetic stimuli via the nervi erigentes to contract bowel muscle and relax the internal sphincter. If the external sphincter is not voluntarily contracted, defaecation will occur.

Digestive processes (see also pp. 153–5)

Mouth

In the mouth, amylase converts starch and glycogen into maltose.

The secretion of saliva is mediated by autonomic nervous stimulation. Salivary mucus provides lubrication for mastication and swallowing. Salivary amylase, on the other hand, initiates the breakdown of starch to maltose.

Stomach

Here pepsin converts proteins into proteoses and peptones.

Gastric secretion is initiated reflexly via the vagus. Once food has entered the stomach the hormone gastrin is released from the antral portion, and is carried in the blood to the parietal (oxyntic) cells of the gastric glands causing the secretion of hydrochloric acid. Hydrochloric acid in turn acts on pepsinogen in the chief cells, converting it into the proteolytic enzyme pepsin. Pepsin further acts on pepsinogen in the presence of acid, so enhancing its own production.

Mucus in the stomach comes from glands around the pylorus and protects the mucosa from the extreme acidity (pH 1.0). Gastric lipase and amylase are of little quantitative importance. In infants, rennin causes the milk to curd, so delaying its emptying from the stomach with subsequent early digestion of casein.

Duodenum and pancreas

Pancreatic trypsin and chymotrypsin convert protein and proteoses into polypeptides and dipeptides. Carboxypeptidase converts polypeptides into lower peptides and amino acids. Amylase converts starch and glycogen into maltose. Lipase converts fats into fatty acids and glycerol.

Bile salts emulsify fats into micelles. Chyle in the duodenum causes the release of the hormone secretin which induces the pancreas to produce large volumes of fluid rich in bicarbonate, but lacking in enzymes. A second hormone cholecystokinin-pancreozymin has the effect of releasing pancreatic enzymes and inducing the gall bladder to contract. Nervous stimulation of the pancreas occurs to a limited extent.

The endocrine function of the pancreas is described on pages 215–6.

Small intestine

The reactions in the small intestine are as follows:

1. Aminopeptidase converts polypeptides into lower peptides and amino acids
2. Dipeptidases converts dipeptides into amino acids
3. Sucrase converts sucrose into fructose and glucose
4. Maltase converts maltose into glucose
5. Lactase converts lactose into glucose and galactose.

Small intestine secretions are mainly induced by reflexes triggered off by food stimulating local nerve endings. Brunner's glands secrete mucus while the crypts of Lieberkühn exude a neutral fluid which is thought to aid absorption of chyle through the epithelial cells of the mucosa where the constituent substances of chyle are acted on by proteolytic, lipolytic and glycolytic enzymes.

Large intestine

Mucus from the goblet cells is produced under normal conditions by the direct contact of food stimulating local myenteric reflexes. Extreme irritation of the bowel wall, e.g. by infection, will result in the secretion of water and electrolytes, so resulting in diarrhoea. Under conditions of stress, parasympathetic stimulation of the *nervi erigentes* results in copious mucus secretion, which may also cause frequent bowel actions, but often without any concomitant faecal material.

NUTRITION

Calorimetry

It is important to appreciate, firstly, certain definitions relating to heat and energy:

1 calorie (cal) = heat required to raise the temperature of water 1°C (e.g. from 15 to 16°C)

1000 calories = 1 Cal or 1 kilocalorie (kcal)

1 joule (J) = energy required to move a force of 1 newton (N) a distance of 1 m

1 newton = the force required to accelerate a 1 kg mass by 1 m/s^2.

For energy conversion a factor of 4.2 is used and thus 1 kcal = 4.2 kilojoules (kJ).

The calorific values of the basic constituents of foodstuffs are:

Carbohydrate	4 kcal/g
Fat	9 kcal/g
Protein	4 kcal/g.

Daily dietary intake should be:

Non-pregnant	2200 kcal
Pregnant	2400 kcal
Lactation	2800 kcal.

Foodstuffs

Protein (see also pp. 135–40)

The normal daily requirement is 1–1.5 g/kg body weight per day and during pregnancy and lactation it should be 1.5–2 g/kg body weight per day.

An average protein diet contains 16% nitrogen and 84% carbon, hydrogen and sulphur. The dietary value of protein depends on the content of essential amino acids; the greater the proportion of essential amino acids, the nutritionally superior is the protein.

Essential amino acids are defined as those not synthesised by the animal organism out of the material ordinarily available at a speed commensurate with normal growth. They are:

Threonine	Valine	Histidine
Lysine	Phenylalanine	Arginine.
Methionine	Leucine	
Tryptophan	Isoleucine	

Histidine and arginine are not strictly essential but are required for normal growth. Complete proteins contain all essential amino acids, an example being lactalbumin. Partial proteins lack certain amino acids; maize, for example, lacks tryptophan and lysine. Animal proteins tend to be more complete than do vegetable proteins. Nitrogen excretion depends on intake; obligatory excretion from tissue breakdown (e.g. on a zero-protein diet) is 2–3 g of urinary nitrogen per day (= 12–18 g protein/day). Menstrual nitrogen loss is 2–3 g/month.

Carbohydrate (see Table 6.5)

Carbohydrates act as protein sparers in the diet as they are metabolised for energy in preference to protein. The average dietary intake is about 400 g/day, which is 50% of the energy value of most diets. In diabetics on a controlled diet the intake is about 200 g/day.

Deficiency of dietary carbohydrate or uncontrolled diabetes leads to ketosis in the following manner:

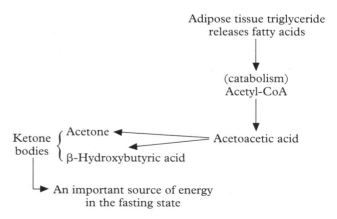

Table 6.5 Main dietary carbohydrates

Dietary source	Carbohydrate	End-product
Cereal, potatoes, peas	Starch	Glucose
Cane sugar	Sucrose	Glucose and fructose[a]
Milk	Lactose	Glucose
Fruit juice	Glucose	Glucose
Honey	Fructose	Fructose[a]

[a] Further partially metabolised to glucose

Fats

Animal fats are predominantly saturated while vegetable fats are predominantly unsaturated. An average Western diet contains about 100 g fat/day, which is important for the following reasons:

1. Its high energy value
2. As a vehicle for fat-soluble vitamins A, D, E and K
3. It contains the essential fatty acids linoleic and linolenic, which are both unsaturated.

In conditions of carbohydrate starvation, such as extreme dieting or uncontrolled diabetes, up to 2.5 g/kg body weight per day of fat may be catabolised without ketone bodies accumulating in the blood stream.

Vitamins (see also pp. 152–3)

Vitamins are substances in foodstuffs required by the body in small amounts. They are either water- or fat soluble. In the B complex group, some vitamins are given numbers, while others are not; this makes for confusion with regard to classification.

The functions of the different vitamins vary widely and our knowledge is incomplete. For the most part the actions of vitamins manifest themselves most strikingly when deficiency occurs but exactly what constitutes deficiency is often a matter for debate. Recent evidence suggests that vitamin deficiency in the mother during the first trimester may predispose to neural tube defects in the fetus. Folic acid, in particular, appears to be important in this respect.

The recommended daily intake of vitamins is shown in Table 6.6. For easy assimilation the important facts concerning vitamins will be given in summary form.

Vitamin A (retinol). Fat soluble.

Plasma level:	200–500 μg/l
Source:	Liver fat (especially cod and halibut liver oils)
	Milk fat — butter, cream, cheese
	Eggs
	Yellow vegetables, especially carrots, contain β-carotene, which is converted into vitamin A in the intestinal wall
Storage:	Liver — up to 9 months supply
Function:	Maintenance of epithelial tissues
	Formation of rhodopsin (visual purple) in the rods of the retina on entering a dark environment), viz. opsin (protein) + vitamin A → rhodopsin
Deficiency:	Xerophthalmia — early signs are depressed dark adaptation (night blindness). Skin changes — dryness and papular eruptions
	Predisposition to infection of epithelial surfaces, e.g. cornea, renal and respiratory tracts
Toxicity:	Drowsiness, headache, hair loss, muscle and joint pains, hepatosplenomegaly. Teratogenic.

Vitamin B₁ (thiamine, aneurin). Water soluble.

Plasma level:	5–10 μg/dl
Sources:	Wheat germ, yeast, wholemeal flour, eggs, pulses and lean meat (especially pork)
Storage:	Minimal (in heart, brain, liver and kidney)
	Excess excreted in urine
Function:	Acts as coenzyme in the metabolism of pyruvate (intermediary in the oxidative breakdown of pyruvate)
Deficiency:	Beri-beri (peripheral neuropathy, cardiac failure, gastrointestinal symptoms, Wernicke's encephalopathy)

Table 6.6 Daily requirements of vitamins

Vitamin	Non-pregnant	Pregnant	Lactation
A (μg)	800	1000	1200
B$_1$ (mg)	1.0	1.3	1.3
B$_2$ (mg)	1.5	1.8	2.0
Niacin (mg)	15	20.0	20.0
B$_6$ (mg)	2.0	2.5	2.5
Pantothenic acid (mg)	5.0	10.0	10.0
B$_{12}$ (μg)	2.0	3.0	3.0
Folic acid (μg)	200	500	400
C (mg)	30.0	60.0	80.0
D (μg)	10.0	10.0	10.0
E (mg)	10.0	12.0	12.0
K	None	None	None

Vitamin B$_2$ (riboflavin). Water soluble.

Plasma level: 100 nmol/l
Source: Yeast, milk, egg yolk, liver, kidney, heart muscle, young green vegetables
Function: Synthesis of two coenzymes, flavin mononucleotide (FMN) and flavin adenine dinucleotide (FAD), which act as hydrogen carriers in oxidative reactions
Deficiency: Cheilosis, dermatitis, keratitis.

Vitamin B, niacin (nicotinic acid, nicotinamide). Water soluble.

Plasma level: 50 μmol/l
Source: Yeast, meat, liver, wholemeal flour, green vegetables
Function: Synthesis of coenzymes nicotinamide adenine dinucleotide (NAD) and nicotinamide adenine dinucleotide phosphate (NADP), which are hydrogen ion acceptors in oxidative reactions
Deficiency: Pellagra (dermatitis, diarrhoea, stomatitis, glossitis, dementia).

Vitamin B$_6$ (pyridoxine). Water soluble.

Source: Yeast, cereal liver, milk, eggs and leafy green vegetables

Function: Coenzyme in transamination for the synthesis of amino acids
Deficiency: Epileptiform convulsions, neuritis, microcytic anaemia, gastrointestinal disturbances.

Vitamin B, pantothenic acid. Water soluble.

Source: Egg yolk, kidney, liver, yeast, vegetables and cereal
Function: No specific features (probably associated with other deficiency states).

Vitamin B$_{12}$ (cyanocobalamin, extrinsic factor). Water soluble.

Plasma level: 250–1000 ng/l
Source: Liver, kidney
Storage: Liver (about 1.5 mg, i.e. 60% of body total)
Function: Synthesis of DNA for cell nuclei maturation
Deficiency: Megaloblastic anaemia, soreness of tongue, peripheral neuropathy, subacute degeneration of the spinal cord.

Vitamin B, folic acid (pteroylglutamic acid, folacin). Water soluble.

Blood level: Whole blood 160–640 ng/ml
Red cells 0.36–1.44 μmol/L
Plasma 4.8–6.4 nmol/L

Source: Leafy green vegetables, liver
Storage: Liver (25 mg, i.e. 30% of body total)
Function: Synthesis of DNA for cell maturation
Deficiency: Megaloblastic anaemia.

Vitamin C (ascorbic acid). Water soluble.

Plasma level: 30–100 μmol/l
Source: Citrus fruits, berries, tomatoes, green vegetables
Function: Maintenance of intercellular materials especially in cartilage, dentine and bone
Deficiency: Defective formation of collagen fibres (scurvy)
Toxicity: Formation of calcium oxalate stones in urinary tract.

Vitamin D (calciferol). Fat soluble.

Source: Halibut and cod liver oil, oily fish (herrings), egg yolk
Ultraviolet light in skin converts provitamin D to active vitamin D_3
Function: Promotion of calcium and phosphorus absorption from the intestine, and phosphate excretion by the kidney
Deficiency: Rickets
Toxicity: Nephrocalcinosis.

Vitamin E (tocopherol). Fat soluble.

Plasma level: 0.35–0.41 mg/dl

Source: Eggs, meat, fish, vegetable oils
Function: Antioxidant, especially of polyunsaturated fatty acids, which easily forms perioxides
Deficiency: Malabsorption. In animals — testicular degeneration and fetal death
Toxicity: Malaise (over 800 mg/day).

Vitamin K. Fat soluble.

Source: Liver, cheese, egg yolk, green vegetables. Synthesised by bacteria in the colon
Storage: Minimal
Function: Prothrombin formation in the liver. Reversal of oral anticoagulants
Deficiency: Impairment of blood clotting
Toxicity: Hyperbilirubinaemia (neonates).

Minerals

Recommended daily intake of minerals is shown in Table 6.7.

Fibre

Consists of bran, pectin, quargum, gel-forming polysaccharides, cellulose, lignin and cutin. These comprise a heterogeneous collection of substances resistant to digestion.

Table 6.7 Daily requirements of minerals

Mineral	Non-pregnant	Pregnant	Lactation
Calcium (g)	0.8	1.2	1.2
Iron (mg)	12	15	18
Sodium (g)	3	3	3
Chloride (g)	3.5	3.5	3.5
Potassium (g)	1.0	1.0	1.0
Phosphorus (g)	0.8	1.2	1.2
Iodine (μg)	100	125	150
Zinc (mg)	150	200	250
Magnesium (mg)	300	400	450

THE LIVER

Anatomical considerations

The adult liver weighs around 1.3 kg and contains about 100 000 lobules. The neonatal liver at term weighs around 145 g.

Each liver lobule surrounds a central vein as shown in Figure 6.20. The central vein drains to the hepatic vein.

The sinusoids are lined by Kupffer cells which, together with the endothelial cells, are powerfully phagocytic. Each sinusoid has a rich lymphatic supply.

Metabolic functions

The metabolism of carbohydrate and fat is considered in Chapter 5 on biochemistry, pages 143–150.

Carbohydrate

Glycogen storage. Glycogen is synthesised from glucose and stored in the liver by the following reactions:

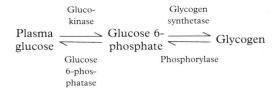

Glycogen synthetase is activated by high plasma glucose and insulin, which thus increase the level of glycogen in the liver and decrease plasma glucose. Phosphorylase is activated by low plasma glucose, adrenaline and glucagon, which therefore raise plasma glucose levels by catabolising glycogen.

Galactose and fructose conversion. Galactose and fructose are both converted to glucose in the liver by the following reactions:

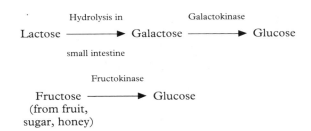

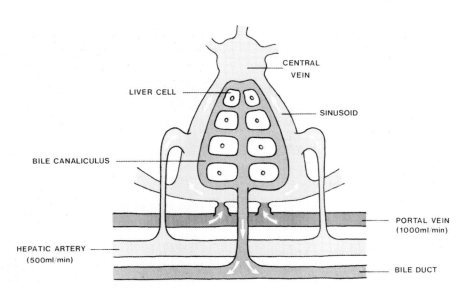

Fig. 6.20 Schematic representation of blood flow through a liver lobule.

Gluconeogenesis. Depletion of body stores of carbohydrate causes the liver to form glucose from glucogenic amino acids, which are derived from protein, and also from glycerol, which is derived from fat. Metabolic pathways are shown below:

(i) Glucogenic amino acids ⟶ Citric acid cycle

(ii) Glycerol (from triglyceride) ⟶

Embden–Meyerhof pathway

⟶ Fructose

⟶ Glucose

Fat

β-oxidation and ketosis. In states of carbohydrate deprivation or juvenile diabetes mellitus, fatty acids are metabolised to ketones as shown below:

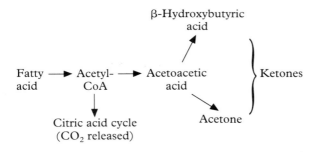

Fatty acid ⟶ Acetyl-CoA ⟶ Acetoacetic acid

β-Hydroxybutyric acid

Acetone

} Ketones

Citric acid cycle (CO_2 released)

Synthesis of triglyceride (lipogenesis). The liver is able to synthesise triglyceride from fatty acids and glycerol, which are both derived from dietary carbohydrate. Triglyceride (neutral fat) is mainly concerned with energy expenditure.

R_1
R_2 +
R_3

CH_2OH
$CHOH$ Esterification
CH_2OH ⇌ Lipolysis

CH_2OR_1
$CHOR_2$
CH_2OR_3

3 fatty acids   Glycerol   Triglyceride

Synthesis of lipoproteins. In particular, the liver synthesises very low-density lipoproteins (VLDL) and pre-β-lipoproteins which are carrier proteins for plasma lipids.

Synthesis of phospholipids. There are three types: lecithins, cephalins and sphingomyelins. Phospholipids are essentially structural lipids of body tissues. Lecithin is a powerful surface-active agent, reducing surface tension in the lung alveolae.

Synthesis of cholesterol. Synthesis is complicated and takes place in several stages whereby acetyl-CoA (CH_3COS-CoA) is built up to form the steroid nucleus

and so to cholesterol.
About 80% of all cholesterol synthesised is converted into bile acids.

Synthesis of fats. This may also occur from excess dietary protein through the conversion of amino acids into acetyl-CoA.

Protein

Deamination of amino acids and urea formation. This occurs by the removal of the amino (—NH_2) group from the amino acid. The ammonia produced by deamination is removed by combining it with carbon dioxide to form urea.

NH_3

NH_3

+ CO_2 ⟶

H_2N
     $\rangle C = O + H_2O$
H_2N

2 molecules of ammonia   Urea

Plasma proteins. Virtually all albumin and fibrinogen are synthesised in the liver. 70% of globulin is synthesised in the liver and the remainder is synthesised in the reticuloendothelial system.

the wall of the Sylvian fissure. Here representation of the body is not so complete, nor so specific.

Fibres from pain and temperature receptors and some other touch receptors also enter the spinal cord via the dorsal root, but synapse with nerves in the substantia gelatinosa of the dorsal horn. Fibres from these neurones cross the midline immediately (cf. spinothalamic tracts) and then ascend in the anterolateral system of the spinal cord (lateral columns) (see Figs 6.25 and 6.26). Touch ascends the ventral spinothalamic tract; pain and temperature ascend the lateral spinothalamic tract. These fibres also project to the thalamus and then synapse with other neurones passing to somatic sensory areas I and II. However, the sensations carried by the anterolateral system are not so exclusively represented in the cerebral cortex as those carried by the spinothalamic tracts. Experimental ablation, or observations on patients with spontaneously occurring lesions, show that proprioception and fine touch (spinothalamic tract) are most affected by cortical lesions. Temperature sensation is less affected and pain sensation (lateral columns) is barely affected at all.

The 'gate' theory accounts for the observation that individuals' perception of pain varies enormously both between individuals and within individuals on different occasions. Many external and internal influences, such as hypnosis, acupuncture and analgesic drugs, can affect pain perception, and probably do so by influencing transmission of impulses from pain receptors at many sites within the central nervous system. One site that has been extensively investigated is in the substantia gelatinosa of the spinal cord (Fig. 6.26) where pain afferent neurones synapse with fibres that will ascend in the lateral columns. Transmission here can be inhibited by stimulation of other fibres, mediating touch or proprioception in the adjacent spinothalamic tract. Stimulation of these fibres has been used clinically in the relief of pain. The fibres may either be stimulated in the skin (as in the treatment of trigeminal neuralgia using an electrical stimulator) or by implantation of chronic stimulators in the dorsal columns.

Reticular activating system

Apart from the classical projection of sensory input to the cortex, some sensory fibres activate the reticular activating system. This is a diffuse system of nerve fibres in the ventral portion of the midbrain and medulla which appears to be responsible for consciousness and to require sensory input to maintain consciousness (see Fig. 6.27). Thus, blunting of sensory input, either ex-

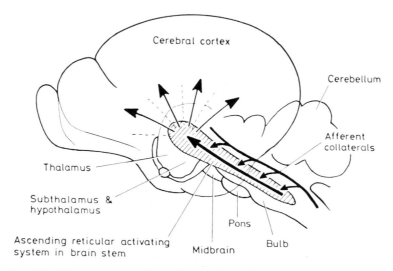

Fig. 6.27 Diagram of ascending reticular activating system (Reproduced with permission from Starozl et al., 1951, A lateral afferent excitation of reticular formation of brain stem, *Journal of Neurophysiology*.)

perimentally or when, for example, prisoners are 'hooded' for interrogation purposes, is associated with disturbed states of consciousness and hallucinations. Patients with tumours that interrupt the reticular activating system are usually unconscious and, if the tumours are small, may be comatose without any other clinical signs. It appears that the reticular activating system integrates all sensory inputs, and that sensory specificity is therefore not important for its function. The reticular activating system contains the respiratory and cardiovascular centres, and can up or down regulate sensation, motor activity, the electrical activity of the cortex, and many endocrine activities via its hypothalamic connections.

The autonomic nervous system

Like the somatic nervous system, the autonomic nervous system has afferent nerves from receptors, central integrating areas (vasomotor centre and respiratory centre) and efferent neurones which run to effector organs. The receptors may be specific to stimuli, such as pressure (carotid sinus baroreceptor) or Po_2 (carotid body chemoreceptor); there are also non-specific receptors in the viscera which respond to pain. Afferents reach the central nervous system via the facial, glossopharyngeal and vagus cranial nerves, and via the dorsal roots from T7 to L2 and from S2 to S4.

The efferent tract of the autonomic nervous system consists of preganglionic fibres followed by postganglionic fibres. The parasympathetic outflow to the visceral structures of the head is via cranial nerves III, VII and IX, to the thorax and upper abdomen via the vagus nerve, and to the pelvis via the sacral outflow, S2–S4. The preganglionic fibres end in, or very near, the viscus that is innervated. These synapse with short postganglionic fibres that run directly to the effector organ (see Fig. 6.28).

By contrast, the sympathetic nervous system is characterised by a chain of ganglia that run outside the spinal cord, but adjacent to it from T1 to L5. The chain is extended towards the head to form three additional cervical ganglia, the superior, middle and inferior or stellate ganglia. The axons of the preganglionic sympathetic nerves leave the

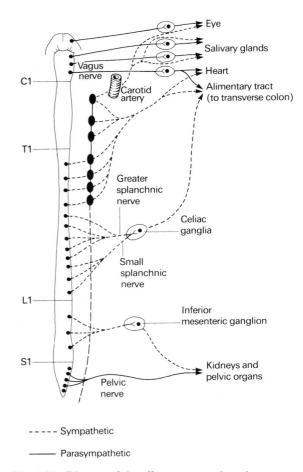

----- Sympathetic

——— Parasympathetic

Fig. 6.28 Diagram of the efferent autonomic pathways.

spinal cord in the ventral roots of the spinal nerves, and pass via the white *rami communicantes* to the paravertebral sympathetic ganglion chain. There they synapse with the postganglionic fibres, which run to the viscera. Some postganglionic fibres return to the spinal nerves, via the grey *rami communicantes*, and then are distributed with the spinal nerves to the autonomic effectors in the appropriate somatic structures innervated by these spinal nerves. Other sympathetic preganglionic fibres do not end in the paravertebral chain, but pass through it to collateral ganglia (coeliac ganglion, superior and inferior mesenteric ganglia) near the viscera that they innervate. Short postganglionic fibres then run to each viscus.

The uterus is unusual in that the preganglionic sympathetic fibres run all the way to the uterus and anastomose there with postganglionic fibres. The adrenal medulla is also atypical in that it is innervated by preganglionic sympathetic nerves that pass to it through the coeliac ganglion without synapsing. Alternatively, the adrenal medulla may be considered as a specialised postganglionic nerve that secretes adrenaline, as well as noradrenalin, directly into the blood stream, rather than secreting noradrenalin at the postganglionic nerve ending.

CHEMICAL TRANSMISSION IN THE AUTONOMIC NERVOUS SYSTEM AND AUTONOMIC PHARMACOLOGY

The parasympathetic nervous system

Chemical transmission at ganglia and at the ends of postganglionic fibres stimulating smooth muscle and glands is by acetylcholine. The postganglionic effects of acetylcholine are mimicked by the alkaloid muscarine, and these are therefore known as the muscarine actions of acetylcholine. They are blocked by atropine. Transmission at the ganglia is mimicked by nicotine, the nicotine action of acetylcholine, and this is not blocked by atropine. It is blocked by very high concentrations of acetylcholine. The acetylcholine is metabolised by cholinesterase. Drugs that interfere with cholinesterase activity, e.g. physostigmine, will potentiate transmission at the autonomic ganglia, and at the postganglionic nerve ending. (These drugs will also potentiate somatic neuromuscular transmission.)

The sympathetic nervous system

Transmission at the ganglia is by the nicotinic action of acetylcholine. Transmission at most postganglionic nerve endings is by noradrenalin (norepinephrine). Some drugs, such as tyramine, or ephedrine, increase sympathetic activity by enhancing noradrenalin release at the postganglionic nerve ending.

Those sympathetic postganglionic neurones which innervate sweat glands are cholinergic (acetylcholine as a transmitter), and so are the sympathetic postganglionic fibres which cause vasodilatation in smooth muscle.

Noradrenalin is one of a group of substances, the catecholamines. The other principal catecholamine found outside the central nervous system is adrenaline (epinephrine) secreted by the adrenal medulla. Dopamine is on the metabolic pathway of adrenaline and noradrenalin. So far it has mainly been studied within the central nervous system and hypothalamopituitary axis, where, for example, dopamine inhibits prolactin release. However, it is likely that dopamine also has peripheral actions, perhaps, for example, being involved in the control of renal blood flow.

The receptors to catecholamine have been divided into α and β receptors on the basis of the drugs which block transmission at the receptor site. α receptors blocked by phentolamine and phenoxybenzamine can be separated from β receptors, blocked by propranolol.

In general, α receptors are excitatory (vasoconstriction, pupillary constriction) and β receptors are inhibitory (bronchodilatation, decreased uterine activity). An important exception is the heart, where β receptors are excitatory. Not all β receptors are the same. Some β-adrenergic blocking drugs chiefly affect the heart; these are β_1-adrenergic blocking agents, or cardioselective beta blocking agents, of which the prototype was practolol. Less toxic agents in current clinical usage are metoprolol and atenolol. Other β receptors are designated as β_2 receptors. These are found in the bronchi and the uterus, and nonselective β-adrenergic blocking agents (e.g. propranolol) block both β_1 and β_2 receptors. The development of specific α-, β_1- and β_2-receptor-blocking agents, allowed the differentiation of both naturally occurring and synthetic catecholamines into α, β_1 and β_2 agonists. Thus adrenaline and noradrenalin stimulate both α and β_1 receptors, but adrenaline also stimulates β_2 receptors. Metaraminol and phenylephrine are specific α agonists. Isoprenaline is a specific β agonist which stimulates both β_1 and β_2 receptors. Salbutamol, orciprenaline, terbutaline and ritodrine, all of which have been used for the treatment of premature labour, stimulate β_2 receptors more than β_1 and so cause relaxation of the

Table 6.8 Responses of organs to cholinergic and adrenergic stimuli

Organ	Response	
	Adrenergic(α/β)	Cholinergic
Pupil	Constriction (α) Dilatation (β)	Constriction
Salivary glands	Scanty viscid secretion (α)	Copious watery secretion
Blood vessels		
Heart	Constrictor (α) Dilator (β_2)	Dilator
Skin	Constrictor (α)	
Muscle	Constrictor (α) Dilator (β_2)	Dilator
Pulmonary	Constrictor (α)	
Kidney	Constrictor (α)	
Lung		
Bronchi	Relaxation (β_2)	Constriction
Bronchial glands		Increased secretion
Heart		
Rate, contractility, conduction velocity	Increased (β_1)	Decrease
Kidney		
Renin secretion	Increased (β_2)	
Sweating	Localised, e.g. palms of hands (α)	Generalised
Pregnant uterus	Decreased contraction (β_2) Increased contraction (α)	

uterus. In addition, these drugs cause bronchial dilatation, and most have been used and were developed for the treatment of asthma. (The exception is ritodrine.)

A list of adrenergic (sympathetic) and cholinergic (mainly parasympathetic) activity is given in Table 6.8. Table 6.9 shows some of the drugs that influence autonomic activity. See also page 235 for metabolic actions of catecholamines.

THE BLOOD

Iron metabolism

Iron is abundant in most soils and waters of the earth's surface. It is easily and reversibly oxidised or reduced. It has been incorporated into numerous proteins of critical importance for the sustenance of both plant and animal life.

The total body iron content of a normal adult male is approximately 50 mg/kg, of an adult women about 38 mg/kg. This difference merely reflects the high incidence of reduced iron stores in women; there are no fundamental differences in iron metabolism between the sexes.

The iron is distributed in several physiologically and chemically distinct forms (Table 6.10).

Haemoglobin iron comprises about 70% of the total body iron and is the largest iron-containing compartment.

The other haem-containing molecule is myoglobin, a protein present in muscle. It is said to provide a reserve of available oxygen in sudden strenuous exercise.

Storage iron is held available for use, as needed, in the macrophages of the reticuloendothelial system and is in two forms — ferritin, which is a glycoprotein detectable by chemical analysis, and aggregates of ferritin, which form haemosoderin.

A very small amount of iron is contained in the enzymes — cytochromes, catalases and peroxidases essential for metabolism of all cells in the body.

A minute portion of the total iron (0.19%) is bound to a specific plasma protein — transferrin (Table 6.10).

Table 6.9 Some drugs influencing autonomic activity

Site of action	Agents decreasing activity	Agents increasing activity
Sympathetic and parasympathetic ganglia	High concentration of acetylcholine Ganglion-blocking agents: 　Hexamethonium 　Mecamylamine 　Pentolinium 　Trimetaphan	Acetylcholine Carbachol Nicotine Anticholinesterase drugs, e.g. 　Physostigmine
Endings of parasympathetic neurones	Atropine Scopolamine Probanthine	Anticholinesterase drugs: 　Acetylcholine 　Carbachol 　Muscarine 　Pilocarpine
Sympathetic postganglionic nerve endings	Reserpine Guanethidine	Drugs releasing noradrenalin: 　Ephedrine 　Amphetamines 　Tyrosine
β_1 receptors	Propranolol Atenolol Metoprolol Practolol } Also block β_2 receptors to a lesser extent	Isoprenaline Adrenaline Noradrenalin
β_2 receptors	Propranolol	Adrenaline Isoprenaline Salbutamol Orciprenaline } Also β_1 but mainly β_2 Terbutaline Ritodrine
α receptors	Phenoxybenzamine Phentolamine	Noradrenalin Adrenaline Metaraminol Methoxamine Phenylephrine

Table 6.10 Distribution of iron

Location	Form	Distribution (%)
Haemoglobin iron		70
Tissue iron		30
Storage iron	Haemosiderin Ferritin	
Essential iron	Myoglobin Enzymes 　Cytochromes 　Peroxidases 　Catalases	
Plasma transport iron	Transferrin	0.19

The total iron content of the body tends to remain fixed within narrow limits, otherwise iron excess (siderosis) or deficiency occurs. Iron is not excreted in the usual sense of the word; it is lost from the body only when cells are lost, especially epithelial cells from the gastrointestinal tract. Urinary iron amounts to less than 0.05 mg/day in desquamated cells. In women, menstrual flow constitutes an important additional route of iron loss. Average daily loss has been estimated to be about 1.0 mg/day in normal adult men and non-menstruating women. About twice this amount is lost in menstruating women.

In normal situations these losses are balanced by an equivalent amount of iron absorbed from the diet.

Therefore, iron balance is unique in that it is achieved by control of absorption rather than control of excretion.

Iron absorption

Since the total body iron content depends so greatly on absorption of iron, the mechanisms by which the rate of absorption is regulated are of critical importance.

Iron is absorbed chiefly in portions of the intestine proximal to the jejunum. Maximum absorption occurs in the duodenum.

Two factors are of prime importance in determining absorptive rate:

1. The amount of storage iron. When it is depleted, iron absorption is increased. When it is excessive, iron absorption is decreased.
2. The rate of erythropoiesis. Iron absorption goes up when red cell production rate is increased and down when production is decreased.

Iron absorption takes place in two distinct steps:

1. Mucosal uptake
2. Transfer of iron from mucosal cell to plasma.

The uptake of iron by the mucosa is influenced by the overall composition of the diet which determines how much iron is available for absorption (see below).

A normal mixed diet supplies about 14 mg of iron each day, of which only 1–2 mg is absorbed. The availability in food is quite variable. In most foods inorganic iron is in the ferric form and has to be converted to the ferrous form before absorption can take place. In foods derived from grain, iron often forms a stable complex with phytates and only small amounts can be converted to a soluble form. The iron in eggs is poorly absorbed because of binding with phosphates present in the yolk. Milk, particularly cows' milk, is poor in iron content. Tea inhibits the absorption of iron.

Haem iron derived from haemoglobin and myoglobin of animal origin is more effectively absorbed than non-haem iron. Factors interfering with or promoting the absorption of inorganic iron have no effect on the absorption of haem iron. This puts vegetarians at a disadvantage in terms of iron sufficiency.

Iron cycle

The metabolism of iron is dominated by its role in haemoglobin synthesis. In this process iron is utilised repeatedly so that the internal movements of iron may be described as a cycle (Fig. 6.29).

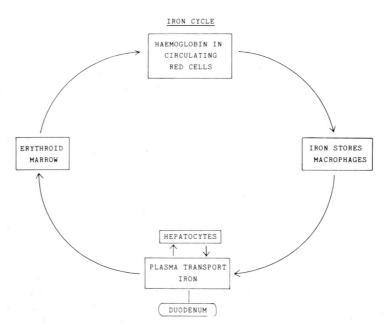

Fig. 6.29 The iron cycle.

Central to this cycle is the plasma compartment in which iron is bound to a transport protein — transferrin. Iron moves from plasma to cells that have the capacity to make haemoglobin. At the end of the red cells' 120-day lifespan, they are ingested by macrophages of the reticuloendothelial system. There, iron is extracted from haemoglobin, delivered to the plasma and bound to transferrin, completing the cycle. A small amount of iron, probably less than 2.0 mg, leaves the plasma each day to enter the hepatic cells and other tissues. Here the iron is utilised to make tissue haem proteins such as myoglobin and the cytochromes.

Haemopoiesis and iron metabolism in pregnancy

There is increased erythropoiesis from early pregnancy due to increased erythropoietin production and possibly due to other hormones such as placental lactogen. In spite of this, some degree of anaemia, as judged by normal non-pregnant standards, is manifest by the end of the second trimester. This is due to haemodilution and occurs because the increase in plasma volume exceeds that of the red cell mass. The haemoglobin reaches its lowest level at 32 weeks of gestation when the haemodilution is maximal (see pp. 169–70).

In pregnancy the demand for iron is increased to meet mainly the needs of the expanded red cell mass and, to a lesser extent, the requirements of the developing fetus and placenta. The fetus derives its iron from the maternal serum by active transport across the placenta predominantly in the last 4 weeks of pregnancy. The total requirement of iron is about 700–1400 mg. Overall, the requirement is 4 mg/day, but this rises from 2.8 mg in the non-pregnant to 6.6 mg/day in the last few weeks of pregnancy. This can be met only by mobilising iron stores in addition to achieving maximum absorption of dietary iron.

Iron absorption is increased when there is erythroid hyperplasia — rapid iron turnover — and a high concentration of unsaturated transferrin, both of which are part of the physiological response in the healthy pregnant woman. There is evidence that absorption of dietary iron is enhanced in the latter half of pregnancy, but this still does not provide enough iron for the needs of pregnancy and puerperium for a woman on a normal mixed diet.

The amount of iron absorbed will depend very much on the extent of the iron stores, the content of the diet and whether or not iron supplements are given.

The commonest haematological problem in pregnancy is anaemia resulting from iron deficiency.

Iron deficiency in pregnancy

Haemoglobin concentration

The changes in blood volume and haemodilution are so variable that the normal range of haemoglobin concentration in healthy pregnancy at 30 weeks' gestation in women who have received parenteral iron is 10.5–14.5 g/dl. However, haemoglobin values of less than 10.5 g/dl in the second and third trimesters are probably abnormal and require further investigation.

Red cell indices

The appearance of red cells on a stained film is a relatively insensitive gauge of iron status in pregnancy. Many hospital laboratories now possess electronic counters, allowing accurate red cell counts to be performed. The size of the red cell (mean cell volume, MCV), its haemoglobin content (mean corpuscular haemoglobin, MCH) and haemoglobin concentration (MCHC) can be calculated from the red cell count (red blood cell count, RBC), haemoglobin concentration and packed cell volume (PCV).

A better guide to the diagnosis of iron deficiency in pregnancy is the examination of these red cell indices. The earliest effect of iron deficiency on the erythrocyte is a reduction in cell size, MCV, and, in pregnancy, with the dramatic changes in red cell mass and plasma volume, this is the most sensitive indicator of underlying iron deficiency. Hypochromia and a fall in the MCHC only appear with more severe degrees of iron depletion.

Some women start pregnancy with already established anaemia due to iron deficiency or with grossly depleted iron stores and they will quickly develop florid anaemia with reduced MCV, MCH and MCHC.

Serum iron and total iron-binding capacity (TIBC)

The serum iron of healthy, adult non-pregnant women lies between 13–27 μmol/l. Serum iron levels vary markedly and even fluctuate from hour to hour. The TIBC in the non-pregnant state lies in the range 45–72 μmol/l. It is raised in association with iron deficiency and is low in chronic inflammatory states. In the non-anaemic individual the TIBC is approximately one-third saturated with iron.

In pregnancy there is a fall in the serum iron and percentage saturation of the TIBC; the fall in serum iron can be largely prevented by iron supplements. Serum iron, even in combination with the TIBC, is not a reliable indication of iron stores because it fluctuates so widely and because it is affected by recent ingestion of iron or factors such as infection which are not directly involved with iron metabolism. With these major reservations, a serum iron of less than 12 μmol/l and a TIBC saturation of less than 15% indicate iron deficiency in pregnancy.

Ferritin

Ferritin is a high-molecular-weight glycoprotein, which circulates in the plasma. The normal plasma concentration is 15–300 μg/l. It is stable and not affected by recent ingestion of iron. It appears to reflect the iron stores accurately and quantitatively, particularly in the lower range associated with iron deficiency which is so important in pregnancy.

Haemostasis

Haemostatic mechanisms have two functions:

1. To confine the circulating blood to the vascular bed
2. To arrest bleeding from injured vessels.

Both these aspects of haemostasis probably depend on:

1. Normal vasculature
2. Platelets — number and function
3. Coagulation factors
4. Healthy fibrinolysis.

Haemostasis and pregnancy

Normal pregnancy is accompanied by dramatic changes in the coagulation and fibrinolytic systems. There is a marked increase in some of the coagulation factors, particularly fibrinogen. Fibrin is laid down in the uteroplacental vessel walls and fibrinolysis is suppressed. These changes, together with the increased blood volume, help to combat the hazard of haemorrhage at placental separation but play only a secondary role to the unique process of myometrial contraction, which reduces blood flow to the placental site. They also produce a vulnerable state for intravascular clotting and a whole spectrum of disorders involving coagulation which may occur in pregnancy; these fall into two main groups — thromboembolism and bleeding due to disseminated intravascular coagulation.

A short account of haemostasis during pregnancy and how it differs from non-pregnant haemostasis follows.

Vascular integrity

It is not known how vascular integrity is normally maintained but it is clear that the platelets have a key role to play because conditions in which their number is depleted or function abnormal are characterised by widespread spontaneous capillary haemorrhages. In health, the platelets are constantly sealing microdefects of the vasculature, minifibrin clots being formed; the unwanted fibrin is then removed by a process of fibrinolysis.

Prostacyclin (PGI_2) is an unstable prostaglandin first discovered in 1976. It is the principal prostanoid synthesised by blood vessels and is a powerful vasodilator and potent inhibitor of platelet aggregation. It has been proposed that there is a balance between the production of PGI_2 and thromboxane, a powerful platelet-aggregating agent and vasoconstrictor. Prostacyclin prevents aggregation at much lower concentrations than is needed to prevent adhesion. Therefore, vascular damage leads to platelet adhesion but not necessarily to aggregation and thrombus formation.

When the injury is minor, small platelet thrombi form and are washed away by the circulation as described above, but the extent of the injury is an important determinant of the size of the thrombus and whether or not platelet aggregation is stimulated. Prostacyclin synthetase is abundant in the intima and progressively decreases in concentration from the intima to the adventitia. In contrast the pro-aggregating elements increase in concentration from the subendothelium to the adventitia. It follows that severe vessel damage or physical detachment of the endothelium will lead to the development of a large thrombus rather than simple platelet adherence.

Deficiency of prostacyclin production has been suggested in platelet consumption syndromes such as the haemolytic uraemic syndrome and thrombocytopenic purpura.

Prostacyclin production has been shown to be reduced in fetal and placental tissue from pre-eclamptic pregnancies and the current role of prostacyclin in pathogenesis of this disease and potential for treatment in hypertension of pregnancy is undergoing active investigation.

There have been several conflicting reports concerning the platelet count during pregnancy. There is probably no significant change in uncomplicated, healthy pregnancy even towards term, but a decrease in the platelet count has been observed in pregnancies with fetal growth retardation, whether or not pre-eclampsia was implicated. There is no evidence of changes in platelet function, or differences in platelet lifespan, between healthy non-pregnant and pregnant women, although the lifespan is shortened significantly in pre-eclampsia.

Arrest of bleeding after trauma

An essential function of the haemostatic system is a rapid reaction to injury, which remains confined to the area of damage. This requires control mechanisms which will stimulate coagulation after trauma and limit the extent of the response. The substances involved in the formation of the haemostatic plug normally circulate in an inert form until activated at the site of injury or by some factor released into the circulation which will trigger off intravascular coagulation.

Local response

Platelets adhere to collagen on the injured basement membrane. This initiates a series of changes in the platelets themselves, including a change in shape and release of ADP (adenosine diphosphate) and other substances. ADP release stimulates further aggregation of platelets, the coagulation cascade is triggered off and the action of thrombin leads to the formation of fibrin, which converts the loose platelet plug into a firm, stable wound seal. The role of platelets is of less importance in injury involving large vessels because platelet aggregates are of insufficient size and strength to breach the defect. The coagulation mechanism is of major importance here, together with vascular contraction.

Coagulation system

The end result of blood coagulation is the formation of an insoluble fibrin clot from the soluble precursor fibrinogen in the plasma. This involves a complex interaction of clotting factors and a sequential activation of a series of proenzymes, which has been termed the coagulation cascade (Fig. 6.30). When a blood vessel is injured, blood coagulation is initiated by activation of factor XII by collagen (intrinsic mechanism) and activation of factor VII by thromboplastin release (extrinsic mechanism from the damaged tissue). But the intrinsic and extrinsic mechanisms are activated by components of the vessel wall and both are required for normal haemostasis.

Strict divisions between the two pathways do not exist and interactions between activated factors in both pathways have been shown. They share a common pathway following activation of factor X.

The intrinsic pathway, or contact system, proceeds spontaneously and is relatively slow, requiring from 5 to 20 minutes for visible fibrin formation. All tissues contain a specific lipoprotein, thromboplastin, which markedly increases the rate at which blood clots. It is particularly concentrated in the lung and brain. The placenta is also very rich in tissue factor, which will produce fibrin formation within 12 seconds, the acceleration of coagulation being brought about by by-passing the reactions involving the contact (intrinsic) system.

Blood coagulation is strictly confined to the site of tissue injury in normal circumstances. Powerful control mechanisms must act to prevent dissemination of coagulation beyond the site of trauma.

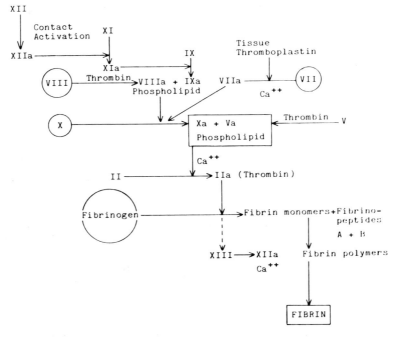

Fig. 6.30   The factors involved in blood coagulation and their interactions. The circled factors show significant increases in pregnancy. (Reproduced with permission from F. Hytten, G. Chamberlain, *Clinical Physiology in Obstetrics*, Blackwell Scientific Publications.)

The action of thrombin in vivo is controlled by a number of mechanisms, particularly its absorption onto the locally formed fibrin, and the presence of a potent inhibitor, antithrombin III, an α_2-globulin, which destroys thrombin acivity. Heparin, which potentiates the action of anti-X^a, may be similar to antithrombin III. This is the rationale for low-dose heparin therapy as prophylaxis in patients at risk for thromboembolic phenomena postoperatively, and in pregnancy and the puerperium.

Normal pregnancy is accompanied by major changes in the coagulation system with increases in the levels of factors VII, VIII and X, and a particularly marked increase in the level of plasma fibrinogen (Fig. 6.30). The increased fibrinogen concentration is probably the chief cause of the accelerated erythrocyte sedimentation rate observed during pregnancy.

The effect of pregnancy on the coagulation factors can be detected from about the 3rd month of gestation. In late pregnancy the fibrinogen concentration is at least double that of the non-pregnant state.

Fibrinolysis

Fibrinolytic activity is an essential part of the dynamic interacting haemostatic mechanism and is dependent on plasminogen activator in the blood (Fig. 6.31). Fibrin and fibrinogen are digested by plasmin, a proenzyme derived from an inactive plasma precursor, plasminogen.

Increased amounts of activator are found in the plasma after strenuous exercise, emotional stress, surgical operations and other trauma.

Tissue activator can be extracted from most human organs with the exception of the placenta.

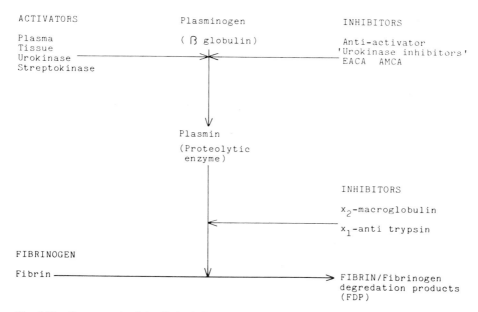

ACTIVATORS   Plasminogen   INHIBITORS

Plasma
Tissue   (β globulin)   Anti-activator
Urokinase   'Urokinase inhibitors'
Streptokinase   EACA AMCA

Plasmin
(Proteolytic
enzyme)

INHIBITORS

x_2-macroglobulin

x_1-anti trypsin

FIBRINOGEN

Fibrin   FIBRIN/Fibrinogen
degradation products
(FDP)

Fig. 6.31 Components of the fibrinolytic system. (Reproduced with permission from F. Hytten, G. Chamberlain, *Clinical Physiology in Obstetrics*, Blackwell Scientific Publications.)

Tissues especially rich in activator include the uterus, ovaries, prostate, heart, lungs, thyroid, adrenal glands and lymph nodes. Activity in tissues is concentrated mainly around blood vessels, veins showing greater activity than arteries. Venous occlusion of the limbs will stimulate fibrinolytic activity, a fact which should be remembered if tourniquets are applied for any length of time before blood is drawn for measurement of fibrin degradation products (FDPs).

The inhibitors of fibrinolytic activity are of two types — anti-activators (antiplasminogens) and the antiplasmins.

Antiplasminogens include ε-aminocaproic acid (EACA) and tranexamic acid (AMCA). Aprotonin (trasylol) is another antiplasminogen which is commercially prepared from bovine lung.

Platelets, plasma and serum exert a strong inhibitory action on plasmin. Normally plasma antiplasmin levels exceed levels of plasminogen, and hence the levels of potential plasmin; otherwise we would dissolve away our connecting cement!

When fibrinogen or fibrin is broken down by plasmin, fibrin degradation products are formed which comprise the high-molecular-weight split products X and Y and smaller fragments A, B, C, D and E (Fig. 6.32). When a fibrin clot is formed, 70% of fragment X is retained in the clot, Y, D and E being retained to a somewhat lesser extent. Therefore, serum, under normal circumstances, can contain small amounts of fragment X and larger amounts of Y, D and E. All of these components have antigenic determinants in common with fibrinogen and will be recognised by fibrinogen antisera. It is important to be aware of this fact when examining blood for the presence of FDPs. Blood should be taken by clean venepuncture and the tourniquet should not be left on too long (see above). The blood should be allowed to clot in the presence of an antifibrinolytic agent such as EACA to stop the process of fibrinolysis which would otherwise continue *in vitro*.

Plasma fibrinolytic activity is decreased during pregnancy, remains low during labour and delivery, and returns to normal within 1 hour of placental delivery.

The rapid return of systemic fibrinolytic activity to normal following delivery of the placenta, and the fact that the placenta has been shown to contain inhibitors which block fibrinolysis, suggest

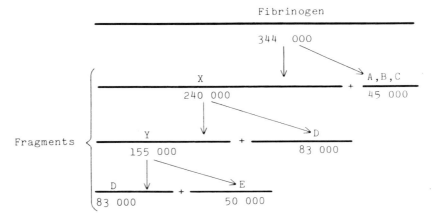

Fig. 6.32 Fibrin degradation products (FDPs) produced by the action of plasma on fibronogen. The molecular weights are shown. (Reproduced with permission from F. Hytten, G. Chamberlain, *Clinical Physiology in Obstetrics*, Blackwell Scientific Publications.)

that inhibition of fibrinolysis during pregnancy is mediated through the placenta.

Summary of changes in haemostasis in pregnancy

The changes in the coagulation system in normal pregnancy are consistent with a continuing low-grade process of coagulant activity. Using electron microscopy, fibrin deposition can be demonstrated in the intervillous space of the placenta and in all the walls of the spiral arteries supplying the placenta. As pregnancy advances, the elastic lamina and smooth muscle of these spiral arteries are replaced by a matrix containing fibrin. This allows expansion of the lumen to accommodate an increasing blood flow and reduces the pressure in arterial blood flowing to the placenta. At placental separation, a blood flow of 500–800 ml/min has to be staunched within seconds, or a serious haemorrhage will occur. Myometrial contraction plays a vital role in securing haemostasis by reducing the blood flow to the placental site. Rapid closure of the terminal part of the spiral arteries will be further facilitated by the structural changes within their walls.

The placental site is rapidly covered by a fibrin mesh following delivery. The increased levels of fibrinogen and other coagulation factors will meet the sudden demand for haemostatic components at placental separation.

Thromboembolism

The dramatic changes described above facilitate arrest of bleeding from the placental site at delivery but carry with them an increased risk of thromboembolism.

The 1991 Confidential Maternal Mortality Survey shows that pulmonary embolism remains the most frequent cause of maternal mortality, responsible for about 10 deaths a year in the United Kingdom.

Thromboembolism was previously regarded as a disease of the puerperium but we now know that a third of the deaths occur in the antenatal period.

Disseminated intravascular coagulation

The changes in the haemostatic system during pregnancy and the local activation of the clotting system during parturition carry with them a risk, not only of thromboembolism, but of disseminated intravascular coagulation (DIC), consumption of clotting factors and platelets leading to severe bleeding — particularly uterine and sometimes generalised. Despite the advances in obstetric care and highly developed blood transfusion services, haemorrhage still constitutes a major factor in maternal mortality and morbidity.

The first problem with DIC is its definition. It is never primary, but always secondary to some general stimulation of coagulation activity by

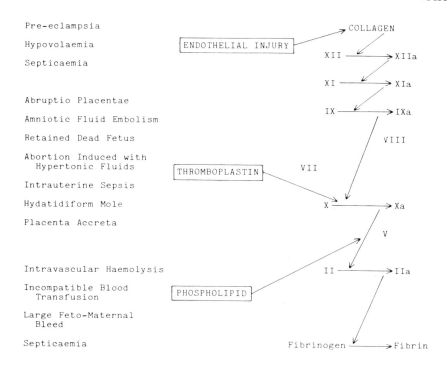

Pre-eclampsia

Hypovolaemia

Septicaemia

Abruptio Placentae

Amniotic Fluid Embolism

Retained Dead Fetus

Abortion Induced with
    Hypertonic Fluids

Intrauterine Sepsis

Hydatidiform Mole

Placenta Accreta

Intravascular Haemolysis

Incompatible Blood
    Transfusion

Large Feto-Maternal
    Bleed

Septicaemia

Interactions of the trigger mechanisms
occur in many of these obstetric
complications

Fig. 6.33 Trigger mechanisms of DIC in pregnancy. (Reproduced with permission from M. de Swiet, *Medical Disorders in Pregnancy*, Blackwell Scientific Publications.)

release of procoagulant substances into the blood (Fig. 6.33). Hypothetical triggers of this process in pregnancy include the leaking of placental tissue fragments, amniotic fluid, incompatible red cells or bacterial products into the maternal circulation. There is a great spectrum of manifestations of the process of DIC, ranging from a compensated state with no clinical manifestation, but evidence of increased production and breakdown of coagulation factors, to the condition of massive uncontrollable haemorrhage with very low concentrations of plasma fibrinogen, pathological raised levels of FDPs and variable degrees of thrombocytopenia.

Fibrinolysis is stimulated by DIC, and FDPs resulting from the process interfere with the formation of firm fibrin clots. A vicious circle is established which results in further severe bleeding.

Obstetric conditions classically associated with

DIC include placental abruption, amniotic fluid embolism, septic abortion and other intrauterine infection, retained dead fetus, hydatidiform mole, placenta accreta, pre-eclampsia and eclampsia and prolonged shock from any cause (Fig. 6.33).

RHESUS INCOMPATIBILITY

In the late 1930s it was discovered that red cells from Rhesus monkeys injected into guinea-pigs and rabbits produced an antibody in the animals' sera which reacted strongly with the red cells of 85% of Caucasians. Those individuals whose red cells were agglutinated strongly with the Rhesus (Rh) antibody were called Rh positive and the remaining 15% were termed Rh negative.

Soon after the recognition of the Rh factor it was shown that this antigen had important clinical significance in terms of haemolytic disease of the newborn and transfusion reactions.

The Rh negative recipients of Rh positive transfusions could suffer haemolytic transfusion reactions and Rh positive babies carried by Rh negative mothers were frequently affected by haemolytic anaemia in utero and in the postnatal period.

An immediate recommendation was that Rh negative female recipients in or below childbearing years should be transfused with Rh negative blood.

However, there were differences in the specificities of the antibodies produced by the sensitised Rh negative mothers, and it became clear that the Rh factor was complex and it would be more reasonable to use the term Rh blood group system.

For a basic understanding of the Rh system only six of the 26 or more Rh antigens recognised need to be considered, namely C, c̄, D, d, E, ē.

There are antisera to identify five of these antigens, but there is no antiserum as yet which can recognise the d antigen.

These Rh antigens are under the control of three closely linked genes with the alleles C and c̄, D and d, and E and ē.

The main combination of genes of the three loci are:

CDē or R_1	
c̄DE or R_2	Rh(D)positive
CDE or R_z	
c̄Dē or R_0	

c̄dē or r	
Cdē or r^1	Rh(D)negative.
c̄dE or r^{11}	
CdE or r_y	

This classification follows the convention that possession of a D gene and antigen is termed Rh positive whereas absence of a D gene and antigen is termed Rh negative:

DD	homozygous	Rh positive
Dd	heterozygous	
dd		Rh negative.

It follows that any Rh positive offspring of an Rh negative mother has to be heterozygous (Dd), having received a D antigen from the father but a d antigen from the mother.

It also follows that if the father is homozygous Rh(DD) positive, then he can only have Rhesus positive children, whereas if he is heterozygous Rh(Dd) positive then there is a 50:50 chance of him fathering a Rh negative baby with a Rh negative spouse which will not be affected by maternal anti-D antibody.

D^u antigen. A few individuals have antigens on their cells which react weakly and variably with the various forms of anti-D antisera — these are termed group D^u. For transfusion purposes an individual with the blood group D^u should be regarded as Rh(D) negative when receiving blood but as Rh(D) positive when donating blood.

Haemolytic disease of the newborn

Haemolytic disease of the newborn (HDN) is a condition in which the lifespan of the infant's red cells is shortened by the action of specific antibodies derived from the mother. The immune antibodies in the maternal plasma are small molecular immunoglobulins of the IgG subclass and therefore, unlike the large molecule, naturally occurring antibodies of the ABO blood group systems (IgM) are able to cross the placenta.

Although HDN can occur in several situations where the mother lacks an antigen which her baby carries on its red cells, there is no doubt that, prior to the introduction of the specific immunoglobulin for the prevention of Rh(D) haemolytic disease, Rh(D) HDN was by far the most important form of HDN in terms of clinical severity and frequency in Caucasian populations. Other Rh antibodies which can cause HDN are anti-E and anti-c̄, in which case the mother is usually Rh(D) positive.

Outside the Rh blood group system the most frequently observed immune-induced antibody is anti-Kell. This is more usually transfusion provoked, 95% of the Caucasian population being Kell negative. Occasionally, this antibody can cause severe HDN where the father is Kell positive (heterozygous or homozygous) and he has transmitted the Kell positive gene to his offspring.

HDN begins in intrauterine life and may result in death in utero. In liveborn infants the haemolytic process is maximal at the time of birth and thereafter diminishes as the concentration of maternal antibody in the infant's circulation declines.

During pregnancy the fetal and maternal circulations are separate. Red cells are not thought to cross the placental barrier in significant numbers in normal circumstances. Oxygen, nutrient and waste exchange takes place by diffusion across the intervillous space. IgG antibodies cross the placenta freely, carrying protection (passive immunity) for the fetus against infective agents to which the mother has had a healthy immune response.

Following delivery and placental separation, rupture of the placental villi and connective tissue allows escape of fetal blood cells into the maternal circulation, prior to constriction of the open maternal vessels. This is when sensitisation takes place in the majority of cases unless prevented (see below).

The incompatible Rh(D) fetal cells enter the maternal spleen and the foreign antigen on the fetal red cell triggers off an immune response causing production of antibody.

In a subsequent pregnancy with an Rh(D) positive fetus, the immune IgG anti-D maternal antibody will cross the placenta and attach to the specific D antigen sites on the fetal red cell. IgG-coated red cells do not have a normal lifespan. They are particularly sensitive to cells of the reticuloendothelial system and are removed from the circulation prematurely. Progressive anaemia in utero occurs from about the 4th month of pregnancy and, in the most severe cases, intrauterine death has been recorded from the 20th week of pregnancy, although it is uncommon before the 24th week. Many of the stillborn infants are grossly oedematous and are then described as having *hydrops foetalis*. Hydropic infants are occasionally born alive and are found to be severely anaemic with cord haemoglobins as low as 3.5 g/dl. There is a great increase in the number of nucleated red cells in the circulating blood, hence the term *erythroblastosis foetalis* is sometimes used to describe the haematological condition.

Jaundice does not occur before delivery because bilirubin produced by the breakdown of cells in the fetal spleen passes via the placenta to the maternal circulation. Albumin transports the fetal bilirubin to the maternal liver where glucuronyl transferase converts it to excretable, direct-reacting bilirubin. The liver of the neonate does not produce glucuronyl transferase and cannot convert bilirubin to an excretable form. Consequently, bilirubin accumulates and if not removed (by exchange transfusion) will collect in the tissues causing jaundice and brain damage. Deeply jaundiced infants often exhibit signs of damage to the central nervous system. These signs usually develop after the age of 36 hours.

It has been shown that the brain contains lipid which takes up the unconjugated bilirubin but does not take up conjugated bilirubin. In kernicterus, the yellow-staining material has been shown to be unconjugated bilirubin.

Detection of Rh anti-D antibody

Direct antiglobulin (Coombs') test (baby's red blood cells, one-stage test)

When a neonate suffers from HDN the red cells are coated with immune IgG antibody. This is known as incomplete antibody. These cells do not agglutinate but if an anti-IgG antiserum is added to a mixture of sensitised cells the gap is bridged between antibody on individual red cells and visible agglutination occurs. This is known as a positive direct Coombs' test.

Indirect antiglobulin (Coombs') Test (maternal serum, two-stage test)

The mother produces antibody against the Rh(D) positive fetal cells. The antibody is free in her serum because her Rh(D) negative red cells do not carry the appropriate antigen. If her serum is incubated with Rh(D) positive cells the antibodies will attach to them but, as it is an IgG, agglutination does not occur. However, if anti-IgG antiserum is then added to the sensitised cells (cf. direct Coombs' test), visible agglutination will occur. This is known as the indirect Coombs' test and is used routinely to detect the presence of anti-Rh and other immune antibodies in maternal serum during pregnancy. By serial dilution of maternal serum and reporting the weakest dilution of the serum at which a reaction with the Rh(D) positive red cell takes place, a crude estimation of the concentration of the antibody can be made. Serial estimations will give an indication of the rate of increase of antibody in a particular pregnancy.

With the advent of automation in blood transfusion laboratories, it has now become routine in large centres to estimate the Rh(D) antibody in international units based on an automated system using the Coombs' test principle.

Amniocentesis

Although measurement of antenatal anti-D concentration has become more exact, correlation between antibody levels and severity of the haemolytic process in the fetus is not sufficient to plan management during pregnancy.

By estimation of the bilirubin concentration in the amniotic fluid, the degree of haemolysis of the infant's red cells can be predicted with greater accuracy.

Several methods are in current usage but the most popular is the spectrophotometric measurement of the bilirubin 'bulge' at a wavelength of 450–460 nm. A decision can then be taken on the need for intrauterine transfusion prior to premature delivery and exchange transfusion, or allowing the pregnancy to go to term. Amniocentesis gives valuable information from 20 to 22 weeks gestation onwards. However fetal blood sampling is becoming the method of choice to determine the degree to which the fetus is affected.

Prevention of Rh(D) HDN

The stimulus for primary induction of antibody formation has been shown to be Rh(D) positive fetal cells entering the maternal circulation at delivery. If Rh anti-D immunoglobulin is injected into the mother within 2–3 days of delivery the antibody coats the fetal Rh positive antigen sites and the coated cells are rapidly removed from the maternal circulation by cells of the reticuloendothelial system. Maternal immune system cells are prevented from producing antibody against the fetal Rh(D) positive cells in the presence of adequate antibody.

Fetal cells in the maternal circulation can be identified and quantitated crudely using the Kleihauer test.

The Kleihauer test depends on the fact that cells (such as neonatal and fetal cells) containing large amounts of fetal haemoglobin have different chemical properties to cells with a high proportion of adult haemoglobin (maternal cells).

Fetal haemoglobin is more stable than adult haemoglobin and resists alkali denaturation and acid elution. In the Kleihauer test a film of maternal blood is stained and flooded with strong acid. Any fetal cells present will retain their haemoglobin and be detectable in a sea of ghost-like maternal cells which will have lost their adult hemoglobin.

Fetal cells probably occur in the circulation of about half of the Rh(D) negative mothers delivered of an Rh(D) positive child. The volumes of fetal blood are up to 0.1 ml in 25–30% of mothers, from 0.1 to 5 ml in 20–25% and over 5 ml in just under 1%. In about one in every 400 pregnancies a massive transplacental haemorrhage of the order of 50 ml or so occurs.

The overwhelming majority of mothers receive less than 5.0 ml into the circulation.

It has been calculated that 100 μg of anti-D is sufficient to cover this volume of fetal cells escaping into the maternal circulation. This 100 μg of anti-D is the standard dose administrated but the volume of fetal cells must always be quantitated using the Kleihauer technique so that the dose can be increased if there has been a fetal bleed greater than 5.0 ml into the maternal circulation.

Other situations in which Rh sensitisation may occur and in which anti-D should be given

1. Women may be sensitised by fetal red cells entering the circulation at termination of pregnancy. It is recommended to give 50 μg of anti-D following all terminations in a Rh(D) negative mother.

2. Rh(D) negative women should be given anti-D following amniocentesis and a Kleihauer test performed. The standard minimum dose is 50 μg up to 22 weeks' gestation and 100 μg thereafter.

3. Other obstetric manoeuvres such as external version should also be covered by a standard dose of anti-D.

4. Threatened abortion may have to be covered with repeated anti-D administration, 50 μg at 4/52 intervals, if bleeding continues over some weeks.

5. Accidental haemorrhage due to abruptio placentae should be treated with a standard dose of anti-D.

7. Endocrinology

THE PANCREAS

The pancreas is made up of two types of tissue, glandular acini and the islets of Langerhans. The glandular acini are responsible for the secretion of bicarbonate and digestive enzymes (see p. 188). The islets of Langerhans are made up of three types of cells: α cells, which produce glucagon, β cells, which produce insulin and δ cells, which produce somatostatin.

Glucagon is a polypeptide consisting of 29 amino acids. Its molecular weight is 3485. It may be synthesised commercially. Glucagon release is stimulated by hypoglycaemia, exercise and adrenaline. Glucagon release is inhibited by free fatty acids.

The release of glucagon results in the rapid mobilisation of hepatic glucose by glycogenolysis. Glucagon also acts on adipose tissue to release fatty acids and may stimulate gluconeogenesis from amino acids and lactate.

Insulin is a polypeptide molecule, molecular weight 5734, in which the total of 51 amino acid residues form two chains, A and B, chain A comprising 21 amino acids. Chains A and B are joined by two disulphide bridges. Insulin can be syn-thesised by recombinant DNA technology.

Proinsulin is the precursor of insulin in the β cells. Zinc is needed for the crystallisation of insulin.

The pancreas stores about 250 units of insulin at any one time, of which about 50 units are needed per day, except in pregnancy when the insulin response to glucose is increased three-fold.

The fasting plasma level of insulin is about 10 μU/ml and rises to a level of 60–100 μU/ml after a standard 75 g glucose load. Insulin levels can be measured by radioimmunoassay which has a sensitivity of less than 1 μU/ml.

Insulin release is stimulated by glucose, amino acids and free fatty acids. Oral glucose results in a greater release of insulin than does intravenous glucose because of the effect of intestinal hormones (gastrin, secretin and pancreozymin) which act on the pancreas. Insulin release is inhibited by adrenaline and noradrenalin.

In muscle and adipose tissue, insulin facilitates transport of small molecules across cell membranes by binding with specific receptor sites in the membrane. This applies particularly to glucose, but insulin will also promote the transport of amino acids and certain ions such as potassium, calcium and phosphate. In fatty tissue only, insulin inhibits lipolysis. In the liver there is no barrier to glucose entering hepatic cells and, there, insulin is concerned with promoting the induction of enzymes such as glucokinase, phosphofructokinase and pyruvate kinase and increasing glycogen and protein synthesis.

Insulin is degraded in the liver and kidneys by the enzyme glutathione insulin transhydrogenase, which breaks the disulphide bonds between the A and B chains. The half-life of insulin is less than 20 minutes.

Little is known of the precise function of somatostatin, a polypeptide which inhibits both insulin and glucagon release. It also has an inhibitory effect on gut motility. In addition, somatostatin is secreted by the hypothalamus and inhibits growth hormone release.

THE HYPOTHALAMUS, PITUITARY, OVARY AND MENSTRUAL CYCLE

The hypothalamus

Situation

The hypothalamus lies in the lower part of the lateral wall of the third ventricle. Its boundaries are:

Anteriorly — the optic chiasma
Posteriorly — the mamillary bodies
Laterally — it extends for a distance of about
  1 cm on each side of the third ventricle
Superiorly — the thalamus
Inferiorly — the tuber cinereum, which is
  formed by the converging walls of the third
  ventricle (Fig. 7.1)

Structure

The hypothalamus is composed of neural tissue. It is divided into medial and lateral regions. The medial region contains groups of important nuclei located in three areas (Fig. 7.2):

1. The supraoptic area in which are to be found the paraventricular, supraoptic and preoptic nuclei

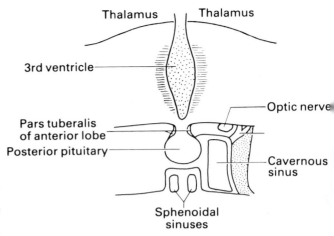

Fig. 7.1   The relations of the hypothalamus.

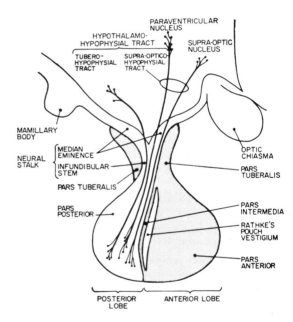

Fig. 7.2   Diagrammatic representation of the hypothalamus and pituitary. The connections of the posterior lobe of the gland with the hypothalamus are indicated. (This figure and Figs 7.3–7.5 by courtesy of the editors of *A Companion to Medical Studies* and Blackwell Scientific Publications.)

2. The tuberal region where the ventromedial, dorsomedial and posterior nuclei are found

3. The mamillary region in which are the mamillary bodies.

The lateral region of the hypothalamus shows no similar distinct nuclear areas. Its cells are separated by the fibres of the median forebrain bundle which passes from the higher centres to the nuclei of the medial region.

Connections

1. To higher centres. The hypothalamus is connected to higher centres by afferent fibres from parts of the frontal lobes and the medial aspects of the temporal lobes. Efferent fibres arise in the hypothalamic nuclei and mamillary bodies and pass to the thalamus and then to higher cortical areas. These connections make up the limbic system which includes the hippocampus, amygdala, cingulate and hippocampal gyri and the pyriform area.

2. To the pituitary. (See Fig. 7.2)
a. The hypothalamus is physically connected to the pituitary by the pituitary stalk. Within this the anterior pituitary (adenohypophysis) is connected to the hypothalamus by the pituitary portal system. In this system, vessels from the carotid and posterior communicating arteries form a capillary loop system in the tuberal part of the hypothalamus. From this loop a primary plexus of vessels forms in the region of the median eminence; these vessels come together as larger venous trunks which pass down the pituitary stalk into the substance of the anterior portion of the pituitary. The blood passing down these trunks enters a sinusoidal system, which, in turn, enters a secondary plexus which empties into the systemic veins draining the area (Fig. 7.3).
b. The posterior pituitary (neurohypophysis) is connected to the supraoptic and paraventricular nuclei of the hypothalamus by a rich plexus of nerves in the interior of the pituitary stalk.

Functions

The hypothalamus produces pituitary-regulating hormones which pass down the pituitary portal system to regulate the production of pituitary trophic hormones by the anterior pituitary. In addition, vasopressin and oxytocin are elaborated in the supraoptic and paraventricular nuclei, whence they pass down the axons of the nerves connecting these structures to the posterior pituitary where the two hormones are stored.

Reference is frequently made to tonic and cyclic control in the hypothalamus. The former is regarded as responsible for the day-to-day constant production of gonadotrophins, the latter for the surges of luteinising hormone (LH) and follicle-stimulating hormone (FSH) activity, which lead to ovulation. Tonic control is mainly under negative feedback control, the cyclic one under positive feedback control.

By its connections with the limbic system, the hypothalamus functions as a centre in which external stimuli reaching the body are converted into the appropriate emotional response such as rage, fear, anger, temperature regulation, feeding and behaviour.

Regulating hormones

The hypothalamic regulating hormones are:

Luteinising hormone-releasing hormone
  (LH-RH), also known as
  gonadotrophin-releasing hormone (GnRH)
Corticotrophin-releasing hormone (CRH)
Growth hormone-releasing hormone (GH-RH)
Growth hormone-release-inhibiting hormone —
  somatostatin
Thyrotrophin-releasing hormone (TRH)
Prolactin-inhibiting factor (PIF) (dopamine).

LH-RH is a decapeptide and somastatin a tetradecapeptide; TRH is a tripeptide. CRH and GH-RH are larger peptides (41 and 44 amino acids respectively).

Mode of production of regulating hormones

The mode of production of the regulating hormones is a neurosecretory one. The hypothalamic nerve cells act both as neurones and as endocrine cells. The hormones are synthesised in the cytoplasm of the neurone and then passed along the nerve axon to the nerve terminal, from which they are released into the hypophyseal portal blood vessels passing to the anterior pituitary (Fig. 7.3).

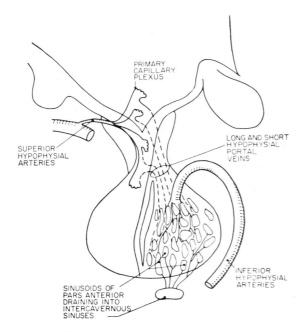

Fig. 7.3 The pituitary portal system and its connections.

The pineal gland

The activity of the hypothalamus may also be influenced by the pineal gland although it must be admitted that most of the information concerning the activity of this curious structure is from animal sources.

The pineal is a small gland which lies deep in the interior of the brain at the posterior part of the hypothalamus. It arises as an upgrowth of the third ventricle roof, but loses all neural connections with the brain. Its neural pathway is a very complex one which originates in the retina and passes through the median forebrain bundle to the upper part of the spinal cord. From there, sympathetic preganglionic fibres pass to the superior cervical ganglion from which postganglionic fibres run directly to the pineal.

The pineal cells are the pinealocytes which produce melatonin under the influence of light and darkness. Melatonin is produced from serotonin through the activity of the enzyme hydroxyindole-*o*-methyltransferase (HIOMT). This synthesis of melatonin is facilitated by darkness and inhibited by light. The absence of light leads to sympathetic stimulation, the liberation of noradrenalin at the nerve endings on the pineal cells and to melatonin production. The pineal body also contains neuroglial cells especially in its stalk.

It seems likely, from animal experiments, that the pineal gland has a part to play in regulating reproductive activity. The rat, subjected to persistent light, for example, produces less melatonin, the ovaries increase in size and the animal remains in constant oestrus. Darkness has the opposite effect. It is probable that this results from interaction between the pineal and the hypothalamus and not by direct pineal/pituitary activity. Pituitary implantation of pineal substances in animals is without effect whereas the implantation of melatonin into the median eminence gives rise to decreased LH stores in the pituitary, and the implantation of serotonin to decreased FSH stores.

The part the pineal might play in normal human reproductive hormone activity, however, remains a matter of speculation and we have no direct evidence on the matter.

Tanycytes

Any activity the pineal might have could be via the function of tanycytes. These are specialised ependymal cells with ciliated borders which line the third ventricle over the site of the median eminence. The anticiliary pole of the tanycytes ends on the portal vessels and this may be the mechanism of pineal–hypothalamic interaction.

The pituitary

Anatomy

The pituitary, or hypophysis, is connected to the hypothalamus by the pituitary stalk. The gland is divided into an anterior and a posterior portion with widely differing functions which reflect their separate embryological development.

The anterior pituitary arises as an upward fold of the ectoderm of the primitive mouth, or stomodeum (Rathke's pouch) (Fig. 7.4). The posterior pituitary arises as a similar down-growth of the neuro ectoderm of the floor of the midbrain; this process — the infundibular process — becomes solid by a proliferation of cells within its

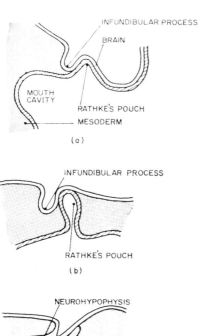

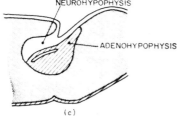

Fig. 7.4 The development of the pituitary.

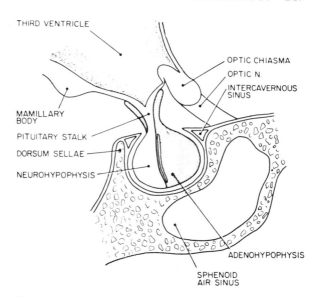

Fig. 7.5 Relations of the pituitary.

cavity. The fold of Rathke's pouch, however, retains a vestigial cavity in its centre, as illustrated; this slit-like cavity becomes separated from the posterior pituitary by a narrow portion of the anterior lobe known as the pars intermedia. Another extension of the anterior lobe, the pars tuberalis, surrounds the infundibulum, which constitutes the neural portion of the pituitary stalk.

Relations (Fig. 7.5)

The pituitary lies within the sella turcica of the sphenoid. Anteriorly and posteriorly the inter--cavernous sinuses lie within the anterior and posterior clinoid processes of that bone; laterally lie the cavernous sinuses and their contained structures, namely the internal carotid artery and the sixth cranial nerve. Superiorly the pituitary is continuous with the hypothalamus as described; in front of the hypothalamus and superior to the anterior lobe of the pituitary lie the optic chiasma and the optic nerves.

The pia and arachnoid blend with the capsule of the pituitary and cannot be identified as separate structures. Above the gland is the diaphragma sellae, a fold of dura mater, through which the pituitary stalk passes.

Structure of the pituitary

Anterior pituitary. The epithelial cells of the anterior pituitary may be divided into three main groups depending upon their reaction to staining with haemotoxylin and eosin. These cells are:

1. Chromophobes which stain only lightly and contain no granules.
2. Chromophils which stain well and contain granules. From their reaction to the stain it is possible to divide chromophil cells into two groups:

    a. Acidophils, which stain red
    b. Basophils, which stain blue.

Both acidophils and basophils contain granules and appear to be the active secretory cells of the anterior lobe.

The precise relationship of these cells to the trophic hormone production of the anterior pituitary is not yet known. The chromophobes are probably reserve cells or resting cells, capable of developing into acidophils and basophils. Recent immunoenzyme histochemical techniques of staining show that the chromophil cells can be divided into a greater number of cell types called α, β_1, β_2, δ_1 and δ_2. The α cells are the acidophils, as described above: they are thought to be responsible for the production of growth hormone and prolactin. β_1 cells are heavily granulated and their granules are strong PAS (periodic acid–Schiff) positive; β_2 cells have granules which stain a blackish colour with aldehyde thionin; they are believed to produce TSH. The δ cells are smaller and are the possible source of gonadotrophins: the δ_1 cell granules also stain with aldehyde thionin; the δ_2 cell granules are PAS positive also, but being smaller than the β_1 cell can be differentiated from it. FSH and LH are contained in the same cells, which are situated towards the anterior and ventral portion of the lobe; the remaining trophic hormones are situated in separate cells scattered in groups throughout the gland. No nerve elements are detectable in the anterior lobe of the pituitary.

Posterior pituitary. This part of the pituitary has a whitish colour which contrasts with the brownish tint of the anterior lobe. It is composed of numerous glial cells known as pituicytes, which are plentiful in the main part of the lobe and less so in the infundibulum. The remainder of the posterior lobe is composed of a multitude of nerves connecting the gland to the nuclei of the hypothalamus.

The hormones of the anterior pituitary

The anterior pituitary produces a number of important trophic hormones:

1. FSH
2. LH
3. Prolactin
4. Adrenocorticotrophic hormone (ACTH)
5. Thyroid-stimulating hormone (TSH), sometimes called thyrotrophin
6. Growth hormone (GH).

All are proteins or complex associations of sugars and polypeptides (glycoproteins). The molecular weights are of the order of 20 000–40 000.

FSH and LH. These hormones have an important combined action on the ovary. In the female, FSH, as its name suggests, is responsible for early development of the Graafian follicle. LH may contribute to follicular growth and oestrogen production but its principle actions are to cause ovulation and to convert the ruptured Graafian follicle to a corpus luteum. In the male, FSH is concerned with maintenance and growth of the germinal epithelium of the seminiferous tubules and with sperm production. Interstitial cell-stimulating hormone stimulates the interstitial cells which produce androgens.

FSH and LH are glycoproteins of molecular weight about 30 000. Each consists of two non-identical subunits — α and β. The α unit is similar in all pituitary glycoproteins of the same species and human chorionic gonadotrophin (hCG); the β units differ and give each hormone its specifity.

Feedback control. FSH and LH are hormones produced during reproductive life in a rhythmic fashion and they interact with the hormones of the ovary to give rise to regular ovulation (Fig. 7.6).

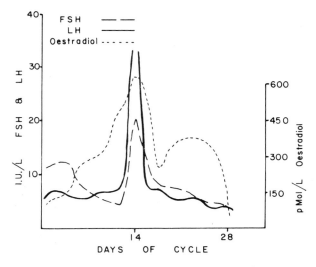

Fig. 7.6 Diagrammatic representation of changes in hormone levels during the menstrual cycle. The LH peak is left open since it is subject to great variation.

The interaction of these substances is the result of an important system of feedback control. Four feedback control mechanisms appear to exist:

1. The long negative-feedback system. As the production of oestrogen by the Graafian follicle rises, the further production of FSH is inhibited and the development of other follicles is temporarily suspended. This long negative-control system probably exerts its principal effect on the hypothalamus, reducing LH-RH production and so causing a fall in FSH. There may be a direct negative action on the pituitary, however.

2. The long positive-feedback mechanism. As oestrogen levels continue to rise, they eventually reach a sufficiently high level to stimulate LH production and to a lesser extent FSH production, and a surge in the production of both hormones results in ovulation. Again, this positive feedback action is thought to be mainly at pituitary level but there may be a direct hypothalamic effect also.

The temporary fall in oestrogen production, which is caused by ovulation, shuts off the positive-feedback effect but maintains a negative one. FSH and LH production therefore remain reduced until the corpus luteum declines and the oestrogen and progesterone values wane. The hypothalamus, and to a lesser extent, probably, the pituitary, are released from inhibition and FSH levels rise again.

3. The short feedback mechanism. The rise in production of FSH and LH by the pituitary exerts a negative-feedback effect on the hypothalamic production of LH-RH.

4. An ultrashort feedback system appears to exist which is concerned with the self-inhibition of hypothalamic regulating hormones as their production rises.

Diagrams such as Fig. 7.6, which illustrates the production of FSH and LH during the menstrual cycle, give the impression that the actual production rate of these hormones is constant. They are, in reality, released in pulsatile bursts of brief duration.

Growth hormone. This hormone is produced by the α cells of the anterior pituitary under the influence of GHRH and somatostatin. It is a protein hormone and the sequence of amino acids which make up its structure has a great deal in common with prolactin and human placental lactogen (HPL). Here it is sufficient to say that its actions comprise:

1. Maintenance of the rate of protein synthesis
2. Reduction in amino acid breakdown so leading to a positive nitrogen balance (this action is dependent upon insulin)
3. Mobilisation of fat stores
4. Inhibition of the oxidation of carbohydrates in the tissues.

The level of the GH in plasma shows marked fluctuations from 60 μg/l down to scarcely detectable levels (< 1 μg/l).

Its control is concerned with food ingestion. This raises the level of glucose which in turn inhibits the production of GHRH and decreases GH production. Hypoglycaemia has the opposite effect. GH secretion is also influenced by exercise, where it appears to have an action leading to the mobilisation of fat stores to meet energy needs.

Prolactin. The existence of this hormone was suspected for many years before it became a reality. It is a protein hormone which possesses 190 amino acid residues and has a molecular weight of about 22 000. Its similarity to GH and HPL has already been mentioned; 80% of its amino acid residues are shared with HPL and 20% with GH.

Prolactin is produced by cells of the anterior pituitary and by special staining techniques it can be shown to arise from different α cells from those secreting GH. These prolactin-secreting cells are present in comparatively small numbers in the non-pregnant subject, but they increase markedly in number during pregnancy.

Prolactin is evidently not stored in the pituitary to any extent, being released once it is synthesised. It is transported in the plasma in a free state and has only a short half-life of 15–20 minutes, its inactivation being in the liver. The action of the hormone is predominantly on the breast in the initiation of lactation (see p. 222). In animals prolactin has a role in promoting corpus luteum development but there is little evidence that this activity is important in man.

The secretion of prolactin by the pituitary is the result of reduction in the amount of prolactin-inhibiting factor (PIF) by which the hypothalamus keeps the hormone in a state of tonic inhibition. It is known, however, that TRH can increase prolactin secretion, which has led to speculation that there may be a prolactin-releasing hormone which is similar to, or even the same as, TRH. There is no confirmation of such a releasing hormone as yet.

A wide variety of stimuli influence prolactin production. Suckling is a powerful stimulant (see below). Other events which may increase its production significantly are general anaesthesia, a surgical operation, coitus and physical exercise. Several drugs raise prolactin production by interfering with dopamine function; these include phenothiazines, reserpine, antihistamines, diazepam, tricyclic-antidepressants and haloperidol. Oestrogens, natural and synthetic, also stimulate prolactin production.

The substances which inhibit prolactin production include L-dopa and dopamine agonists, of which the most important are drugs of the ergot group, including 2-bromalphaergocriptine.

ACTH. This hormone stimulates the adrenal cortex to produce corticosteroids. The relationship of this production to the levels of steroids required and produced is described on page 234.

TSH. The function of this hormone is described on pages 237–8.

Hormones of the posterior pituitary gland

Two hormones — oxytocin and vasopressin (antidiuretic hormone, ADH) — are produced by the sequential action of the hypothalamus (paraventricular and supraoptic nuclei) and the posterior pituitary lobe. Hormones are synthesised in the nerve cells of these hypothalamic nuclei, combined to protein carrier molecules (neurophysins), and transported down the axons of the nerve tracts in the pituitary stalk leading to the posterior lobe. Here they are stored and are visible as granular particles. Their release is controlled by nerve impulses which similarly arise in the hypothalamus and pass down the same nerve tracts to the posterior pituitary.

Oxytocin and vasopressin possess a similar structure. Both are nonapeptides and they show a difference of only two amino acids.

Vasopressin has its primary action on the kidney where it increases the permeability of the cells on the collecting tubules so that water is reabsorbed in greater quantities. If vasopressin cannot be produced in sufficient quantities, because of disease of the posterior lobe, the individual develops diabetes insipidus and passes large quantities of very dilute urine.

Vasopressin is released in response to alterations in plasma volume and osmolality. Oxytocin is produced in a similar fashion to vasopressin. It is apparently released into the blood stream as a result of neurogenic stimuli, notably from the uterus or breast. Oxytocin has, of course, a marked stimulatory action on the amplitude and frequency of uterine contraction. Uterine sensitivity to oxytocin, however, varies greatly; in early pregnancy the uterus is relatively insensitive and will only respond to the administration of high doses whereas its sensitivity considerably increases towards term. We do not unfortunately yet know the precise role this hormone plays in normal parturition. One important effect of oxytocin, however, is to aid the milk ejection reflex; this action is discussed below.

Lactation. Lactation is the result of a variety of influences on the breast. Breast development itself is, of course, primarily due to oestrogen stimulation. The increase in breast size during pregnancy may, however, be the result of other hormonal stimulation as well as that of oestrogen, notably by progesterone and human placental lactogen.

Prolactin is essential for lactation and this hormone increases steadily in the blood throughout pregnancy. For the period of pregnancy, however, and for the first 3 or 4 days of the puerperium, colostrum, not milk, is produced. The failure of milk production during this time may be due to the inhibition of the alveoli in the breast by oestrogen. When oestrogen levels fall after delivery, this inhibition is withdrawn and milk begins to be produced. The different composition of milk and colostrum is shown in Table 7.1.

Once these hormonal changes have initiated lactation, its continuation is due to a complex reflex action which begins with suckling. Suckling initiates nervous impulses in the nipple which

Table 7.1 The components of milk and colostrum

	Protein	Fat	Carbohydrate	Water
Colostrum	8.6	2.3	3.2	85.6
Milk	1.25	3.3	7.5	87.0

pass to the supraoptic area of the hypothalamus. Further impulses then pass down the supraopticohypophyseal tract and stimulate the production of oxytocin from the posterior pituitary. Oxytocin causes contraction of the myoepithelial fibres which surround the milk ducts in the breast and milk is ejected. Without suckling, breast engorgement results in cessation of milk production; if suckling is continued, lactation can be prolonged for 2–3 years as sometimes happens in primitive societies.

The menstrual cycle

FSH–LH–ovarian relationships

The action of FSH and LH on the ovary and the ovarian response to stimulation will now be discussed more fully.

At the beginning of the menstrual cycle, FSH production has been allowed to rise by the fall in oestrogen production from the previous waning corpus luteum. This FSH stimulates follicle growth in the ovary. Many follicles respond — perhaps as many as a 1000 per cycle on average; only one or, rarely, two, however, fully develop and ovulate, the remainder undergo atresia at an early stage.

When the primary follicles begin this process of development they consist of an oocyte which is surrounded by a single layer of granulosa cells. These cells quickly multiply and in the dominant follicle many layers of granulosa cells are produced. During this process a fluid, liquor folliculi, is secreted into the centre of the follicle which becomes a fluid-filled cavity (Fig. 7.7). The granulosa layers around this cavity are now called the membrana granulosa. At one point there is localised proliferation of granulosa cells — the discus proligerous or cumulus oophorus — in the depths of which the oocyte is to be found. Outside the granulosa layer the stromal cells become formed into the theca interna, which is composed of a layer of spindle cells, outside which is the theca externa, where the cells are more flattened. As the Graafian follicle increases in size, it makes its way towards the periphery of the ovary with the discus proligerous facing the ovarian surface.

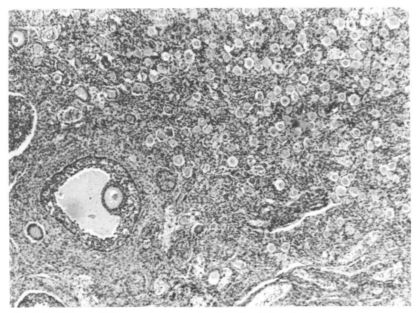

Fig. 7.7 Primary follicles and a developing Graafian follicle in the ovary.

The movement towards the periphery of the ovary is facilitated by the formation of a cone-shaped development of theca interna cells. Ovulation occurs when full follicle maturation has been achieved.

Immediately following ovulation the follicle collapses round a small quantity of blood and fluid which has been left behind. It is then transformed into a corpus luteum (Fig. 7.8). Both granulosa and theca interna cells increase in size and take on a swollen appearance by a process known as luteinisation. In this process, fluid rich in carotene is deposited within the cell cytoplasm giving the corpus luteum its characteristic yellow colour. As

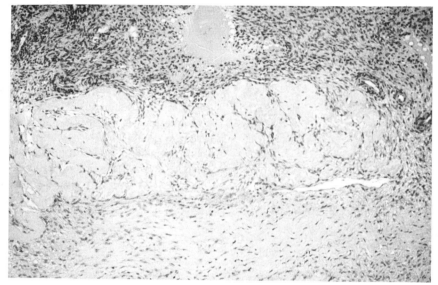

Fig. 7.8   A corpus luteum showing its characteristic folded appearance.

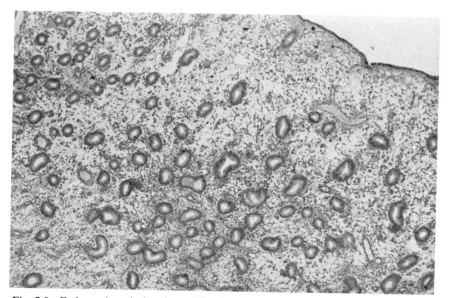

Fig. 7.9   Endometrium during the proliferative phase.

the cells of the corpus luteum collapse into the empty cavity they are thrown into folds, giving it the characteristic histological appearance shown in Figure 7.8.

The uterine response

Very important endometrial changes accompany the hormone changes just described. At the end of the menstrual period the endometrium is thin, its glands straight and narrow and lined by cuboidal epithelium and its stroma is compact. The first action of oestrogen during follicle development is to produce growth of all the elements of the endometrium. The glands remain straight but become longer and their epithelial lining becomes tall and columnar, the nuclei taking up a basal position (Fig. 7.9). At the same time there is an increase in the number of stromal cells, which become more loosely packed together. Blood vessels grow freely throughout the area, giving the endometrium a highly vascular appearance.

The addition of progesterone activity to the oestrogen effect just described is to convert the endometrium into a secretory one. The glands, once straight, become tortuous and convoluted (Fig. 7.10). The epithelium lining then goes through a series of changes, during which the nuclei move from their basal position towards the centre of the cell by the formation of vacuoles beneath the nuclei — subnuclear vacuole formation. Within the lumina of the glands more and more secretion collects, reaching a maximum about day 24 or 25 of the 28-day cycle. This secretion is rich in glycogen. There is further increase in size of the stromal cells, which are more loosely arranged, giving the whole an oedematous appearance.

The endometrial arterioles adopt a spiral course directly upwards towards the cavity of the uterus from the arteries which supply the basal portion of the endometrium; as the cycle proceeds, these arterioles become more and more coiled.

When the corpus luteum begins to regress, levels of oestrogen and progesterone fall and the endometrium can no longer be maintained. Shrinkage occurs first when constriction of the spiral arteries is evident giving rise to stasis which leads to necrosis and bleeding. The deeper basal layers of the endometrium are able to maintain their blood supply but the superficial layers break down and are cast off as menstrual flow.

Cervical mucus changes

Important changes in cervical mucus also take place throughout the menstrual cycle. In the first

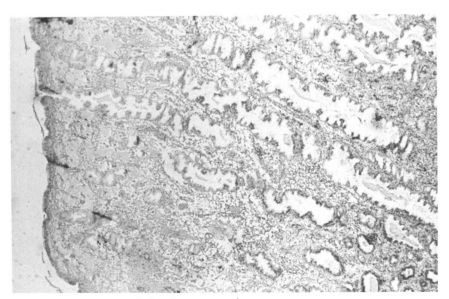

Fig. 7.10 Endometrium during the secretory phase.

few days following menstruation the mucus is thick, opaque and small in quantity. The mucus secretion increases during the proliferative phase and reaches a peak shortly before ovulation. In addition to the increase in quantity there is an important change in quality, for the mucus at the time of ovulation becomes thin and watery and permits the passage of spermatozoa readily. The mucus at this time shows the property known as spinnbarkeit which refers to its ability to be drawn out in long threads. Also evident at that time is arborisation, which is a fern-like formation visible when a drop of mucus is placed on a glass slide and allowed to dry and examined under a microscope. During the secretory phase of the cycle, the mucus again becomes thick and tenacious and prevents the passage of spermatozoa and the fern-like pattern disappears.

Vaginal changes also take place during the menstrual cycle and are recognisable by exfoliative cytology. Four types of cell may be seen lining the vagina. These are basal cells closely attached to the basement membrane which do not exfoliate; more superficial to these are parabasal cells followed by intermediate cells and superficial cells. When oestrogen production is at its height, large numbers of superficial cells exfoliate and may be seen on a slide, staining pink with Papanicolaou's stain. When progesterone is the predominant hormone, a large number of intermediate cells, which stain either pink or blue with Papanicolaou's stain, may be seen in the smear. After the menstrual period, when oestrogen levels are low, there is a preponderance of parabasal cells staining blue.

Ovarian steroidogenesis

Steroidogenesis probably takes place in three separate parts of the ovary:

1. The follicle, which synthesises mainly oestradiol with small amounts of progesterone.
2. The corpus luteum, producing mainly progesterone but continuing oestradiol production.
3. The stroma, which is evidently capable of synthesising androstenedione, testosterone, dehydroepiandrosterone and very small amounts of oestradiol and progesterone.

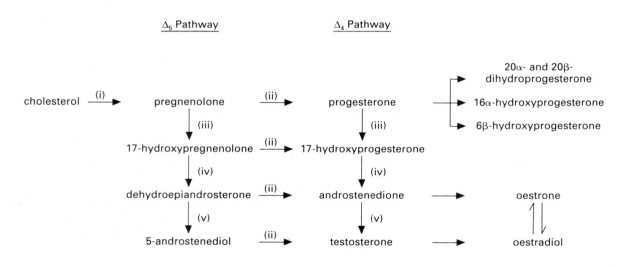

Enzymes: (i)   20,22-desmolase
          (ii) 3β-hydroxysteroid dehydrogenase
          (iii) 17α-hydroxylase
          (iv) 17,20-desmolase
          (v)   17β-hydroxysteroid dehydrogenase

Fig. 7.11 Pathways of biosynthesis of gonadal steroids.

height velocity is reached, and growth then rapidly declines and stops altogether. Peak height velocity is generally reached about the age of 12 years in Great Britain, but there is much individual variation around this mean.

The menarche, i.e. the first menstrual period, occurs between the ages of 11 and 15 years in more than 90% of girls in Western Europe and the USA, and most of the remainder will menstruate between the ages of 10 and 16 years.

The first menstrual period occurs at a variable time after the earliest sign of puberty, the average being 2.3 years. Although the menarche is not closely related to chronological age, it is more closely related to bone age. Most girls menstruate for the first time between the bone ages of 13 and 14 years, and the majority of the remainder between 12.5 and 14.5 years. It is usual for the menarche to occur after peak height velocity has been attained and between breast stages IV and V.

Whether the menarche is early or late, it is evidently concerned with nutrition and with the environmental conditions in which a girl lives. Better nutrition and freedom from chronic disease lead to an earlier menarche by promoting growth and a larger body size at an earlier age. It has been suggested that girls require to obtain a body weight of 47 kg for the menarche to take place, but although there is general agreement that early growth and weight gain promote early puberty, this figure has not been universally accepted.

The improvement in standards of living which have occurred in most countries has in general led to a lowering of the mean menarcheal age throughout the world during this century.

Early menstrual cycles soon after the menarche are often irregular, this irregularity persisting in many instances for a year or more. Ovulation does not usually occur until some time after the menarche, although early ovulation is occasionally seen. It seems probable that more than 2 years elapse before ovulation becomes at all regular.

Important changes characterise the genital organs. The ovaries change shape, the elongated ovary of the child becoming the fatter oval structure of the adult. This change is not the result of an increase in the number of follicles. The number actually falls. The ovaries have their maximum number of follicles at about 5 months of fetal life,

when there are almost 7 million present. By birth, this number has fallen to 1–2 million, and to 250 000–300 000 or so around the menarche. It is the development of many more of these primary follicles into Graafian follicles at various stages of development which increases ovarian bulk.

The uterus, too, changes at puberty. At birth, the uterus is relatively large because of placental steroids which have affected it. The cervix is large and thick walled, and comprises two-thirds of the size of the whole organ. Within a few weeks of birth, rapid shrinkage occurs as placental steroids are withdrawn. Uterine growth is very slow throughout childhood, but close to puberty there is much greater growth at this time affecting the body of the uterus to a greater extent than the cervix so that when the menarche occurs the uterine body is equal in length to the cervix (ratio 1:1). This proliferation of the myometrium in the uterine body continues for the next year or so, so that soon the uterine body becomes twice the length of cervix (ratio of body to cervix 2:1). The vaginal changes are very marked. The thin, non-stimulated epithelium of the vagina — only a few layers thick in the child — greatly increases to become the stratified squamous epithelium many layers thick of the pubertal girl; the cells are rich in glycogen. Glycogen is acted upon by Döderlein's bacillus to produce lactic acid and the pH of the vagina becomes acidic.

The vulva, too, reacts to the increasing hormone levels of puberty but to a less marked extent.

The endocrinology of puberty

The endocrinology of puberty need not be discussed at length. In general, it may be said that by modern methods of endocrinological assay it is possible to detect all the sex hormones in any child of any age. Towards puberty, there is an increase in the previous low levels and adult levels are reached soon after puberty is complete.

Attention may be drawn to certain specific matters. One of the earliest changes to be evident is an increase in adrenal androgens, which may be related to a decrease in the sensitivity of the hypothalamus and pituitary to oestrogen inhibitory feedback (see below). The pattern of FSH and LH production is curious, and different from that of other hormones. Both FSH and LH are elevated in the plasma during early life, FSH levels remaining high from 2 to 4 years and LH levels high for some 6 months. Levels then fall until close to puberty, when a gradual rise can be discerned. Progesterone remains at a low level until ovulation is established on a regular basis, which is some 2 years or more after the menarche. It must be emphasised that there is much day-to-day variation in the levels of all these hormones.

The initiation of puberty

For many years there has been speculation upon the timing of puberty. Why does it occur when it does, and not sooner or later? Recent work has shown that the hypothalmus and pituitary are capable of activity long before puberty, and the ovary is certainly capable of response to stimulation. The process of puberty appears to be kept in abeyance, and the principal reason for this seems to be the unusual sensitivity of the hypothalmus and pituitary to inhibitory feedback. The very low levels of oestrogen produced by the child's ovary are sufficient to inhibit hypothalamic and pituitary activity until, as puberty approaches, this sensitivity becomes less and puberty changes can appear. The early activity of adrenal androgens has been thought possibly to be concerned with the diminution of hypothalamic pituitary sensitivity.

Higher centres may also be concerned in the inhibition of puberty changes in the young child. The limbic system and the pineal body appear to exercise some inhibitory function in the experimental animal, but it is not known to what extent they do so in the human.

THE MENOPAUSE

The menopause occurs because the ovary no longer has any follicles to respond to hypothalamic/pituitary stimulation. It has been mentioned that, at the menarche, there are some 250 000–300 000 oocytes present, which are gradually used up in the succession of menstrual cycles from that time until around 50 years of age, which is the average age for the menopause in the

Table 7.4   The effects of oestrogen deficiency at the menopause

Release of hypothalamic/pituitary inhibition

Genital tract atrophy

The end of ovulation

Menopausal symptoms

Bone demineralisation

Increased risk of cardiovascular disease

Changes in lipid profile

UK. Ovarian activity then effectively ceases and the changes outlined in Table 7.4 occur.

Release of the hypothalamus and the pituitary from inhibition results in raised FSH and LH characteristic of the menopause and well above those seen in the menstrual cycle at times other than the LH surge. These elevated levels persist for 10 years or more, then slowly decline.

The genital organs undergo general atrophic changes. The ovaries become shrunken and fibrous. The uterus and tubes shrink and, in the case of the uterus, the body shrinks to a greater extent than the cervix so that the ratio of the body to cervix becomes 1:1 or even 1:2. The vaginal epithelium shrinks markedly, glycogen disappears from the cells, lactic acid is no longer produced and the environment of the vagina becomes alkaline.

A series of menopausal symptoms arise in many patients, some concerned directly with hormone deficiency, some possibly concerned with ageing, and some emotionally related. Those directly concerned with oestrogen lack are vasomotor symptoms, and vaginal atrophic changes, which can lead to dyspareunia. The extent to which other symptoms are directly associated with oestrogen deprivation is debatable.

Important bone changes occur. Demineralisation of bone is evident and is associated with a rise in serum calcium, phosphate and alkaline phosphatase, whilst the urinary calcium:creatinine ratio and the phosphate:creatinine ratio are also raised. There is a greater diminution in bone mineral mass in women over 50 years of age than in men of the same age, which is reflected in a greater liability to fractures.

Cardiovascular changes are evident too. Premenopausal women appear to have some immunity from coronary thrombosis and anginal attacks, which may be causally related to their different lipid background when compared with men. After the menopause, all lipid levels rise; the level of triglyceride increases by 44% and that of cholesterol by 30%. High-density lipoprotein (HDL) cholesterol (which protects against cardiovascular disease) increases by 11% and low-density lipoprotein (LDL) cholesterol increases by 36%. The oral contraceptive pill which has been incriminated as a risk factor for cardiovascular diseases increases triglyceride concentration by 50% and cholesterol concentration by 5–7%. In combined oral contraception preparations this increase is due to an increase in LDL cholesterol with little change in HDL cholesterol.

THE ADRENAL GLANDS

The adrenal glands consist of two parts, the cortex and medulla, which are embryologically and functionally quite unrelated. Bilateral adrenalectomy is rapidly fatal unless the hormones of the cortex are administered: the medulla is not essential to life.

The adrenal cortex

Structure

The adrenal cortex consists of three distinct zones. The outermost is the zona glomerulosa; the middle one, the zona fasciculata, is the widest and consists of cells filled with lipids (mainly cholesterol esters). The innermost is the zona reticularis which has clear cells. The zona fasciculata and zona reticularis are controlled by ACTH and are concerned with the secretion of cortisol (and other steroids). The zona glomerulosa which produces aldosterone is under the control of the renin-angiotensin system.

Hormones of the adrenal cortex

The steroid hormones of the adrenal cortex are of three types:

1. The glucocorticoids (notably cortisol), which are involved in the control of protein, carbohydrate and lipid metabolism
2. The mineralocorticoids (notably aldosterone), which are involved in electrolyte and water balance
3. Sex steroids — both androgens and oestrogens, which are important at the time of puberty, during reproductive life and after the menopause.

All the steroids have a similar mode of action on their respective target tissue. They first bind to a receptor in the cytosol of the cell. The steroid–receptor complex enters the nucleus and binds to chromatin. RNA synthesis is stimulated and, following this, protein (including enzyme) production is modified. These changes then produce the effects of the hormone.

Biosynthesis of adrenal steroids

All steroid hormones have the same basic ring structure of 17 carbon atoms but with different added groups. Oestrogens have one extra methyl group and androgens, two, to give 18 and 19 carbon atoms respectively. Glucocorticoids and mineralocorticoids all have 21 carbon atoms, as does progesterone. Biosynthesis is from acetate via a complex sequence of reactions leading to cholesterol (with 27 carbon atoms) which is stored in steroid-producing cells. This is converted to pregnenolone and progesterone and thence to other biologically active steroids. Glucocorticoids are built from progesterone by a sequence of hydroxylations — at carbons 17, 21 and 11. Aldosterone is formed by hydroxylation of progesterone at carbons 21 and 11 (not 17) then hydroxylation at carbon 18 followed by oxidation to an aldehyde. The adrenal produces many androgenic steroids, including testosterone and androstenedione, but the main ones are dehydro-epiandrosterone (DHA) and its sulphate (DHAS). DHAS production is particularly important in the fetal adrenal — from the fetal zone which regresses after birth. DHAS is a substrate for oestriol synthesis by the fetoplacental unit in pregnancy. The adrenal cortex also secretes small amounts of oestrogen, particularly oestrone.

Functions of adrenal steroids

1. The glucocorticoids (notably cortisol) have metabolic actions which are, in general, catabolic and antagonistic to those of insulin. In the circulation, the levels of glucose, fatty acids and amino acids are increased. In muscle and fat tissue, glucose uptake and glycolysis are decreased and protein breakdown to amino acids is increased. There is increased lipolysis and decreased lipogenesis in fat tissue. In the liver, gluconeogenesis, protein synthesis and glycogen formation are all increased. In addition to these metabolic effects, the glucocorticoids have other actions: anti-inflammatory, immunosuppressive, on bone (osteoporotic action), and some mineralocorticoid action (to increase sodium reabsorption by the renal tubules).

2. Aldosterone is about 1000 times more active as a mineralocorticoid, than is cortisol. It causes sodium retention and potassium loss by the kidney (see p. 183). Extracellular fluid and blood volumes are increased.

3. Androgens of adrenal origin contribute about half the circulating androgens in normal females. They are particularly important during the initiation of puberty and as a source of oestrogen precursors after the menopause.

Regulation of secretion of adrenal steroids

1. The biosynthesis and release of the corticosteroids is under the control of pituitary ACTH, which in turn is regulated by corticotrophin-releasing hormone (CRH) from the hypothalamus. ACTH stimulates the conversion of cholesterol to progenenolone and also later biosynthetic steps. Pituitary ACTH and hypothalamic CRH are under the negative-feedback control of cortisol: when its secretion is reduced (e.g. in congenital adrenal hyperplasia) then ACTH is increased. There are two controlling factors which are superimposed upon this feedback. There is a basic diurnal rhythm of CRH–ACTH–cortisol secretion, which is maximal in the early hours of the morning and which is entrained by light/dark and activity/rest patterns. Secondly, the hypothalamus–pituitary–adrenal axis is involved in the response to stress (e.g. infection, emotion, hypoglycaemia, surgery).

2. The secretion of aldosterone is increased by sodium lack, potassium excess or a reduction in the extracellular fluid volume. Receptors that detect changes in blood volume are located in the juxtaglomerular apparatus in the walls of afferent arterioles in the kidney. These respond to decreased arterial pressure and renal blood flow and produce an enzyme, renin. This in turn converts a large plasma protein, angiotensinogen, to angiotensin I in plasma; angiotensin I is converted to angiotensin II which stimulates aldosterone secretion from the zona glomerulosa of the adrenal cortex (see also p. 172).

3. Adrenal androgens are to some extent controlled by pituitary ACTH but there may also be other, still unidentified, factors.

Transport and metabolism of adrenal steroids

1. Over 90% of cortisol is bound with high affinity to a circulating globulin, corticosteroid-binding globulin (CBG, transcortin). Only the free, unbound fraction is able to enter cells and it is this fraction which is biologically active and responsible for the negative feedback. CBG is increased by oestrogens (e.g. during pregnancy). Corticosteroids are metabolised in the liver and excreted as water-soluble conjugates (mainly glucuronides) in urine. These metabolities can be measured as 17-oxogenic steroids (17-ketogenic steroids is the former term for the same substances; in the USA the term 17-hydroxycorticoids is used).

2. Aldosterone is also excreted in the urine, partly as metabolites, partly unchanged.

3. The androgens are partly bound to the carrier protein sex hormone-binding globulin (SHBG) and are excreted as metabolites called 17-oxosteroids (17-ketosteroids is the former name for these: they should not be confused with 17-oxogenic steroids).

Test of adrenal function

1. Plasma cortisol levels show a diurnal variation: measurements are made at 08:00

hours and midnight to evaluate this; total cortisol output is measured by estimating 24-hour urinary cortisol.

2. The adrenal responsiveness can be tested by an ACTH stimulation test: this is now done with Synacthen — a synthetic ACTH molecule with a rapid action.

3. Insulin-induced hypoglycaemia is used to test the function of the hypothalamic–pituitary control system.

4. Suppression tests (e.g. with dexamethasone) are used to diagnose conditions of cortisol over-production.

Abnormalities of adrenal function

1. Hypofunction — Addison's disease. In the past, tuberculosis was the most common cause: now it is normally part of an autoimmune disease.

2. Hypersecretion of cortisol causes Cushing's syndrome. This may be of pituitary origin, or caused by an adrenal tumour. Other causes include ectopic ACTH secretion by certain tumours (especially of bronchus) and iatrogenic corticosteroid therapy.

3. Excess androgen secretion can be caused by adrenal tumours (adenomas or, more rarely, carcinomas) or by

4. Congenital adrenal hyperplasia. In this group of conditions there is a congenital lack or deficiency in one of the enzymes involved in cortisol biosynthesis. The most common defect is in the 21-hydroxylase enzyme. The reduced cortisol production leads to excess ACTH secretion (negative feedback is lessened) which stimulates the adrenal gland to produce more steroids especially 17-hydroxyprogesterone, which is the steroid immediately before the 21-hydroxylase block, and androgens which then have a masculinising effect.

The adrenal medulla

Structure

The adrenal medulla is part of the sympathetic nervous system derived from neuroectoderm. The cells are stainable with chromic acid (chromaffin tissue) and are richly supplied with sympathetic nerve fibres from the greater splanchnic nerve.

Hormones of the adrenal medulla

Two catecholamines are present in the adrenal medulla, adrenaline and noradrenalin, in the ratio of about 4:1. These are synthesised from the amino acid tyrosine by the following sequence of reactions:

$$\text{Tyrosine} \rightarrow \text{Dihydroxyphenylalanine (DOPA)} \rightarrow$$
$$\text{Dopamine} \rightarrow \text{Noradrenalin} \rightarrow \text{Adrenaline}$$

The catecholamines are metabolised by two enzyme mechanisms: the monamine oxidase and the catechol-*o*-methyltransferase (COMT). One of the principal metabolities is vanillylmandelic acid (VMA); other metabolites are known collectively as metanephrines.

Actions of adrenaline and noradrenalin

Adrenaline stimulates both α and β receptors in tissues whereas noradrenalin acts almost entirely on α receptors. These are described on pages 201 and 202. In addition these hormones have the following metabolic actions:

1. In the liver, adrenaline increases glycogen breakdown by increasing cyclic adenosine monophosphate (cAMP) levels which results in a conversion of the enzyme phosphorylase from its inactive to active form. This action is similar to, but less potent than, that of glucagon.

2. In muscle, adrenaline has a similar effect on glycogen breakdown (and is much more active than glucagon in the tissue).

3. In fat tissue, adrenaline increases lipolysis and the circulating levels of free fatty acids and glycerol. The fatty acids act as a fuel in muscle and a source of glucose (by gluconeogenesis in the liver).

4. In the pancreas, adrenaline inhibits insulin release.

THE THYROID GLAND

The major role of the thyroid gland is to secrete iodinated thyronines, i.e. thyroxine (T_4) and tri-iodothyronine (T_3). In addition, the C cells produce calcitonin, a hormone which decreases the level of calcium in the blood. Thyroxine has widespread effects in stimulating oxygen consumption and other metabolic processes. In young animals, thyroxine is essential for normal growth and maturation.

The structures of mono- and diiodotyrosine are shown in Fig. 7.16. Of the two isomers of T_4, only L-thyroxine is found in vivo. T_3 is more potent than T_4 (Table 7.5). Although it is present in blood in much smaller quantities than T_4, it is less highly protein bound. This, together with the increased potency of T_3, means that T_3 is responsible for more peripheral activity than is T_4 (Table 7.5).

Iodine metabolism (see Fig. 7.17)

Iodine is absorbed from the gut as iodide. A minimum of 790–1180 nmol/day is necessary to balance urinary loss, and the small amounts secreted in the bile and lost in the faeces.

From the pool of iodide in the blood, about 590 nmol are trapped each day in the thyroid cells, under the influence of TSH. This is a highly efficient system since the thyroid-to-plasma iodide concentration ratio can exceed 100. Within the thyroid gland, iodide is oxidised to iodine under the control of a peroxidase enzyme, and reacts with tyrosine molecules of thryoglobulin in the thyroid colloid. The iodine first reacts with tyrosine to form monoiodotyrosine (MIT) and then another iodine atom reacts with MIT to form diiodotyrosine (DIT) (Fig. 7.16). Two molecules of DIT are condensed to form T_4. One molecule of MIT is condensed with one molecule of DIT to

Table 7.5   Relative binding of T_4 and T_3 to plasma proteins and its effect on their activities

	T_4	T_3
Total in serum	50 nmol/l	1 nmol/l
Fraction bound		
TBG[a]	85%	75%
TBPA[b]	14%	0
Albumin	0.95%	24.5%
Fraction free	0.05%	0.5%
Total free	25 pmol/l	5 pmol/l
Potency of free hormone[c]	1	8
Activity (total free × potency)	25	40

[a] TBG, thyroxine-binding globulin.
[b] TBPA, thyroxine-binding prealbumin.
[c] Potency, calorigenic effect and prevention of goitre in propylthiouracil-treated animals.

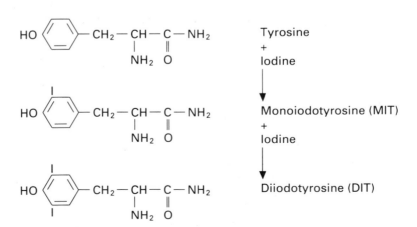

Fig. 7.16   The structure of monoiodotyrosine and diiodotyrosine

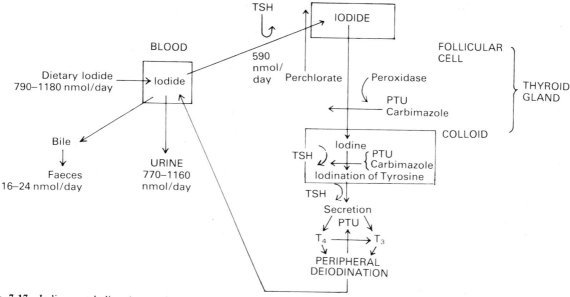

Fig. 7.17   Iodine metabolism (see text).

form T_3. The alternative, reverse T_3, is formed by the condensation of one molecule of DIT with one molecule of MIT. T_4 is the hormone that is secreted in greatest proportion. Reverse T_3 has much less metabolic activity than T_4 and very much less than T_3. It is secreted in large quantities by the fetal thyroid gland; it is not known why the fetus pursues this alternative metabolic pathway. Some peripheral conversion of T_4 to T_3 and to reverse T_3 by deiodination also occurs. Once they are liberated from the thyroid gland, thyroid hormones are very strongly protein bound (see Table 7.5). In somatic cells the hormones are metabolised and the liberated iodide returns to the peripheral pool.

Antithyroid drugs

Antithyroid drugs, such as carbimazole and propylthiouracil, prevent the peroxidase oxidisation of iodide to iodine within the thyroid gland, the iodination of tyrosine, and the release of T_4 and T_3. Propylthiouracil also prevents the peripheral deiodination of T_4. Perchlorate prevents uptake of iodide by the follicular cell. The mechanism whereby large doses of iodine inhibit T_4 and T_3 synthesis in hyperthyroid patients, and cause involution of the thyroid gland, is unknown.

Iodine will only suppress thyroid activity for about 10 days.

Control of thyroid secretion

The thyroid gland is controlled by TSH secreted from the anterior pituitary gland (Fig. 7.18). There is a direct negative-feedback process whereby increasing circulating levels of T_4 and T_3 decrease pituitary TSH secretion and vice versa. In addition, TSH secretion is increased by thyrotrophin-releasing hormone (TRH) passing down the neurohypophysial portal system from the hypothalamus. TSH secretion is decreased by

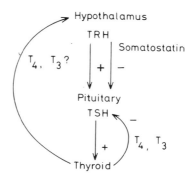

Fig. 7.18   Feedback control mechanisms of the thyroid gland.

somatostatin, also liberated from the hypothalamus. It is not known whether TRH or somatostatin release are affected by T_4 and T_3 levels at the hypothalamus.

Thyroid function tests

The original (out-dated) tests of thyroid function involved measurement of basal metabolic rate (BMR). This was a difficult procedure, and the BMR was affected by numerous other agents than thyroid status. Next came measurement of protein-bound iodide (PBI) and a dynamic assessment of iodine uptake by the thyroid gland, using external counting of γ radiation after administration of an appropriate isotope of iodine, usually[131] I. The PBI which reflected total T_4 and T_3 was very much dependent on the level of thyroxine-binding globulin (TBG), which varies considerably, particularly increasing in pregnancy and in patients taking oestrogen-containing contraceptives. In addition, administration of iodine-containing contrast media, such as are used for intravenous pyelography, will cause a marked elevation of PBI. The PBI and iodine uptake tests have been largely, but not completely, superseded by measurement of the free thyroxine index (FTI), or, more recently, free thyroxine (FT_4).

Radioactive iodine should not be used in pregnancy because of the danger of inducing hypothyroidism in the fetus, or causing carcinoma of the thyroid later in the child's life. Iodide is secreted in high concentration in breast milk, so that radioactive iodine should not be given to lactating mothers.

Measurement of the FTI entails a measurement of total T_4 by radioimmunoassay. The total T_4 is then adjusted to give a free thyroxine index by allowing for the in vitro uptake of T_3 by the patient's red cells. If the quantity of binding protein is increased, there will be more alternative binding sites available for T_3 on red cells. The T_3 uptake test is thus an in vitro compensation, and gives no information about the level of free T_3 in the patient's blood. This can be measured by a separate immunoassay.

Thyroid function in pregnancy

The thyroid gland enlarges in many people during pregnancy. This is largely due to the increased glomerular filtration rate (see p. 185), which increases the amount of iodide secreted in the urine. Plasma inorganic iodide falls, and the thyroid gland increases in size to maintain a normal iodine uptake. This may be entirely due to increased TSH secretion; alternatively, hCG, which has thyroid-stimulating function, may contribute. In the USA, where iodised table salt is commonly used, and in Iceland, where the intake of dietary iodide from fish is very high, plasma inorganic iodide levels do not fall appreciably in pregnancy, and goitre is no more common in the pregnant than the non-pregnant population. Goitre in pregnancy may therefore indicate mild iodine deficiency.

The placenta can also trap iodine, and maintain a placenta-to-plasma iodide concentration ratio of up to 50.

In the fetus, T_4 can be detected in the serum from before 18 weeks' gestation, and TSH in the pituitary gland from 14 weeks. There is a 10-fold increase in TSH levels within minutes of birth, probably due to cold exposure, so that TSH levels are markedly higher in the newborn than in its mother.

The placenta is impermeable to maternal T_4, T_3 and TSH in the second half of pregnancy; therefore, at this time the fetus is autonomous so far as thyroid function is concerned. Cretinism is an irreversible form of mental retardation associated with the congenital absence of the thyroid gland, or very severe maternal iodine deficiency. In addition, antithyroid drugs, such as carbimazole, do cross the placenta, and can cause hypothyroidism, or, in extreme cases, cretinism. Thyroid-stimulating immunoglobulins, thought to be responsible for maternal hyperthyroidism, can also cross the placenta and cause neonatal hyperthyroidism.

Carbimazole is secreted in breast milk and should only be taken with caution by lactating mothers. Propylthiouracil is probably safe, but the newborn infant should still be carefully observed for possible hypothyroidism.

and hypercalcaemia. In addition, it has recently been recognised that impotence is a relatively common side-effect of diuretics.

Vasodilators

Hydralazine

This drug is an arterial vasodilator but the mechanism of its action at a cellular level is not known. Hydralazine is metabolised by acetylation. Patients who are 'slow acetylators' and therefore have higher blood levels of hydralazine are particularly prone to develop the hydralazine-induced lupus syndrome.

Calcium-entry blockers

These drugs reduce calcium flux through voltage-operated channels on the cell membrane by acting at specific receptors. The calcium antagonists are a chemically diverse group of drugs and this is reflected in their differing actions. The dihydropyridines (nifedipine, nicardipine, nimodipine, etc.) have little if any direct action on the heart but are arterial vasodilators. Nimodipine is relatively selective within the arterial system for the cerebral vessels. Verapamil and diltiazem belong to a different chemical group and have more predominant cardiac actions. They have negative inotropic effects and verapamil also has antiarrhythmic properties.

Adverse effects of calcium antagonists are largely predictable from their pharmacological action, e.g. headaches and peripheral oedema. Verapamil should not be given with β blockers since serious conduction defects can result. By contrast, the other calcium antagonists are frequently given with a β blocker in the management of hypertension.

α adrenoceptor antagonists

Drugs in this group include prazosin, terazosin and doxazosin. They act on α_1 receptors in both arteries and veins to produce vasodilation. There are other drugs which produce vasodilatation but not by a direct action on blood vessels.

α_2 receptor agonists

Stimulation of α_2 receptors in the brain stem leads to a reduction in sympathetic outflow. Both methyldopa and clonidine act by this mechanism. Clonidine is itself an α_2 agonist while methyldopa is metabolised to α-methylnoradrenaline, which is also an α_2 agonist. Clonidine is rarely used partly because its abrupt withdrawal can lead to severe rebound hypertension and partly because it causes drowsiness and dry mouth. Methyldopa is not often used in non-obstetric practice but it still has a definite place in hypertensive diseases of pregnancy (see below). It, too, causes drowsiness. In addition, methyldopa can produce postural hypotension, a positive direct antiglobulin test (Coombs' test) and can sometimes produce haemolytic anaemia. It is also a rare cause of hepatitis.

Angiotensin-converting enzyme (ACE) inhibitors

The ACE inhibitors prevent the formation of angiotensin II from angiotensin I by enzyme inhibition (e.g. captopril, enalopril and lisinopril). This leads to vasodilatation by reducing angiotensin II formation (angiotensin is a potent vasoconstrictor). Also, since angiotensin II leads to aldosterone release, the use of ACE inhibitors also results in reduced salt and water retention. The fall in blood pressure produced by ACE inhibitors is not accompanied by a reflex tachycardia, indicating a mechanism of action perhaps more complex than simply reduced angiotensin II formation.

The main adverse effects are a profound fall in blood pressure, which occurs particularly in people who are salt and water depleted, and also a dry cough. ACE inhibitors also have potassium-sparing effects (by reducing aldosterone formation).

The use of ACE inhibitors in pregnancy is contraindicated because of fears about the fetus.

Antimicrobials

Penicillins and cephalosporins

These two drug groups share a common structure — the β-lactam ring — which is responsible for their mechanism of action, which is to inhibit bacterial cell wall synthesis. These drugs are therefore bactericidal.

Both immediate and delayed hypersensitivity can occur with these drugs and there is approximately 10% cross-reactivity between penicillin and cephalosporins in this regard. Diarrhoea is a particularly common side-effect with ampicillin. An unusual side-effect is that most patients with infectious mononucleosis or chronic lymphocytic leukaemia who are put on ampicillin develop a rash. Some of the older cephalosporins, such as cephaloradin, can cause renal damage (and this is potentiated by loop diuretics and aminoglycosides). Cephalosporins can reduce prothrombin concentration. In addition, cephalosporins can cause false-positive urinalysis tests for glucose.

Ampicillin has been reported to cause oral contraceptive failure and to potentiate the anticoagulant effect of warfarin. It is probable that both effects result directly or indirectly from the effect of ampicillin on gut flora.

Aminoglycosides

These drugs are bactericidal and act at the level of the ribosome. They are not absorbed from the normal gastrointestinal tract. Aminoglycosides have two important adverse effects. They are both concentration related. First, the drugs can cause nephrotoxicity by tubular destruction. Secondly, eighth nerve damage can occur. The nephrotoxicity is enhanced by cephaloridine (see above) and the ototoxicity by loop diuretics. Aminoglycosides can lead to neuromuscular blockade after rapid injection (particularly in patients with myasthenia gravis) and can prolong the action of curare.

Other antimicrobials

Suphonamide/trimethoprim combinations inhibit two consecutive steps in folate metabolism: p-amino benzoic acid to folate (sulphonamide) and folate to tetrahydrofolate (trimethoprim). The drugs are therefore bactericidal. Because of the sulphonamide component, these drugs can cause allergic reactions, the Stevens–Johnson syndrome or renal failure, and both constituents can cause blood dyscrasias. Sulphonamides given in the new-born period can displace bilirubin from protein and result in kernicterus. Sulphonamides are important inhibitors of liver enzymes and can potentiate the actions of phenytoin, tolbutamide and warfarin. Sulphonamides can also precipitate methotrexate toxicity by a protein-binding interaction.

Erythromycin has a similar spectrum of activity to penicillin and is therefore used in patients who are penicillin sensitive. It occasionally causes cholestatic jaundice with prolonged use.

The tetracyclines are bacteriostatic. Their most important adverse effect concerns binding to calcium, leading to impaired bone growth and discoloured teeth, both in utero and in children up to the age of around 7 years. Both liver and renal failure have been reported, the former only with parenteral therapy.

Antituberculous drugs

Isoniazid is an enzyme inhibitor (see sulphonamide above). Rifampicin is an enzyme inducer and can reduce the efficacy of oral contraceptives, warfarin and sulphonylureas.

Ethambutol can cause retrobulbar neuritis.

Antiviral drugs

The most important advance in antiviral therapy has been the development of acyclovir, which, unlike previous antiviral drugs, is not uniformly toxic to all cells in the body. Acyclovir is itself inactive but is metabolised by a herpes simplex specified enzyme (thymidine kinase) to acyclovir triphosphate, which prevents further DNA synthesis. Acyclovir therefore only has an effect in cells containing herpes virus. Acyclovir is not teratogenic.

Oral contraceptives

Drugs which contain both oestrogen and progestogen inhibit ovulation: oestrogen inhibits the release of follicle-stimulating hormone and progestogen the release of luteinising hormone. Drugs containing only progestogen alter cervical mucosa and the endometrium but do not inhibit ovulation so effectively.

Oral contraceptives influence the coagulation system by decreasing antithrombin III and plasminogen activator and by increasing platelet activation. The contraceptive pill is associated with both venous and arterial thromboembolism, although the risk factors for this association are different on the two sides of the circulation. The risk of venous thrombosis is increased by increasing oestrogen dose and by immobility such as surgical procedures. The risk of myocardial infarction and stroke is increased by age (particularly in excess of 35 years) and by cigarette smoking. In the case of venous thromboembolism the risk increases soon after starting the pill, stays constant during use and returns to normal very soon after the pill has been stopped. In the case of myocardial infarction and stroke, the risk continues for an undetermined length of time after the pill has been stopped.

There is a statistically significant rise in blood pressure in all women taking oral contraceptive but in the majority of cases this is of no clinical importance. Rarely there is a substantial elevation of blood pressure, which returns to normal 3–6 months after stopping the pill. The pill has various metabolic effects. Glucose tolerance is slightly reduced and high-density lipoproteins are changed (increased by oestrogen and decreased by progestogen). Whether any of these metabolic changes are of clinical significance is unknown.

There are several common but relatively minor side-effects such as irregular bleeding, headaches and changes in mood. Migraine can sometimes get worse in women on the pill and focal migraine is usually an indication for stopping the oral contraceptive because of the risk of residual neurological deficit. Cholestatic jaundice is a rare complication. The pill increases thyroid-binding globulin concentration and therefore increases the total concentration of thyroxine. The free thyroxine level is not affected.

The relationship between oral contraceptives and cancer is controversial. Endometrial and ovarian carcinoma are less frequent in women taking the pill. There is an association between pill use and cervical neoplasia, but a cause–effect relationship is doubted by many, with the number of sexual partners possibly being the major aetiological factor. There have been claims that oral contraceptive use below the age of 20 years can lead to breast carcinoma at a relatively early age but this question is still substantially unresolved.

There are several important drug interactions involving the oral contraceptive. Drugs which can lead to pill failure by enzyme induction include phenytoin, carbamazepine, phenobarbitone, primidone and rifampicin. Note that sodium valproate is not included in this list. Broad-spectrum antibiotics (e.g. ampicillin) can also cause pill failure. This is believed to be the result of interrupting the enterohepatic circulation of the oral contraceptive.

Anticoagulants and antiplatelet drugs

Heparin is a large (molecular weight 15 000) highly acidic molecule. These chemical properties explain why it does not cross the placenta. Low concentrations of heparin, such as those achieved following subcutaneous low-dose administration, enhance antithrombin activity. Larger doses of heparin also bind irreversibly to thrombin. In addition to the obvious side-effect of bleeding (reversed by protamine sulphate), long-term heparin treatment can also produce oesteoporosis.

Warfarin inhibits the synthesis of vitamin K-dependent clotting factors II, VII, IX and X. It is highly protein bound and is eliminated by metabolism; both these factors make it a target for drug interactions. The anticoagulant effect of warfarin is reduced by the enzyme induction effects of rifampicin, griseofulvin, barbiturates, phenytoin and carbamazepine. Vitamin K also reduces the anticoagulant effect. The anticoagulant effect is increased by cimetidine and sulphonamides (enzyme inhibition) and by broad-spectrum antibiotics (reduced vitamin K absorption).

Aspirin covalently and irreversibly binds to the enzyme cyclooxygenase. This action occurs preferentially in platelets, thereby leading to a reduction in thromboxane A_2 production. The same enzyme is responsible in endothelial cells for producing prostacyclin but low-dose aspirin has less effect on this pathway. The reason for this differentiation is unclear at present. Aspirin therefore inhibits platelet aggregation by preventing thromboxane A_2 production. Aspirin undergoes about 50% first-pass metabolism and it is likely that most of this antiplatelet effect occurs in the portal circulation. Even in low doses aspirin can produce gastric erosions and bleeding. This problem is, however, less common than with higher doses.

Note that when used in analgesic doses within 5 days before delivery aspirin can produce haemostatic problems in the neonate.

Dipyridamole is a phosphodiesterase inhibitor which prevents platelet aggregation by increasing cyclic adenosine monophosphate levels. Clinical trials have failed to demonstrate that dipyridamole and aspirin in combination confers any benefit above that of aspirin alone.

ANALGESIA AND ANAESTHESIA

Opioid analgesics

Morphine is an agonist at the μ subtype opioid receptor. In addition to analgesia, morphine produces a sense of euphoria or detachment and it also has sedative properties. Adverse effects associated with acute administration include respiratory depression, hypotension, increase in vasopressin release, decrease in pupil size, nausea and vomiting. The hypotension produced by morphine is more marked on standing and is not accompanied by a reflex tachycardia. Morphine also produces decreased motility in the gastrointestinal tract which produces constipation in long-term use. Morphine causes histamine release: this is probably not relevant to its cardiovascular properties but it may on occasion contribute to some bronchoconstriction.

Diamorphine (heroin) is more potent on a weight-for-weight basis than morphine and has a high lipid solubility.

Codeine is another opioid but considerably less potent than morphine or heroin. Codeine suppresses cough and decreases gut motility.

Pethidine is a synthetic opioid with a more rapid onset and shorter duration than morphine or heroin. It is said to cause less smooth muscle contraction than the other opioids. Pethidine is metabolised to an active metabolite (norpethidine) which undergoes renal excretion and can accumulate in patients with renal disease.

Buprenorphine has antagonist as well as agonist properties at the opioid receptor. It has some interesting differences to the other opioids. In particular, it has less dependence potential and

also its effects on the respiratory system are not so easily reversed by naloxone, as are the effects of the other opioids.

Naloxone is an opioid antagonist, which at the dosage used clinically is specific for the μ receptor. Naloxone is a pure antagonist and has no agonist activity. At the dosage used clinically, naloxone has no pharmacological effects when given on its own.

Local anaesthetics

Lignocaine is a sodium channel blocker which delays nerve conduction by this mechanism. It is also an antiarrhythmic agent. In systemic overdose lignocaine can produce serious problems, including myocardial depression and convulsions.

Other local anaesthetics such as bupivacaine and prilocaine differ from lignocaine largely qualitatively rather than in any fundamental pharmacological manner.

Inhalation anaesthetic agents

Nitrous oxide does not produce surgical anaesthesia on its own and is therefore used in combination with other drugs. It can rarely cause bone marrow depression if used for extended periods.

Halothane can cause myocardial and respiratory depression. Hepatotoxicity is a rare problem, particularly associated with repeated exposures.

Neuromuscular blocking drugs

Suxamethonium prolongs neuromuscular depolarisation. The duration of action is short and the drug is normally broken down by plasma cholinesterase. Some patients have a genetically specified abnormality in this enzyme and in these cases paralysis is considerably prolonged. Suxamethonium can cause bradycardia, painful muscles and an increase in intraocular pressure.

Tubocurarine is a competitive antagonist at the acetylcholine receptor. The drug is eliminated by the kidneys and accumulation can occur in renal impairment. Tubocurarine can cause histamine release, leading to hypotension. The interaction with aminoglycosides has been mentioned above.

DRUGS WHICH INFLUENCE UTERINE ACTIVITY

Prostaglandins

These are 20-carbon-atom polyunsaturated fatty acids which are derived from arachidonic acid. This is converted by cyclooxygenase to an endoperoxide intermediate which can then be converted by different steps to various prostaglandins, including PGE_2, $PGF_{2\alpha}$, thromboxane A_2 and PGI_2 (prostacyclin). Most current scientific interest centres on these last two prostaglandins with respect to their involvement in platelet and vascular function. However, it is the first two which are relevant to uterine contractility.

PGE_2 and $PGF_{2\alpha}$ stimulate myometrial activity, both in the non-pregnant and pregnant uterus. Myometrial sensitivity to prostaglandins increases in the third trimester. Prostaglandins cause disaggregation of collagen fibres in the cervix.

Systemic administration of prostaglandins leads to a variety of unpleasant side-effects, including hypothermia, gastrointestinal cramping, diarrhoea, nausea and vomiting. In high doses, $PGF_{2\alpha}$ has a positive inotropic effect and PGE_2 produces vasodilatation as the predominant cardiovascular action.

Oxytocin

This drug stimulates uterine activity only towards the end of pregnancy, with maximum effects occurring after the membranes have ruptured. It is likely that oxytocin requires the presence of prostaglandins for its myometrial activity.

High doses of oxytocin can lead first to a fall in blood pressure with tachycardia followed by a rise in blood pressure with bradycardia. The drug has antidiuretic properties even at modest doses, probably related to its structural similarity to vasopressin.

β_2 adrenoceptor agonists

This group of drugs suppress myometrial activity and are used in preterm labour. The drugs most commonly used are ritodrine, salbutamol and terbutaline. The last two are also commonly used in aerosol form in the management of asthma. The pharmacological properties of the β_2 agonists are largely predictable. They increase the heart rate (because receptor selectivity is not absolute and there is a good deal of overlap at the β_1 receptor) and they cause peripheral vasodilatation by stimulating the β_2 receptors in the peripheral vasculature. These drugs can also cause tremor. The two major metabolic effects are an increase in serum glucose and a fall in serum potassium, resulting from a shift of potassium from extra- to intracellular sites.

Combination of β_2 agonists with steroids has been responsible for cases of pulmonary oedema, although the exact mechanism has never been elucidated. Prolonged use of β_2 agonists can rarely lead to cardiomyopathy in the mother. The fetal heart rate increases.

DRUGS IN PREGNANCY

Placental transfer

The only commonly used drugs which do *not* cross the placenta are heparin and curare. Heparin is both a large molecule and highly polar, and curare does not cross purely because of its polarity. The rate of transfer across the placenta is relevant only in the case of drugs given during delivery and it is not a consideration when a course of drug treatment is being administered before labour, for under these circumstances most drugs equilibrate between maternal and fetal compartments.

Influence of pregnancy on dose requirements

The physiological changes of pregnancy can influence pharmacokinetics. Fluid retention and decreased protein concentration will tend to increase volume of distribution with consequent decrease in plasma concentration. In addition, some liver metabolic pathways are induced and renal blood flow increases substantially.

Anticonvulsants show the most dramatic changes, with clinically important increases in clearance having been reported for phenytoin, phenobarbitone, carbamazepine and sodium valproate. The main factor involved in anticonvulsant pharmacokinetics is an increase in drug clearance. Plasma levels fall significantly. Since some of the fall is due to a decrease in binding protein, the free and metabolically active concentration of the drug does not fall so much.

Lithium and ampicillin are both eliminated by the kidney and their clearance increases by around 100% during pregnancy with the necessity for increased dose requirements (except obviously in the treatment of urinary tract infections).

Teratogenic drugs

Anticonvulsants that are currently used all appear to be teratogenic. Phenytoin causes a variety of abnormalities, including cleft lip/palate, microcephaly, hypertelorism and fingernail hyperplasia. Growth deficiency also occurs. Phenytoin teratogenicity appears to be at least in part genetically determined, tending to 'run true' in successive pregnancies and occurring in only one of a pair of dizygotic twins. Sodium valproate is associated with neural tube defect. Carbamazepine causes a range of defects similar to those seen with phenytoin, possibly because both drugs are metabolised to the same highly reactive intermediate substances known as arene oxides. The incidence of fetal abnormality with anticonvulsant use does not exceed 10%. There is quite persuasive evidence that epilepsy itself is associated with a higher than normal occurrence of fetal abnormality, irrespective of drug treatment.

Lithium causes cardiac abnormalities when given during the first trimester, of which the most frequent is Ebstein's anomaly.

Warfarin causes problems throughout pregnancy. When given during the first trimester it is associated with chondrodysplasia punctata with abnormalities of bone and cartilage formation. It also causes microcephaly, asplenia and diaphragmatic hernia. Later in pregnancy, intracerebral microhaemorrhage can lead to mental retardation and optic atrophy (blindness).

Retinoic acids are vitamin A analogues used in the treatment of severe systemic acne and other chronic dermatoses. These drugs cause major malformations, including craniofacial, cardiac, thymic and central nervous system defects.

Diethylstilboestrol, when given during pregnancy is associated with adenocarcinoma of the vagina in the female offspring. *Danazol* (which is not a contraceptive agent) causes virilisation of the female fetus.

Drugs given later in pregnancy

Anticonvulsants can cause a neonatal coagulation defect which is thought to be the result of vitamin K deficiency. It can be prevented by giving vitamin K. The coagulation defect is associated with increased levels of a substance called PIVKA (protein induced by vitamin K absence), both in the mother and the neonate.

Heparin can cause osteoporosis in the mother. Heparin in a dose of 10 000 U/day for more than 20 weeks has been associated with radiological features of bone demineralisation during pregnancy and occasionally with symptoms due to rib fracture or vertebral collapse.

Aspirin in analgesic doses can influence haemostasis in the neonate. Aspirin ingestion within 5 days of delivery has been associated with bleeding problems such as pectechiae, haematuria and cephalohaematoma. At the time of writing the use of low-dose aspirin seems not to be associated with this adverse effect.

Indomethacin has been associated with premature closure of ductus arteriosus. Earlier in pregnancy the use of indomethacin as a tocolytic agent has been associated with constriction of the duct, as demonstrated by echocardiography.

Methyldopa has a good safety record in pregnancy, including a paediatric follow-up to 7.5 years.

Drugs and breast feeding

Most commonly used drugs can be safely administered to a mother who is breast feeding, specifically non-narcotic analgesics, pencillins and cephalosporins; methyldopa, β blockers, phenytoin, carbamazepine and sodium valproate should be considered safe.

Some drugs should be avoided during breast feeding: laxatives cause diarrhoea in the neonate; amiodarone (an antiarrhythmic) may adversely affect the neonatal thyroid; indomethacin has been associated with neonatal convulsions; barbiturates can cause drowsiness; benzodiazepines also lead to drowsiness and failure to thrive if given regularly;

lithium has been associated with hypotonia and cyanosis; carbimazole and methimazole can suppress the neonatal thyroid.

Drugs of abuse

Alcohol

Chronic excessive intake of alcohol during pregnancy can cause a fetal syndrome with a broad flat mid-face, flattened nose and short palpebral fissures, pre- and postnatal growth and mental retardation, and sometimes other major anomalies. Most of the cases that have been reported were in the USA and France. Drinking more than 30 ml of ethanol (75 ml of spirits) daily in pregnancy gives the baby some risk of developing the syndrome; with 90 ml of ethanol a day the risk is serious. Suggested mechanisms include the toxic action of the metabolite acetaldehyde, vitamin B deficiency and protein malnutrition. Regular consumption of smaller amounts of alcohol throughout pregnancy may give rise to a small risk of abortion or of intrauterine growth retardation.

Smoking

It is accepted that women who smoke heavily in pregnancy have an increased risk of intrauterine growth retardation and of premature labour; the perinatal mortality is a little increased, probably in consequence. The mechanism may be related to carbon monoxide reducing oxygen carriage or to toxic products, including nicotine itself, in the smoke. The placental vasculature may be affected, and stopping smoking in mid-pregnancy does not improve the fetal prognosis. The chance that the mother may develop pre-eclamptic toxaemia is reduced.

Drugs of addiction

Narcotic addicts have an increased incidence of placental insufficiency, with intrauterine growth retardation and an increase in perinatal mortality. Complete withdrawal in pregnancy gives an increased fetal loss; methadone maintenance improves the fetal prognosis. The newborn baby may suffer from serious withdrawal symptoms. It is difficult to differentiate the effects of a given narcotic from those of other drugs taken concurrently, nutritional deficiencies and virus and other infections to which addicts are liable, and there is no clear evidence that narcotic abuse causes congenital malformations.

For similar reasons it has not been possible to determine whether or not a small number of fetal abnormalities reported in association with lysergic acid diethylamine (LSD) are due to the drug or to associated factors. The minor chromosome abnormalities reported in the newborn of some users of the hallucinogen were not detected in the baby's blood at 3 months of age. There is no evidence that marihuana causes congenital abnormalities in humans.

The evidence with respect to amphetamine abuse and congenital biliary atresia or congenital heart defects is equivocal.

ANTIMITOTIC DRUGS

Introduction

Anticancer drugs are designed to cause cell death, rather than to modify physiological or pathological functions, as do other drugs, and they are frequently toxic—in contrast to, for example, antimicrobial chemotherapy where damage to host cells is usually minimal because of major biochemical differences between host and pathogen.

The alkylating agents

These drugs are derived from a parent substance, nitrogen mustard. They have two (bifunctional) alkylating arms in each molecule, which replace hydrogen atoms in the bases of DNA and can also cause similar alkylation of other cell constituents to inhibit replication.

$$H_3C-N \Big\langle \begin{array}{l} CH_2-CH_2-Cl \\ CH_2-CH_2-Cl \end{array}$$

Nitrogen mustard

Nitrogen mustard is now of very limited use, mainly in the treatment of Hodgkin's disease.

Cyclophosphamide

Cyclophosphamide can be administered intravenously (i.v.) or orally. It is activated by hepatic enzymes and those in the plasma where it has a half-life of 6.5 hours. Excretion is mostly via the faeces but about 27% is excreted into the urine, frequently producing cystitis and occasional haematuria. High-dose intravenous therapy is usually associated with nausea, vomiting and alopecia. It can cause ovarian and testicular destruction which is dose related and its immunosuppressive effects are also used to treat non-malignant conditions such as rheumatoid arthritis. It is of especial interest in its action upon ovarian carcinoma.

Chlorambucil

This is usually given orally. Prolonged continuous administration, as with other alkylating agents, may be associated with profound myelosuppression and even acute leukaemia. Intermittent therapy, e.g. alternate fortnights, reduces these risks considerably. It is well tolerated, with only occasional reports of gastrointestinal upset. Alopecia is uncommon. Its principal uses are in chronic lymphocytic leukaemia and ovarian carcinoma.

Melphalan

L-Phenylalanine mustard was synthesised in the hope of using it against malignant melanoma since phenylalanine is a precursor of melanin. It is administered i.v. or orally with minimal side-effects, except myelosuppression which is common. It has been used extensively in the treatment of myelomatosis, breast and ovarian cancer.

Treosulphan

Treosulphan is converted *in vivo* to L-diepoxybutane and can be administered orally, usually daily in alternate months to minimise myelosuppression and the risk of the development of acute leukaemia, which can occur when any alkylating agent is given continuously for prolonged periods of time. It has shown very good activity in ovarian carcinoma treatment.

Thiotepa

Triethylene thiophosphoramide (thiotepa) acts like an alkylating agent. It is given i.v. and is occasionally given topically, although its intraperitoneal and intrapleural action is not sclerosing and there is little advantage, if any, in this route over the intravenous one. It frequently causes bone marrow suppression, anorexia, nausea and vomiting. It has had widespread use in advanced ovarian cancer, but it has largely been superceded by more effective agents.

Hexamethylmelamine

Although similar in structure to that of the alkylating agent triethylenemelamine, it differs in action. It inhibits the incorporation of precursor into both DNA and RNA. It is orally administered and its main side-effects are nausea, vomiting and diarrhoea. Some patients develop peripheral neuropathies and moderate myelosuppression. It has shown significant activity in the management of ovarian carcinoma, and some activity in tumours of the uterine cervix and endometrium.

Cisplatin

One of a new group of platinum-based cytotoxic agents, *cis*-dichlorodiammineplatinum has a mode of action which is not fully known. It does, however, inhibit DNA synthesis, possibly by cross-linking complementary strands of DNA. In the nucleus it binds preferentially to guanine and therefore might be considered to act like an alkylating agent. It is administered i.v. and is excreted mainly in the urine. Side-effects include nausea and vomiting. Toxicity is dose related and includes moderate myelosuppression and reversible sensory neuropathy. In high doses it will cause kidney damage unless prevented by a forced diuresis during treatment. In combination with vinblastine and bleomycin, it produces prolonged, complete remissions in a large proportion of young men with disseminated testicular tumours. Cisplatin has shown considerable activity in advanced ovarian carcinoma and forms the basis of many treatment schedules for this disease; some potential has been demonstrated for its use in carcinoma of the cervix.

Nitrosoureas

Bischloroethylnitrosourea (BCNU) and cyclohexyl-chloroethylnitrosourea (CCNU) have two chloroethyl arms and act similarly to the bifunctional alkylating agents. They are also myelotoxic and are mainly used in Hodgkin's disease, and because they cross the blood–brain barrier, in intracerebral cancers; they are used infrequently in gynaecological malignancies.

The antimetabolites

Folinic acid analogues

Methotrexate competes with folic acid and inhibits the enzyme dihydrofolate reductase, effectively blocking DNA synthesis. It may be administered orally or i.v. and is excreted in the urine. Reduced renal function increases its concentration and prolongs its half-life. Methotrexate is most useful in fast-replicating tumours, and its toxicity as a consequence results from its effects on the bone marrow and gastrointestinal tract where there are also rapid cell turnovers. High concentrations can be tolerated by patients for a day or so but after 36 hours there is extensive damage to normal tissues. This is often associated with the appearance of diarrhoea and throat ulceration. The duration of effect may be shortened by the administration of folinic acid after about 24 hours, to 'rescue' normal cells. Methotrexate is used extensively in the treatment of trophoblastic disease, and it is of use in advanced carcinoma of the cervix and, occasionally, in vulval carcinoma. In trophoblastic disease, methotrexate administration programmes may be structured around the monitoring of the disease based upon the serum β subunit of human chorionic gonadotrophin levels (Fig. 8.1).

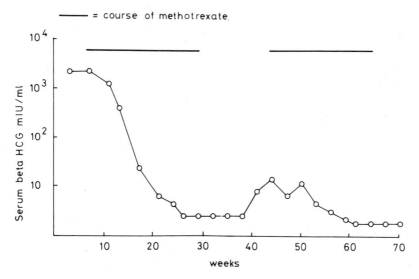

Fig. 8.1 Courses of methotrexate are given depending on the level of the β subunit of human chorionic gonadotrophin (HCG) in the serum. A rise in β-HCG at 40 weeks indicates the necessity for further methotrexate therapy.

Purine analogues

6-Mercaptopurine interferes with the biosynthesis of nucleotides and has use in the treatment of leukaemias. Although unhelpful in the management of solid tumours, its imidazol derivative, azathioprine, has been widely used as an immunosuppressant.

Pyrimidine analogues

5-Fluorouracil blocks the enzyme thymidylate synthetase involved in DNA synthesis. It is administered i.v. or orally and can be applied topically in the form of a paste. Side-effects include nausea, diarrhoea and vomiting, with some alopecia. Toxic effects include bone marrow depression and ulceration of the gastrointestinal tract. 5-Fluorouracil has been used in the palliation of inoperable tumours of the gut and beneficial effects have been reported in advanced tumours of bladder, cervix and ovary.

5-Fluorouracil

Vinca alkaloids

These 'spindle poisons' arrest mitotic division in metaphase by binding to the proteins of the microtubules involved in spindle formation. Administered i.v. the two principal alkaloids have different effects: vinblastine causes marrow depression; vincristine causes neuropathies and is very irritant if extravasated. In combination with other cytotoxics, vinblastine is used in the treatment of Hodgkin's disease, lymphomas, testicular teratoma, and methotrexate resistant chorio-carcinoma whilst vincristine is used in various leukaemias, lymphomas, solid tumours in children, and in cancers of the breast and cervix.

Antibiotics

A variety of antitumour antibiotics have been isolated from *Streptomyces* species.

Actinomycin D

Antinomycin D binds to DNA in the presence of guanine and inhibits RNA synthesis. It is administered i.v.; side-effects include nausea, vomiting, malaise and toxic effects include myelosuppression and gastrointestinal ulceration. It is frequently used in combination with vincristine and cyclophosphamide in the treatment of solid tumours in children, in methotrexate-resistant gestational choriocarcinoma and as an immunosuppressant.

Doxorubicin (adriamycin)

This drug acts by intercalating between base pairs of DNA and inhibiting RNA synthesis by loss of template activity. It is administered i.v. and side-effects include local tissue destruction if extravasated, nausea, vomiting and alopecia. Toxic effects are moderate myelosuppression, and cardiac failure due to cardiomyopathy (dose related). Doxorubicin has shown activity in a wide range of solid tumours, including cancers of the bladder, breast, ovary and cervix.

Bleomycin

The bleomycins are water-soluble glycopeptide antibiotics extracted from cultures of *Streptomyces verticillus*. They cause fractures in single-stranded DNA and inhibit DNA synthesis. Given parenterally, bleomycin causes mucositis, alopecia (10–20% patients), pigmentation of the skin and relatively mild myelosuppression. Pulmonary effects are not uncommon with quite severe fibrosis in some cases. It is used in combination therapy against advanced testicular teratoma and squamous cell carcinomas of the vulva and cervix.

Steroid hormones

Corticosteroids can interfere with DNA synthesis and occasionally find a place in combination therapy against lymphomas, breast cancers, etc. It is known that progestational steroids lower the levels of oestrogen receptors in normal endometrium and in endometrial tumours. More than one-third of patients with advanced endometrial carcinoma show evidence of response following treatment with substances such as medroxyprogesterone acetate.

9. The fetus

FETAL PHYSIOLOGY

Fetal physiology considers the functions of the human body in the first 38 weeks of the continuum of activity starting in the embryonic period with active growth and maturation and then continuing past birth into the physiology of infant and adult. Many of the functions in the fetus mirror those found in extrauterine life but the process of birth is associated with dramatic changes in physiological activity, particularly those concerned with respiration, circulation, barometric homeostasis and temperature control.

Inside the uterus the fetus is well protected, living in a gravity-free environment suspended in amniotic fluid. There is no light, an even temperature, very little touch, sensation or sound. This tranquil existence is separated from the extrauterine life by the tumultuous process of uterine contractions and passage down the vagina — labour. It used to be thought, as recently as 30 years ago, that in the uterus the fetus was dormant and body systems sprang into activity at birth. This is not so and many functions are working from as early as 12 weeks; for example, the heart is contracting, the chest wall moves and limb movements are performed *in utero*. There is a sleeping and waking cycle identical with that of a newborn baby.

It is difficult to measure activities inside the uterus because of the anatomical and physiological barriers which exist between the measurements made in the outside world and the milieu interieur of the fetus. Some functions are measured indirectly from the effects that changes in fetal physiology have on the mother's metabolism; in others, direct physical measurements can be made using methods like ultrasound and Doppler scanning.

Much of the research in human fetal physiology in the past has been based on fetuses born early, between 12 and 28 weeks of gestation. Those delivering so early in pregnancy might not be a representative sample of the larger population of babies, for such fetuses might not have been born soon unless there was some pathological process behind their premature delivery, be it spontaneous or iatrogenic.

The progress of fetal physiology owes much to animal work but extrapolation from one species to another can sometimes be misleading. The simple mathematical concept of apportioning fractions of gestational ages is not logical. For example, the human fetus usually stays 38 weeks in the uterus while that of the rat, 21 days. Hence some would consider that 14 days of rat pregnancy would produce a fetus of equivalent maturity to a human

Table 9.1 Weight of the fetus and mother compared, the ratio between them and the ratio of fetal brain to body weight

Species	Fetal weight (g)	Maternal weight (g)	Fetal/maternal weight at birth (%)	Fetal brain/ body weight (%)
Sheep	4000	70 000	6.0	1.3
Human	3200	56 000	6.0	12.5
Monkey	500	8 000	14.3	12.0
Cat	100	3 000	4.8	3.3
Guinea pig	85	700	8.0	3.0
Rabbit	50	2 500	0.2	2.9
Rat	5	150	3.0	5.0

of 26 weeks of gestation. This is not valid, for variations of maturity between species at all stages of gestation are clearly evident. Indeed, the maturity and development of the newborn animal at birth ranges so widely as to destroy any proportional timing about events in the length of gestation. Table 9.1 shows this in relation to both birth weight as a proportion to the mother's weight and the ratio of fetal brain to the fetal body weight.

Fetal growth

From one cell, produced by an ovum fertilised by a sperm, the human fetus grows in 38 weeks to about 6 billion cells. The rate of growth exceeds that of any other time during the rest of life. Adequate growth depends upon an appropriate supply of nutrients and oxygen being provided for this rapidly growing mass of cells. The development of lower vertebrates is characterised by a large supply of nutrients in the yolk in each egg on which the growing embryo depends but higher mammals and marsupials have an intrauterine development where the fetus depends upon a supply of oxygen and nutrients crossing the placenta from the mother.

The ultimate size attained by the fetus depends upon many factors.

Genetic

Within any species, the offspring of big parents tend to be large themselves. The mating of Shire horses with each other produces larger foals than

that between Shetland ponies. If, however, a Shire stallion is mated with a Shetland mare, the offspring will owe more to the dam's genetic material than the male, for it is through her pelvis that the fetus must pass. In the human species, big subspecies produce big babies and those from smaller races produce smaller ones, e.g. the mean weight and body length at birth for Malaysians is much less than that for Scandinavians.

Placental size and function

At any gestational age, large placentae are associated with a large mean birth weight (Fig. 9.1). The fetal/placental weight ratio increases from 20 weeks, the fetus growing faster than the placenta (Fig. 9.2). Late in pregnancy, fetal growth rate increases while that of the placenta continues to grow at a slower rate, so that while a 32-week fetus is about four times as heavy as the placenta, at 40 weeks it is five or six times as heavy.

In addition to the overall weight of placenta, the surface area presented by the cotyledons is important. In the sheep, cotyledon total surface area can be correlated with the total DNA content of the placenta. Figure 9.3 shows the correlation of one aspect of placental function with DNA as a measure of cotyledon total surface area and Figure 9.4 shows the increase in total DNA with gestational age.

In the human, much of the evidence about fetal and placental size is observational rather than interventional. Placental weights vary greatly with features such as water content, the blood included in the placenta when it is weighed, whether the

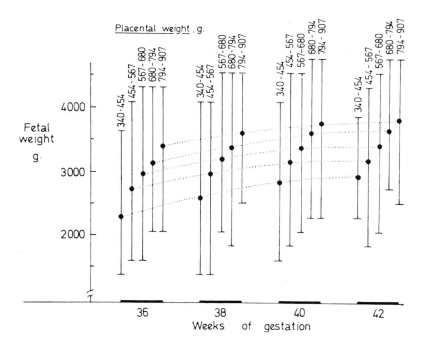

Fig. 9.1 The means and ranges of birthweight by placental weight at certain weeks of gestation. (From A. M. Thomson, Billewicz and F. E. Hytten, 1969, The weight of the placenta in relation to birthweight, *Journal of Obstetrics and Gynaecology of the British Commonwealth* 76: 865–872.)

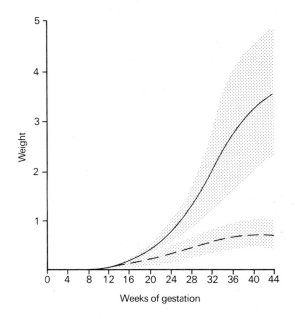

Fig. 9.2 Growth of the fetus and the placenta in man, showing the means and range.

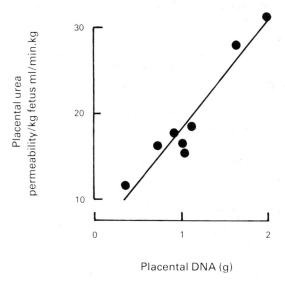

Fig. 9.3 Correlation in the sheep of the permeability of urea to the DNA content of the placenta (see text). (From Kalhanck et al; 1974, *American Journal of Physiology* 226: 1257.)

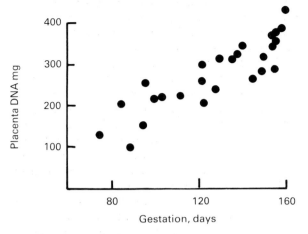

Fig. 9.4   Correlation in the Macaque monkey of total placental DNA and gestation. (From D. E. Hill, 1975, in D. B. Cheek (ed.) *Fetal and Postnatal Cellular Growth*, John Wiley.)

membranes are still attached and the length of cord included. Obviously serial measurements of weight of the placenta and fetus cannot be made in the human or the animal but, more recently, the use of ultrasound has given us another measure of placental volume. This is a non-interventional measurement and so can be repeated longitudinally on the same fetus and placenta several times in pregnancy.

Site of implantation

If the blastocyte should implant close to a better maternal blood supply, fetal growth will probably be faster, particularly in early pregnancy. This factor applies more to species that have several fetuses in their litter, such as the rat or the rabbit, and is less important in the human. However, it is well known that when two or three human fetuses share the same uterus, their individual weights are less, although their total weight is usually more than that of an equivalent singleton in later gestation. For example, the mean combined birth weight in twin pregnancy is about 5 kg, whereas the mean weight of single fetuses born at the same gestation is about 3 kg.

The limitation in size of fetuses in multiple pregnancies is probably due to a reduction in blood flow to the placental bed serving each fetus. Crowding in the myometrial sac and increased pressure from adjacent objects might be important over a long period of time but it is probably not a major feature in the human with one or two fetuses in the uterus. The pregnancy length of human twins is on the average 3 weeks less than that of singletons while triplets have a mean gestational length 6 weeks shorter. Probably, litter size and placental weight are independent variables, either of which could affect fetal growth.

Placental bed

The human placental bed is served by about 200 arteries, all end artery branches of the uterine artery. The flow through these vessels is variable, but by term between 1 and 1.5 l/min jets into the placental pool. Here it circulates around the fronds of villi, which contain the fetal blood vessels. Thus, maternal blood is free in the pool, whereas fetal blood is confined by the fetal capillaries in the villi; between the two is the single layer of syncytiotrophoblast and the thin lining of the capillaries. Exchange, therefore, is very rapid. Maternal blood drains from the placental bed through venules which are not arranged around the disc of the placental bed, as thought previously, but scattered throughout its surface.

In the Western world, probably the principle determinant of fetal growth is the supply of oxygen and nutrients during pregnancy from the maternal blood. The spiral arteries all penetrate through the myometrium and the decidua. Early in pregnancy, waves of trophoblast cell invasion take place so that the inner ends of these arteries are greatly widened to produce deltas. The second wave of trophoblast invasion occurs between 16 and 20 weeks of gestation and this greatly widens out the mouths of the arteries. Should such trophoblastic invasion fail, then the resultant fetal malnutrition leads to intrauterine growth retardation and possibly, in extreme cases, to fetal hypoxia.

The blood flow in these spiral arteries to the placental bed and flow in the umbilical arteries from the fetus can be measured non-invasively by Doppler equipment. A pulse of ultrasonic sound is transmitted onto the flowing column of blood.

Its echo back depends on the blood flow; if the diameter of the vessel can be measured by ultrasound then a rate can be estimated. This method is being used more in obstetrics, so that the flow in the placental bed arteries can be measured serially, allowing longitudinal measurement of the same vessels throughout pregnancy. This may indicate a reduction in the afferent supply of nutrients and oxygen to the fetus. When the flow rate is reduced, the fetus can be in danger and it may be wise to consider delivery.

More acutely, the flow in the umbilical vessels can be measured, and when this starts to diminish (or even reverse at the end of the diastolic phase of flow) the fetus should be delivered very soon, for this is a more precise measure of fetal hazard.

Sex

Until the last few weeks of pregnancy in the human species, both male and female fetuses grow at the same rate; after 32 weeks of gestation, males grow more rapidly so that by 38 weeks the mean is about 150 g heavier than females. There is little or no concomitant increase in placental weight which relates to the sex of the offspring.

Parity

In many cases, babies of successive pregnancies are larger, although this may be counterbalanced by a reduced mean birth weight associated with increasing maternal age. Should pregnancies follow each other quickly, however, the influence of parity is seen in a series of slightly increasing birth weights, features that are important when there are poor contraceptive services and women have babies quickly one after another.

Maternal nutrition

Extreme malnutrition of the mother has been shown to be associated with diminished fetal growth in many species. However, in the human, the times when extreme malnutrition occurs are often associated with other great stresses (e.g. the Dutch famine of 1944–5 and the Leningrad experience in 1943–4). Data from parts of the world where chronic malnutrition still exists are often difficult to interpret for many other features of socio-economic deprivation exist as well as that of just an absence of foodstuffs.

However, intervention studies, where protein and carbohydrates supplements have been given, have shown that malnutrition plays a significant role in addition to other features. In general, the length and severity of nutritional deprivation relate to the diminution in fetal growth. However, such deprivation usually goes on after birth and studies should be of much longer term, involving neonatal and infant measurements also.

In this decade, malnutrition in countries that can make adequate measurements of their obstetrical data is rarely as extensive as that seen in experimental animal studies. The role of minimal food deprivation which is seen commonly in the human is less clear as a factor affecting fetal growth. It may be that some specific aspect of the diet, such as the lower levels of certain vitamins or trace elements, has a special importance, rather than the total overall protein or calorie intake.

Measurements of fetal growth

The measurement of fetal growth by clinical methods such as abdominal palpation is imprecise, although a single observer may be able to detect poor growth if the woman is examined over several weeks. Biochemical estimates do not help as much as do biophysical methods. Of these, X-rays are associated with an increased fetal risk of genetic damage and congenital abnormalities; whilst teratogenesis is in the first 10 weeks of pregnancy, there is evidence that chromosomes, particularly those of the gonads, can be damaged in later weeks of gestation.

Pulsed ultrasound is now widely used in obstetrics. Ultrasound waves in the range of 1–10 million cycles per second (compared with sound waves in the range 30–15 000 cycles per second) are made by passing a current through a synthetic ceramic crystal. This produces a focused beam of ultrasound which is passed through the body, being reflected back from planes between layers of different acoustical density, for example fluid and solid.

Ultrasound can be used to:

1. Identify the number of embryos or fetuses
2. Identify structural abnormalities of the fetus, such as:
   a. The central nervous system (16–20 weeks)
   b. The cardiovascular system (22–26 weeks)
   c. The urinary tract (26–40 weeks)
   d. The alimentary tract (26–40 weeks)
   e. Bony abnormalities of the limbs (16–40 weeks)
3. Measure the fetus in several dimensions such as:
   a. Crown–rump length (8–12 weeks) (Fig. 9.5)
   b. Biparietal diameter (16–30 weeks) (Fig. 9.6)
   c. Abdominal circumference (24–40 weeks)
   d. Femur length (16–40 weeks).

When there is poor perfusion of the placenta, the fetal head and brain may be spared the worse effect and so we need to measure another part of the fetus. The best is the fetal abdominal circumference or area, for these offer an estimate of the

fetal liver size. This organ is proportionately much larger in the fetus than in the adult. In addition, the ratio of head circumference to abdominal circumference or area has a better relationship with subsequent outcome than does either head or abdominal measurement alone. This is now widely used in clinical medicine (Fig. 9.7). Further, a

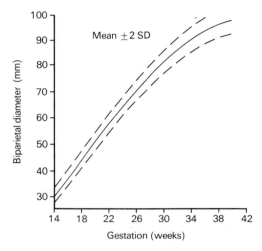

Fig. 9.6 Ultrasound measurement of the biparietal diameter of the fetal head (– – –, ± 2 SD).

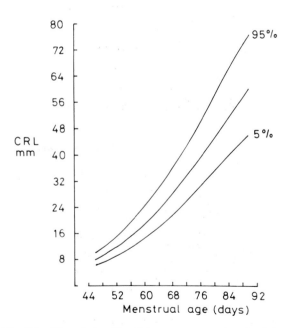

Fig. 9.5 The relationship of the crown–rump length of the fetus to gestational age. (Reproduced with permission from Robinson and Fleming, 1975, A critical evaluation of sonar crown–rump length measurements, *British Journal of Obstetrics and Gynaecology* 82: 702–710.)

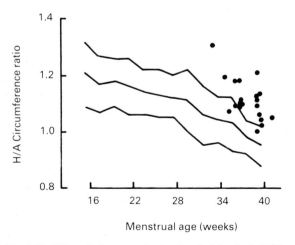

Fig. 9.7 The ratio between the head and abdominal (H/A) circumference by gestation. The mean ± 2 SD of the mean are shown; the dots represent 20 small for dates babies. (Redrawn with permission from S. Campbell, *Placental Transfer*, Pitman Medical.)

close estimate of fetal weight can be obtained from these measures from 24 weeks of gestation. This is helpful to the obstetrician who may need to deliver prematurely.

Ultrasound can also be used to measure the volume of amniotic fluid and detect any abnormal increase (polyhydramnios) or a diminution in volume (oligohydramnios).

Ultrasound is widely used in the identification of structures to guide intrauterine operative procedures such as drawing blood from the umbilical cord (cordocentesis) or chorionic villus biopsy.

Fetal circulation

Introduction

The circulation of blood in the heart within the embryo is one of the earliest systems to function, being present by the age of 21 days. The demands made of this system are different from those in the adult because there is a large extracorporeal organ, the placenta, to perfuse; also, circulating oxygen levels are much lower; an efficient means of distributing nutrition to a rapidly growing organism is required from an early age.

Development

The heart is seen in the 18-day embryo as two tubes originating from splanchnic mesenchyma. These canalise to form the right and left endocardial heart tubes, which then fuse to form a single organ by 22 days. This then elongates and develops varying internal diameters as the different cardiac chambers differentiate. These include the bulbus cordis, ventricle and atrium followed by the truncus arteriosus and sinus venosus (Fig. 9.8). The primitive heart then folds upon itself due to its connections with the surrounding tissues and develops its separate atrial and ventricular chambers. (For further details of development of the heart see Ch. 2.) The heart itself begins to beat by 22 days. The contractions are initially myogenic in origin but by 8 weeks, as it becomes innervated, a loose control is regulated through the sympathetic and parasympathetic nervous systems.

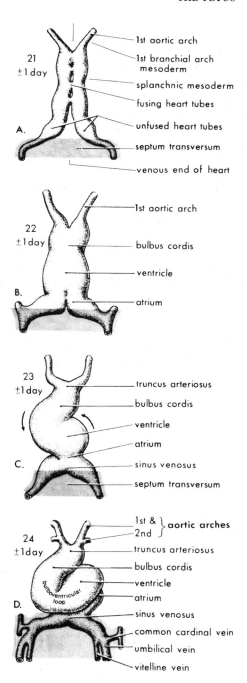

Fig. 9.8 Drawings of the ventricular surface of the developing heart between about 20 and 25 days. The heart tubes fuse to form a single organ which later bends to form a bulboventricular loop as illustrated. (Reproduced with permission from Professor Keith L. Moore and W. B. Saunders.)

Response to stress

The fetal circulation undergoes specific responses in relation to stress during intrauterine life. These lead to preferential redistribution of oxygenated blood to the myocardium, the adrenal glands and the brain, with relative underperfusion of peripheral tissues and other organs including the lung. As the infant matures the aortic chemoreceptors become more active and this further increases the vasoconstrictive response to stress in peripheral tissues. The overall effect of these changes is to cause an elevation of arterial blood pressure and this results in increased blood flow through the placenta, by up to 15% during periods of stress.

Although these responses are beneficial to the fetus, they persist after birth and at this stage become counterproductive since by now the placenta has been removed and the shunting of blood away from the lungs exacerbates any hypoxic insult.

Pattern of circulation

The pattern of circulation in later fetal life is shown in Fig. 9.9. Oxygen is transferred to fetal blood in the capillaries present in the placental villi. The oxygenated blood is returned to the fetus via the placental veins to the umbilical vein, which passes superiorly beneath the anterior abdominal wall and distributes blood in roughly equal proportions between the ductus venosus and branches of the portal venous system. Blood returning via the portal veins passes through the liver into the hepatic veins and thence to the inferior vena cava. The ductus venosus blood enters the inferior vena cava directly although its flow rate is controlled by a sphincter at its entrance.

Most blood entering the heart via the inferior vena cava is streamed through the right atrium directly into the left atrium across the foramen ovale, which is patent in fetal life. This preferentially selects the oxygenated blood returned from the placenta thus directing it to the systemic circulation and bypassing the lungs. The remaining inferior vena cava blood passes through the right atrium to the right ventricle and is ejected into the main pulmonary artery. This vessel, however, has a large fetal channel, the ductus arteriosus, connecting it to the aorta opposite the position of the left subclavian artery. Most of the blood leaving the right ventricle also enters the aorta across the ductus. This leaves only a small proportion to supply the airless lungs along the pulmonary arteries. This is because the pulmonary vascular resistance is very high, a state which is maintained in fetal life, only to be reduced by the sudden aeration of the lungs at birth.

This arrangement of the circulation provides the brain with the most oxygenated blood flowing from the left ventricle and allows the less oxygenated blood which has passed via the ductus arteriosus to supply the lower body via the aorta. Since the placenta has a large volume and relatively low resistance much of the aortic flow is returned via the iliac and umbilical arteries to the placenta itself so facilitating reoxygenation.

The flow of blood along the vessels of the umbilical cord and major fetal arteries can be measured using Doppler imaging of pulsed ultrasound. This gives a guide to the total fetal afferent flow for nutrition and oxygenation or regional flows within individual vessels, e.g. the carotid artery.

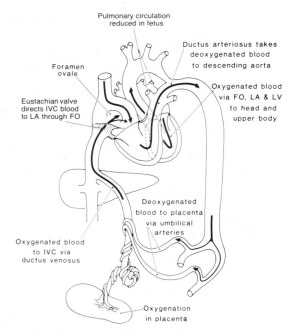

Fig. 9.9 The fetal circulation.

Distribution of blood flow

The most oxygenated blood returning from the placenta through the inferior vena cava accounts for approximately 75% of the venous return to the heart. Some 40–50% of this is shunted directly through the foramen ovale to the left atrium and from there it is distributed mainly to the brain and upper body. The remaining cardiac output is distributed to the rest of the body including the lungs. In fetal life only about 10% of the cardiac output enters the pulmonary arteries with the remaining blood directed to the descending aorta. About 60% of aortic blood flow enters the umbilical arteries and is thus directed to the placenta.

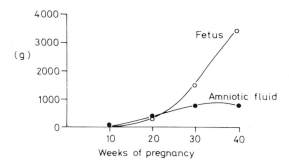

Fig. 9.10   The relationship between fetal weight and the weight of amniotic fluid through pregnancy. (Reproduced with permission from F. Hytten and G. Chamberlain, Blackwell Scientific Publications.)

Changes at birth

Immediately after birth the umbilical vessels are occluded by spasm and, in humans, more recently by clamping; this produces a sudden and large reduction in venous return to the right heart. The major consequence is that pressure in the right atrium drops and the foramen ovale closes. Simultaneously aeration of the lungs during the first breath produces pulmonary arteriolar vasodilation and so lowers pressures in the pulmonary circulation. Right ventricular output is therefore directed increasingly into the pulmonary arteries so contributing to redistribution of blood flow to an adult pattern. As these changes proceed, the ductus arteriosus closes, chiefly in response to the increasing arterial oxygen concentration as breathing is established. In most healthy infants the foramen ovale and ductus arteriosus close functionally soon after birth so that a stable adult circulatory pattern is established within a few hours of delivery. More permanent closure is by fibrosis, days later. The ductus arteriosus is also sensitive to prostaglandins which in theory could delay closure. Prostaglandin synthetase inhibitors (e.g. indomethacin) accelerate duct closure.

Renal function

The kidneys like the lungs do not have a vital role during intrauterine life. After delivery and removal of the placenta they must be capable of excreting nitrogen waste products and controlling electrolyte and water balance very soon.

Fetal clearance rates increase with gestation, probably correlating better with fetal size and kidney weight than with gestational maturity; hence improved renal function is a reflection of growth. Once the fetus has been delivered there is a dramatic increase in glomerular filtration rate and renal blood flow. Nevertheless, at birth the fetal kidney is still relatively immature; in particular, it is unable to conserve sodium efficiently.

The fetal urine is excreted into the amniotic cavity so that by later pregnancy, the fetal kidney is one of the principal sources of amniotic fluid (see p. 50). Fetal urine production rates can be measured by ultrasound and in late pregnancy a normal fetus passes 500–700 ml/day; production is reduced in growth-retarded fetuses. This concords with the common clinical finding of oligohydramnios encountered in those with intrauterine growth retardation. The relationship of amniotic fluid volume to fetal weight is shown in Fig. 9.10. In late pregnancy, amniotic fluid osmolality falls (probably due to a fall in sodium levels) while creatinine concentrations rise.

Central nervous system

The central nervous system develops early in fetal life (see p. 37). There is a critical time between 12 and 16 weeks of gestation when the nerve cell processes appear and nuclei cease to increase in volume. This histological change corresponds with an increase in biochemical activity of many enzymes in the central nervous system and the functional response of muscle to cortical stimulation. Just after this, spontaneous electroencephalographic activity can be first detected.

Despite the relatively early development of the cortex, at birth the central nervous system of the human offspring is relatively immature; the full reflex responses are not complete but appear later. This is not always a factor of the length of gestation or stage of development at birth but is more a feature of the length of time since delivery, thus implying facilitation with usage.

The blood flow to the fetal brain is regulated to maintain a constant oxygen delivery, despite varying oxygen tensions. During hypoxia, the blood flow increases; in the rat, for example, over a maternal arterial Po_2 range of 23–140 mmHg and an arterial content of 2.1–9.9 mmol/l, constant tissue oxygen concentration can be maintained. This is due to a combination of dilatation of the vessels in the cerebral circulation and an increased blood flow brought about by greater cardiac output associated with sympathetic stimulation; this is reflected in the tachycardia noted in the early stages of hypoxia in clinical obstetrics. Compensatory constriction of the intravascular space in other fetal tissues and altered flow in the fetal circulation also maintain cerebral blood flow.

Peripheral nervous system

Ganglia and nerves appear in the human embryo between 28 and 35 days. Nerve fibres with enlargements at their growing tips appear amongst the myeloblasts at 35 days but they lack end plates. Motor and sensory nerve endings are found later (12–16 weeks). However, muscle contractions can be elicited at 8 weeks by direct stimulation of the muscle.

The sensory endings in the skin of the human fetus appear between 12 and 16 weeks but structural alterations continue throughout fetal life. It is doubtful if pain or temperature appreciation exists in prenatal life but touch and stretch response do. A brisk response will come from the fetus who receives a touch stimulus from an external source in late pregnancy.

The autonomic nervous system, regulating the response of the milieu interieur to the external environment, is little required in utero but must be ready to work soon after birth. Pulmonary reflexes and baroreceptor mechanisms maintaining blood pressure will be required immediately after delivery; both are functional in the last weeks of pregnancy. The reflexes initiated by the stimulation of the bronchioles are present well before birth and the lung inflation stimulates these. Baroreceptor stimulation of the aortic branches of the vagus nerve results in bradycardia. Chemoreceptors in the carotid body respond in utero to alterations of pH; alterations of the Pco_2 level can be appreciated directly in the midbrain.

All these reflex mechanisms mature in the last weeks of gestation so that the changes in heart trace of a 28-week fetus in response to hypoxia are very different and less reactive than are those of a fully mature fetus. This is a practical and important point when monitoring labour in the mid- or early third trimester.

Skin physiology

Skin is a major organ of water balance in early pregnancy. Until about 20 weeks of gestation, fluid passes freely along physical gradients; there is a net loss by transudation of water across this thin multicellular membrane. After this time, keratinisation appears and slows exchange, but still at the end of pregnancy the skin has some contribution to amniotic fluid production. Sweat glands do not function very early, despite the development of a lumen by 28 weeks but the sebaceous glands are obviously working in the immature infant, being responsible for the production of vernix caseosa.

Alimentary tract

During intrauterine life, nutrition is provided through the placenta and the alimentary tract has no immediate function. However, immediately after birth it must be prepared to receive water and nutrients. Amniotic fluid is swallowed by the fetus as early as 12 weeks of gestation and the rate of swallowing increases with age. The fetal skin cells can be found in the lumen of the intestine and by term as much as 250 ml of fluid is taken in by this route each 24 hours. Anencephalic fetuses swallow much less. This may be one of the reasons for the commonly associated polyhydramnios.

The nutritional value of this fluid and its contained cells is doubtful. Sweetening the fluid with saccharin causes an increased rate of swallowing; some have tried adding simple proteins and amino acids to the amniotic fluid to help improve the nutritional intake of the fetus by a route which bypasses the placenta. These experiments have shown no significant improvement in growth in the human.

The villi and glands of the intestine are laid down early and digestive enzymes are found by 16–20 weeks. Liver and pancreatic secretions begin about the same time but glycogen storage in the liver does not occur until very much later.

Meconium is a sterile odourless substance whose dark colour comes from the bile pigments — it is very pale in congenital atresia of the bile ducts. Meconium contains secretions of intestinal glands and the stomach as well as amniotic fluid swallowed by the fetus; microscopy will reveal hair, vernix and epithelial cells. The motor activities of the gut are under no central control at first although isolated movements of the small intestine can be seen by 11 weeks in the human fetus. Sympathetic nerves must grow from the mesenteric plexuses before any coordinated movements can be shown.

During hypoxia, peristaltic intestinal movements change — tone is reduced, while movements and rhythmical segmentation appear. Then, defaecation follows contraction of the large bowel and relaxation of the anal sphincter mechanisms. Meconium appears in the amniotic fluid and, if the membranes are ruptured, as in labour, meconium can also be seen in the vagina.

Initiation of respiration

The initiation of respiration at birth is a very complex process dependent on a number of powerful stimuli which occur at this time. It depends on an intact nervous system, mature enough to react to the afferent mechanical and chemical inputs and with sufficient efferent drive to maintain regular respiration when breathing is established. At the same time, adequate aeration of the lungs associated with simultaneous absorption of lung fluid must occur in order to produce a stable resting lung volume or functional residual capacity after the first few breaths. As these changes take place, the fetal circulation alters in a major way with loss of placental return of oxygenated blood and a marked increase in pulmonary blood flow due to massive pulmonary vasodilatation as breathing is initiated. The role of each system in this complex process will be discussed separately.

Central nervous system

Breathing movements are present in the fetus from as early as 11 weeks of gestational age. These are irregular at first but become more regular as gestation increases, usually being associated with rapid eye movement sleep in experimental animals. As labour approaches, fetal breathing decreases. Stress to the fetus at this time may result in deeper gasping inspiratory movements at a much slower rate. These responses are probably mediated through the central nervous system but by different mechanisms.

At the time of the first breath a number of changes occur which affect the activity of the respiratory centres in the brain stem. These include the enormous number of touch stimuli and the drop in skin temperature which occur at the moment of birth; chemoreceptor stimuli caused by hypoxia and hypercapnia following the closure of the placental circulation are added to an efferent input from stretch receptors within the lung itself. Light, sound and the sensation of gravity produces other changes in cerebral activity during the first few minutes of life. Regular respiration is established within a few minutes in the normal infant although irregular patterns continue to occur for months during rapid eye movement sleep. The most important stimuli to the first breath are thought to be tactile and thermal but, thereafter, chemical changes in the blood and cerebrospinal fluid are prominent in the stabilisation and maintenance of regular breathing patterns.

The lungs

Although gasping movements of the chest wall will occur in a fetus of less than 24 weeks of gestation, regular breathing cannot be sustained until there is adequate alveolar development to maintain a stable resting lung volume at the end of expiration. This process is also dependent on the presence of a mature pulmonary surfactant system, which stabilises the alveolar wall at low lung volumes. The final or alveolar phase of lung development occurs from 23 weeks onwards and consists of acinar budding and thinning of the type I alveolar lining cells, which facilitate gas exchange across the alveolar wall. At the same time the type II alveolar lining cells, which synthesise pulmonary surfactants, also mature.

Pulmonary surfactants are a complex group of materials which are largely phospholipid in origin (about 70%) and also contain other lipids and some proteins. Their function is to maintain the surface tension of the alveolar wall at low lung volumes thus preventing alveolar collapse or atelectasis once breathing is established. The level of these substances has been related to the incidence of respiratory distress syndrome in the newborn infant. This is most commonly expressed as the ratio of lecithin to sphingomyelin (L/S ratio) in amniotic fluid (Fig. 9.11, Table 9.2).

During the process of birth, some of the fluid filling the lungs is squeezed out through the pharynx as intrathoracic pressure increases. As the first breath is taken fluid is absorbed across the alveolar wall directly into the capillaries and lymphatics of adjacent lung tissue. As the thoracic wall expands on delivery air passes into the chest and a cycle of breathing is established (Fig. 9.12). The first breaths may be associated with large respiratory excursions and expiratory grunting or crying. Intrathoracic pressures up to −70 cm H$_2$O have been recorded during this phase, so estab-

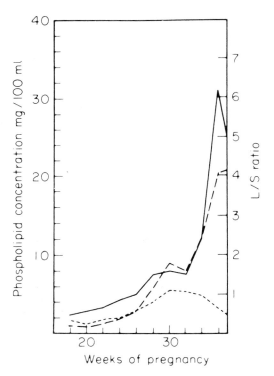

Fig. 9.11 Concentrations of acetone precipitable (surface active) lecithin (———) and sphingomyelin (- - -) in amniotic fluid are comparable until 30–32 weeks of gestation (L/S ratio, – – –.) After 32 weeks of gestation, the concentration of lecithin increases sharply, while sphingomyelin decreases steadily until term. The lung is usually mature when lecithin concentration reaches 10 mg/100 ml or the L/S ratio is over 2. (Reproduced with permission from Dewhurst (ed.) *Obstetrics and Gynaecology for Postgraduates*, Blackwell Scientific Publications.)

lishing functional residual capacity within a few breaths. In a number of babies this process is performed with smaller breaths and lower pressure changes. Babies born by caesarean section have lower resting lung volumes in the first few hours as the thoracic cage is not so compressed as it would have been during vaginal delivery.

The volume of the first breath varies between 10 and 60 ml; the normal tidal volume during quiet breathing is about 6 ml/kg body weight (about 20 ml in a 3 kg baby). Functional residual capacity averages 30 ml/kg within 30 minutes of birth (about 100 ml in a 3 kg baby) (see the section on respiration in Ch. 6 for a definition of functional residual capacity).

Table 9.2 Incidence of respiratory distress syndrome (RDS) related to the lecithin/sphingomyelin ratio

L/S ratio	RDS	No RDS	Total
>2:1	40 (1.8%)	2089 (98.2%)	2139
<2:1	163 (48%)	178 (52%)	341

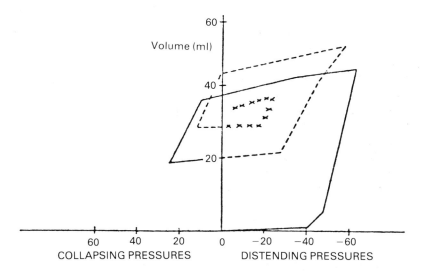

Fig. 9.12 Diagrammatic representation of the pressure–volume changes during the first three breaths: —, first breath; – –, second breath; XXX, third breath. (Redrawn from Hytten and Chamberlain (eds), *Clinical Physiology in Obstetrics*, Blackwell Scientific Publications.)

Pulmonary circulation

The pulmonary circulation is intimately involved with the fetal circulation as a whole and has already been considered in detail. When the cord is clamped and placental circulation is lost, the fall in pressure on the right side of the heart promotes closure of the foramen ovale and diminished blood flow through the ductus arteriosus. The acute changes in blood gases occurring as a result of the cessation of cord circulation stimulate the peripheral chemoreceptors to promote the establishment of regular respiration.

When breathing commences, the arterial Po_2 rises rapidly and the pH falls as carbon dioxide is excreted through the lung. Both of these changes are potent stimuli to the relaxation of tone in the arteriolar muscles in the pulmonary vascular bed. This leads to a large reduction in pulmonary vascular resistance so promoting a large increase in pulmonary blood flow. These changes serve to match perfusion of the lung with the increasing ventilation which is occurring as breathing is established.

The initiation of respiration is thus a complicated sequence of events which begins some time before birth itself and which relies on close integration between the central nervous system, the lungs and the pulmonary circulation.

PLACENTAL TRANSFER

All anabolites needed for fetal metabolism come from the mother's blood across the placenta while fetal catabolites are passed back into the mother's circulation whence they are disposed of to the milieu exterieur through the mother's kidneys, skin and lungs. The placenta used to be considered a passive filter; physiologists in the past used to classify the number of layers of tissue interposed between the maternal and fetal circulations and consider that the speed of transfer depended upon these. The concept of a placental barrier was built up. In fact, in time most substances would cross the placenta provided a high enough concentration is maintained in the maternal blood. The placenta is only a relative barrier which is greatest to substances of larger molecular weight and low lipid solubility.

The transfer capacity of the placenta depends mostly upon the surface area exposed to maternal blood in the placental bed and on maternal blood flow. There is generally an increase in placental mass during pregnancy up to about the 37th week of gestation, after which there is little further growth.

The surface area of the villi also increases until about 37 weeks and so the capacity of the placenta to exchange will probably increase until this time. After 37 weeks, the metabolic capacity of the placenta can be shown to be diminished (e.g. human placental lactogen levels and oestrogen secretion are reduced); it is probable that the exchange functions are similarly affected.

There is a natural placental reserve which is greater than was previously thought; as much as 50% of the placental surface can be impaired yet adequate exchange of nutrients and oxygen for the fetus can still be achieved. Such a change is seen in association with maternal hypertensive disease when both the maternal vessels to the placenta bed and the fetal blood vessels leaving it become grossly changed and are in danger of reducing fetal exchange; despite this dramatic histology, the fetus still survives. Not so relevant are the gross placental infarcts seen with the naked eye. It used to be considered that fetal growth was limited by the size of the placenta; this would imply that the placenta had been working at nearly full capacity. This is probably incorrect; possibly the small placenta associated with the smaller fetus is not the cause of the small baby but the effect of it, for the placenta is a fetal organ and small babies have small organs.

Water transfer

Water transport between the mother, the fetus, the placenta and amniotic fluid occurs both by perfusion exchange and osmotic transfer. Between 3 and 4 litres of water are exchanged each hour. Such a volume is so great that a small change in the rate of exchange would alter the total volume of amniotic fluid rapidly and could also affect the fetus. Perfusion exchange increases during pregnancy (Fig. 9.13). In late pregnancy, exchange may be reduced, possibly due to deposition of fibrin over the surface of the villi.

The rate of net accumulation of water on behalf of the products of conception is shown in Figure

9.14. The net movement of water between mother and fetus is in response to the differences of osmotic pressure in the two compartments. There is a tendency for such osmotic pressure differences to equalise throughout all body compartments but there is invariably some lag; therefore the fetus will always share in, but respond more slowly to, any dehydration or overhydration of the mother. These may happen respectively with prolonged vomiting and diarrhoea or after the large intravenous fluid load which accompanies higher doses of oxytocic drugs given in labour.

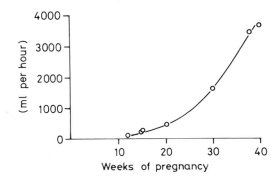

Fig. 9.13   Transfer rate of labelled water between mother and fetus. (Redrawn with permission from F. Hytten, G. Chamberlain, *Clinical Physiology in Obstetrics*, Blackwell Scientific Publications.)

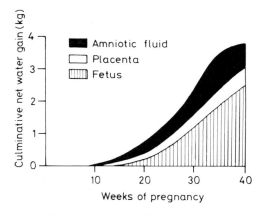

Fig. 9.14   The cumulative net gain of water by the fetus, placenta and amniotic fluid. (Redrawn with permission from F. Hytten, G. Chamberlain, *Clinical Physiology in Obstetrics*, Blackwell Scientific Publications.)

Gas transfer

Respiratory gases (oxygen and carbon dioxide) cross the placenta by simple diffusion. They are small molecules; the rate and quantity of gas transferred depends upon the concentration of each gas on either side of the placenta. Hence the capacity of maternal and fetal blood to carry oxygen and carbon dioxide are important. The dissociation curves in both maternal and fetal blood and the supply of blood to each side of the placenta alter the rates of gas exchange.

For example, fetal red cells have a greater affinity for oxygen than maternal red cells; thus the oxygen dissociation curve is shifted so that of the fetus is to the left of that in maternal blood (Fig. 9.15).

At term, the amount of oxygen carried by the maternal and fetal bloods will be different. A woman with a haemoglobin of 12 g/dl is exposed to air (20% oxygen and 80% nitrogen approximately). The partial pressure of oxygen is a fifth of the total pressure or about 150 mmHg. After exchange in the lungs, the arterial P_{O_2} is 100 mmHg and the blood is 95% saturated with oxygen. In consequence, 100 ml of maternal blood carries about 15 ml of oxygen.

The blood of the fetus has a haemoglobin of about 17 g/dl. Even though the P_{O_2} in the placental pool is only 45 mmHg, the greater fetal haemoglobin affinity for oxygen and the increased total amount of haemoglobin per decilitre allows the fetal blood to carry 25 ml of oxygen per 100 ml of blood. This is a measure of the differential from fetal and maternal blood oxygen-carrying capacities.

Carbon dioxide is very soluble and once in the blood soon passes into the red cells (see p. 178) where about 30% combines with haemoglobin to form carboxyhaemoglobin. About 10% of the rest of the carbon dioxide is in physical solution and 60% combines with water to carbonic acid, which ionises almost immediately; the hydrogen ion is buffered by fetal haemoglobin so there is only a slight drop in the pH and the fetus is enabled to carry more carbon dioxide. The bicarbonate ion passes out of the red cell. Because of the high haemoglobin content in fetal blood, there are smaller pH changes for any given increase in the P_{CO_2}.

At the placental surface, maternal blood releases oxygen and so its haemoglobin is free to attach to the hydrogen ion formed from the two-thirds of the carbon dioxide in the ionised state of H^+ and HCO_3^-. At the same time in fetal blood, oxygen is binding to the HbF molecule and carbon dioxide is released without any alteration in P_{CO_2}. This is a double Haldane effect and only occurs in the placenta because of the relative positions of fetal and maternal oxygen dissociation curves relating to their different haemoglobins.

Fetal hypoxia

Fetal hypoxia is due to both diminution of oxygen levels and an increase in carbon dioxide concentration. In addition, in the fetus, anaerobic respiratory mechanisms take over rapidly. The breakdown product of glucose is usually pyruvate, which is normally reduced to carbon dioxide and oxygen in the Krebs cycle. In hypoxia, it is converted to lactate, which accumulates in fetal tissues producing a metabolic acidosis. The high energy links released during this latter mechanism are only one-fifteenth of those of aerobic respiration and it is, therefore, a less efficient energy process.

A hypoxic fetus thus develops both respiratory and metabolic acidosis. The fetus which has become deficient in oxygen has compensating mechanisms for acute acidosis. Fetal haemoglobin is a major buffer and in acidosis the oxygen dissociation curve shifts to the right so that for any

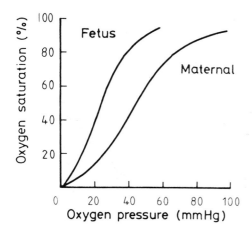

Fig. 9.15 Haemoglobin oxygen dissociation curves for fetal and maternal blood in the sheep. (Redrawn with permission from Bancroft *Research in Prenatal Life*, Blackwell Scientific Publications.)

given Po_2 the oxygen saturation falls; this releases oxygen for use in the tissues and makes more fetal haemoglobin available for buffering (deoxygenated haemoglobin is a better buffer than oxygenated haemoglobin — see p. 177).

Carbohydrate transfer

Glucose is a major substrate for energy production and metabolism in the fetus. It is also a precursor for the lipids required by the baby after birth. Facilitated diffusion from the mother to the fetus takes place in the face of adverse concentration gradients; such exchange requires energy. There is possibly a protein carrier in the membranes of the placental cells, which produces a lipid-soluble complex diffusing across the membrane itself and releasing glucose into the fetal blood.

Amino acid transfer

The amino acid levels in fetal blood are often higher than those in the maternal circulation.

Transfer must be facilitated against the biochemical concentration gradient which may be as high as 3 to 1 for the acidic branch chain and basal groups of amino acids. Transfer may be through intercellular channels directly or maternal plasma. Proteins also can join the free pool in the membrane itself; from here they pass to the fetal plasma.

Fat transfer

Fats are insoluble in water; they are carried in the blood stream as free fatty acids bound to albumin or as lipoprotein. They are probably not transferred selectively across the placenta but according to the concentration which they present on the maternal side. Fatty acids and certain phospholipids are picked up by the placenta and converted to simpler forms in the membranes. There is great species variation in fatty acid transfer and little is known of the human system although most fetal fats are probably anabolised by liponeogenesis from carbohydrates.

10. Statistics

INTRODUCTION

Statistics is a branch of applied mathematics which is finding increasing application in all sectors of medical research and community medicine. It is concerned with the numerical properties of groups of individuals; a single item of information on an individual patient is not, in general, of much interest to a statistician. In contrast, a clinician would be eager to know all the relevant information about an individual, particularly if that individual were his patient.

Why should an obstetrician or gynaecologist need to know anything about statistics? There may be administrative applications. For example, if it were necessary to plan the provision of maternity hospital beds for a community it would be necessary to determine: the size of the community within the catchment area; what proportion of the community were women of childbearing age; how many of these would be likely to have babies in a given year; how many would require hospitalisation; how long the mother should stay in hospital after the birth of the baby. These data would improve the use of hospital confinements while simultaneously minimising the risks to mothers and babies. These are problems whose solutions require numerical information, that is, statistics.

A rather different problem arises in research. We might, for example, be interested in comparing two drugs A and B for the treatment of severe idiopathic respiratory distress syndrome. If we took two infants with this syndrome and treated one with drug A and the other with drug B, the comparison of the outcomes of these two treatments would not provide a very useful indication of the relative efficacy of the drugs. Clearly what is required here is a group of infants treated with A and another group treated with B. Then it may be possible to make a valid comparison of, say, survival rates for infants treated with each drug. How many infants would be required for this trial? How should the outcome of the treatments be assessed for comparison? Statistics also plays an important role in many medical specialities, for example epidemiology. The methodology of both descriptive and analytic epidemiology is based on a solid foundation of mathematical statistics.

Finally, it is becoming increasingly difficult to read the research literature of obstetrics and gynaecology critically without at least some knowledge of the language of statistics.

DATA SUMMARISING

Statistical data is usually of two types, either quantitative or qualitative. Data derived from quantitative variables have numerical values; examples are birthweight (kilograms) or age at menarche (years), while qualitative variables indicate the presence or absence of a characteristic; for example, a woman is either pregnant or not pregnant, a baby is either born alive or born dead. The first

Table 10.1 Example of frequency distributions

(a) *A qualitative variable. Outcome of 1827 pregnancies*

Outcome	Frequency	%
Spontaneous abortion	54	2.95
Induced abortion	148	8.10
Stillbirth	22	1.20
Live birth	1603	87.74
Total	1827	99.99

(b) *A quantitative variable. Parity distribution of mothers of 1 469 086 births of which 18 847 were stillbirths. England and Wales 1969–70*

Parity	Total births	%	Stillbirths	%	Stillbirth rate/1000
0	564 003	38.39	8032	42.62	14.24
1	482 074	32.81	4707	24.97	9.76
2	234 732	15.98	2853	15.14	12.15
3	101 167	6.89	1494	7.93	14.77
4	44 553	3.03	819	4.35	18.38
5–9	41 144	2.80	887	4.71	21.56
10	1413	0.10	55	0.29	38.92
Total	1 469 086	100.00	18 847	100.01	12.83

stage in summarising any data is to construct a frequency distribution such as those in Table 10.1.

There are situations where it is not particularly useful to construct frequency distributions, for example the sample size might be very small; then it is usual to summarize the data even further by concentrating on just one or two measures. For quantitative data, it is usual to calculate the sample *mean* and the *standard deviation*, while for qualitative data it is usual to calculate the sample proportion p with the characteristic or equivalently the percentage.

The sample mean or, as it is often called, the average value is calculated by adding up all the observations and dividing by the total number of observations. Algebraically this calculation would be written as

$$\bar{x} = \frac{\Sigma x}{n}$$

where $\bar{x}$ is the symbol used to denote the sample mean, Σx means the sum of all the observed values and n is the sample size. While the sample mean is a measure of the overall magnitude of the observations, the standard deviation, denoted by the symbol s, is a measure of the variability of the ob-

servations about their mean value. The algebraic formula for the standard deviation is

$$s = \sqrt{\frac{\Sigma(x - \bar{x})^2}{n - 1}}$$

which, with some algebraic juggling, can be rearranged to ease calculation to give

$$s = \sqrt{\frac{\Sigma x^2 - (\Sigma \bar{x})^2/n}{n - 1}}$$

Nowadays, the calculation is programmed into many electronic calculators. To interpret the magnitude of the standard deviation a simple rule is that the interval $\bar{x} \pm 2s$ should include about 95% of all the observations. The interval mean $\pm$ two standard deviations is often called the *normal range* of values. For comparison $\bar{x} \pm s$ includes 68% of all the observations. $\bar{x} \pm 3s$ includes over 99% of all the observations.

POPULATIONS AND SAMPLE

In sampling, a part of a population is chosen to provide information which can be generalised to the whole population. In this context, the population is any defined group of individuals which is of interest in a particular study. It may be a population of people, for example pregnant women living in a defined geographical area at a particular time, but in general the population might be hospitals, medical records or stillbirths. Sampling is adopted to reduce labour and hence costs, but by taking a sample rather than studying the whole population there is a loss of precision.

In general, a parameter of the population is to be estimated using the information provided by the sample. This population parameter could be, for example, the mean value of some measurement or the proportion of the population with some characteristic. If a sample is used, the conclusions about the population parameter may involve error; that is, a sample mean or sample proportion is unlikely to equal exactly the population mean or population proportion.

It is useful to distinguish between two sorts of error, sampling error and bias. Sampling errors arise because only a part of the population has been observed. Sampling errors get less important as sample size increases. In contrast, a bias does not necessarily get less important as sample size increases. A bias arises if the sample is systematically unrepresentative of the population. Non-random sampling is perhaps the most important cause of bias but there may be many other sources of bias in any particular study. For example, a tendency to forget early spontaneous abortions may bias a study involving reproductive histories; a patient's refusal to participate in a study may cause a bias if the reasons for refusal are related to the interests of the study.

While bias may be important in a particular study, the causes and control of bias are dependent on the study itself and, apart from emphasising the importance of random selection for the sample, general rules cannot be laid down. In contrast, although sampling error cannot be calculated for a sample estimate, it is possible to estimate the maximum likely value of sampling error. If, for example, a population mean μ is to be estimated from a sample of size n, the sample mean $\bar{x} = \Sigma x/n$ is calculated. The actual sampling error is $\bar{x} - \mu$ and this cannot be calculated because μ is clearly unknown. The standard error of a sample estimate is a measure of the precision

of the estimate and, in general, the maximum likely value of $\bar{x} - \mu$ is twice the standard error. In this context likely corresponds to a probability (P) of about 0.95 or 95%.

Thus, if an interval, defined by the value of an estimate $\pm$ twice the standard error of the estimate, is calculated, this interval is called a 95% confidence interval and has a 95% chance of including the value of the population parameter. Some examples are:

1. Estimation of a population mean. Take a random sample of n individuals and calculate the sample mean $\bar{x}$ and the standard deviation s. The estimated standard error of the sample mean is $s/\sqrt{n}$ and $\bar{x} \pm 2 \times s/\sqrt{n}$ is a 95% confidence interval for the population mean. It is assumed that n is greater than about 30.

2. Estimation of a population proportion. Take a random sample of n individuals, count the number with the characteristic of interest r and the sample proportion $p = r/n$. The estimated standard error of the sample proportion is

$$\sqrt{\frac{p(1-p)}{n}}$$

and

$$p \pm 2 \times \sqrt{\frac{p(1-p)}{n}}$$

is a 95% confidence interval for the population proportion with the characteristic.

3. Estimation of the difference between two population means. Take a random sample of n_1 individuals from the first population and n_2 individuals from the second population and calculate their means $\bar{x}_1$ and $\bar{x}_2$ and standard deviations s_1 and s_2. Then $\bar{x}_1 - \bar{x}_2$ is the estimate of the difference between the two population means. The estimated standard error of $(\bar{x}_1 - \bar{x}_2)$ is

$$\sqrt{\frac{s^2}{n_1} + \frac{s^2}{n_2}}$$

where

$$s^2 = \frac{(n_1 - 1)\, s_1^2 + (n_2 - 1)\, s_2^2}{n_1 + n_2 - 2}$$

and

$$\bar{x}_1 - \bar{x}_2 \pm 2 \times \sqrt{\frac{s^2}{n_2} + \frac{s^2}{n_2}}$$

is a 95% confidence interval for the difference between two population means. It is assumed that $n_1 + n_2$ is greater than about 30.

4. Estimation of the difference between two population proportions. Take a sample of n_1 individuals from the first population and n_2 individuals from the second population and calculate the two sample proportions $p_1 = r_1/n_1$ and $p_2 = r_2/n_2$ and the overall proportion $p = (r_1 + r_2)/(n_1 + n_2)$. Then $p_1 - p_2$ is the estimate of the difference between the two population proportions. The standard error of $(p_1 - p_2)$ is

$$\sqrt{p(1 - p)\left(\frac{1}{n_1} + \frac{1}{n_2}\right)}$$

and

$$p_1 - p_2 \pm 2 \times \sqrt{p(1 - p)\left(\frac{1}{n_1} + \frac{1}{n_2}\right)}$$

is a 95% confidence interval for the difference between the two population proportions.

SIGNIFICANCE TESTS

A significance test is a test of a hypothesis which specifies a value of a population parameter. In its simplest form a significance test is achieved by considering a confidence interval. For example, if the hypothesis were that the mean value of some variable in a population were say, μ_0, then if the 95% confidence interval included the value μ_0 it would be argued that the sample provided no strong evidence against the value μ_0. If, on the other hand, μ_0 were outside the limits of the confidence interval, it would be stated that μ_0 is an unlikely value for the population mean, and the difference between the value μ_0 proposed by the hypothesis and the sample mean $\bar{x}$ is significant at the $P < 0.05$ or 5% level. The 0.05 or 5% here is the probability that the confidence interval does not include the population mean μ.

By a similar argument, two sample means can be compared. Here the hypothesis is that the difference between the two population means is zero. If the 95% confidence interval for the difference between the two population means includes zero then it would imply that the samples provide no strong evidence of a difference between the

population means. If the interval does not include zero then it is concluded that the difference between $\bar{x}_1$ and $\bar{x}_2$ is significant at the $P < 0.05$ or 5% level (see (3) above).

The same arguments can be applied to significance tests of a single sample proportion and the difference between two sample proportions.

The t test and the χ^2 tests of these hypotheses are refinements of the test procedures outlined above and further details can be found in standard textbooks.

LINEAR REGRESSION AND CORRELATION

It often happens, in modern surveys, that more than one measurement is made on each individual. For example, in a study of diastolic blood pressure in pregnant women, for each woman examined there may be several measurements apart from blood pressure, such as gestational stage, age, weight, weekly tobacco consumption. One object of such a study might be to see how the *response* or *dependent* variable, blood pressure, varies with the *explanatory* or *independent* variables, age, weight.

Consider the simplest situation in which there is one response or dependent variable conventionally denoted by y, and one explanatory or independent variable x, and assume the relationship between them is linear.

If there are n pairs of observations (x_1, y_1), $(x_2, y_2) \ldots (x_n, y_n)$, to see how y varies with x a scatter diagram should be drawn with y on the vertical axis and x on the horizontal axis.

If the points lie fairly closely on a straight line, it may be adequate to fit the line by eye, but an *objective* method of fitting a straight line through the set of points on the scatter diagram should be used for a full analysis.

A straight line can be described algebraically in the form

$$y = \alpha + \beta x.$$

The problem is to find estimates of α and β (which we will call a and b) from the data such that the line fits the points on the scatter diagram as closely as possible. Suppose the scatter diagram

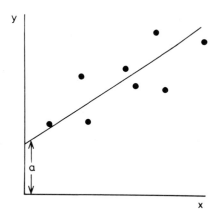

Fig. 10.1 An example of a scatter diagram with the best-fitting straight line.

and the closest-fitting line looks like that in Fig. 10.1.

If we call the vertical distance of the points from the line d, we choose estimates of α and β which minimise Σd^2. These estimates are called *least squares* estimates.

The use of differential calculus shows straightforwardly that the expressions for a and b, our sample estimates of α and β, which satisfy this condition, are

$$a = \bar{y} - \frac{S_{xy}\bar{x}}{S_{xx}}$$

and

$$b = \frac{S_{xy}}{S_{xx}}$$

where

$$S_{xx} = \Sigma(x - \bar{x})^2 = \Sigma x^2 - \frac{(\Sigma x)^2}{\sqrt{n}}$$

and

$$S_{xy} = \Sigma(x - \bar{x})(y - \bar{y}) = \Sigma xy - \frac{(\Sigma x)(\Sigma y)}{\sqrt{n}}.$$

We will also use, later,

$$S_{yy} = \Sigma(y - \bar{y})^2 = \Sigma y^2 - \frac{(\Sigma y)^2}{\sqrt{n}}$$

Thus a and b can be calculated and the straight line drawn on the scatter diagram.

The quantity a (the sample estimate of α) is called the intercept because it is the value of y when the line crosses the y axis (i.e. since $y = a + bx$, $y = a$ when $x = 0$).

The quantity b (the sample estimate of β) is called the estimated regression coefficient and is very important because it measures the average increase in y per unit increase in x, i.e. b is the estimated slope of the line.

The concept of correlation arises in attempting to measure the association which exists between quantitative variables. The degrees and kinds of correlation are best illustrated diagrammatically in the case of two variables conventionally denoted by x and y.

Figure 10.2 shows a perfect linear relation between x and y in which y increases as x does and vice versa. This situation is an ideal one, but close approximations to it occur in some experiments in the physical sciences. It rarely, if ever, occurs in biological work.

The situation in Fig. 10.3 is similar to that in Fig. 10.2 but, in this case, as one variable increases the other decreases. We say that Fig. 10.2 shows perfect positive correlation and Fig. 10.3 shows perfect negative correlation. This is again an ideal case occurring in the same restricted situations as in Fig. 10.2.

Figure 10.4 with Figures 10.5 and 10.6 shows the type of association which is usually encountered in practice. In Fig. 10.4 there is a tendency for one variable to increase as the other

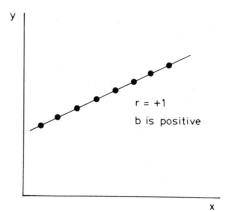

Fig. 10.2 Perfect positive correlation.

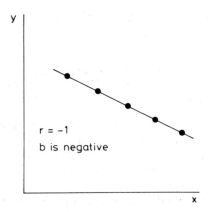

Fig. 10.3 Perfect negative correlation.

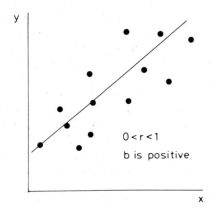

Fig. 10.4 Some degree of positive correlation.

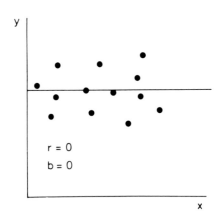

Fig. 10.6 No association between y and x.

does, but there is no certainty about the increase. All we can say is that the average value of y for a given value of x tends to increase as x increases, and vice versa. There is some degree of positive correlation.

Figure 10.5 shows the same sort of situation as Fig. 10.4, but the tendency here is for one variable to decrease as the other increases. There is some degree of negative correlation and the average value of y for a given value of x decreases as x increases.

Figure 10.6 shows the situation where there is no association at all. As x increases there is no tendency for the average value of y to increase or decrease, i.e. neither variable sheds any light on the behaviour of the other, as it does in Figures 10.2–10.5.

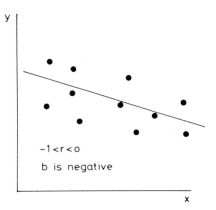

Fig. 10.5 Some degree of negative correlation.

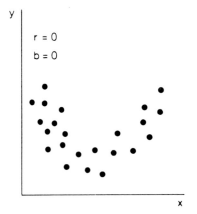

Fig. 10.7 No linear association between x and y.

Figure 10.7 shows a fairly strong association, but the relationship between x and y is non-linear. This situation is important when we have to interpret zero values of the correlation coefficient, shortly to be defined.

Supposing n pairs (x_1, y_1), (x_2, y_2) . . . (x_n, y_n) form a sample of size n. Then the (product-moment) correlation coefficient of x and y in the sample is denoted by r and defined by

$$r = \frac{S_{xy}}{\sqrt{S_{xx} \; S_{yy}}}$$

The properties of this coefficient are as follows (NB always take the positive square root in the denominator):

1. The sign of r is the same as the sign of S_{xy}. If S_{xy} is positive, so is r; if S_{xy} is negative, so is r.

2. r can never be less than -1 or greater than $+1$.

3. If $r = \pm 1$ then all the pairs lie on a line. This has a positive slope if $r = +1$ and a negative slope if $r = -1$. In other words, r $= +1$ corresponds to perfect positive correlation and $r = -1$ to perfect negative correlation.

4. If $r = 0$ this *can* mean that there is no association between the two variables but this is not necessarily the case. Given that $r = 0$ we can deduce nothing about the extent of association between x and y. This is shown by Fig. 10.6 and 10.7 above, where in both cases $r = 0$. We can say, however, that the association, if any, between x and y is not linear.

INTERPRETATION OF THE REGRESSION COEFFICIENT AND THE COEFFICIENT OF CORRELATION

The regression coefficient b is a measure of the average change in y for a unit change in x. If all the points on the scatter diagram lay on the regression line it would be reasonably certain that y would increase by exactly b for a unit increase in x. There would be an exact or perfect relationship between x and y. In practice this is not the case, and y can vary independently of x, so that two observations of the same x could produce differing values of y. Given any particular value of x, however, the *expected* value of y can be calculated but, since factors other than x may affect y, the observed value of y cannot be predicted exactly.

Thus the regression equation expresses only the average relationship between x and y. It does not measure the closeness of the association between the two variables. When the points lie close to the regression line a strong association is implied, but if they are scattered widely about the line, the regression line will still show the average relationship between the two variables, but the association is weaker.

The coefficient of correlation is a measure of the closeness of association between the two variables.

11. Physics

DIAGNOSTIC ULTRASOUND

Very high-frequency sound, or ultrasound, is useful in diagnosis because it can be directed and will penetrate the body like X-rays but it does not cause ionisation at the energy levels used. Frequencies are in the range of 1–10 MHz, the most common being around 3 MHz, about 200 times the highest frequency the average adult can hear. Sound waves cause particles of the medium through which they are travelling to move a minute distance back and forth along the direction of their path. Such waves are called longitudinal

to indicate the direction of displacement of the particles supporting the wave.

The power to produce these waves is generated electrically and the device that transforms it into sound power is called a transducer. A common form of transducer uses a thin slice of piezoelectric ceramic or quartz. These materials alter their thickness according to the voltage (V) applied between their faces. The change in thickness is small, only a few micrometres in the highest-powered machines, producing waves with displacements of about 1 nm which travel through tissues at about 1540 m/s (Fig. 11.1).

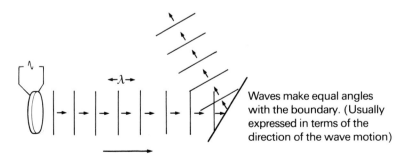

Waves make equal angles with the boundary. (Usually expressed in terms of the direction of the wave motion)

Wave crests move at about 1540 m/sec in tissue

$$\lambda = \text{distance between crests} = \frac{1540}{\text{Ultrasonic frequency}}$$

Fig. 11.1 Ultrasound generation and reflection.

Intensity

Intensity describes how much energy is passing through a certain cross-sectional area, usually 1 cm^2. It is usually defined in watts per square centimetre (W/cm^2).

Characteristic impedance and reflections

The characteristic impedance of a material describes how it resists being moved in response to a given sound pressure wave. For soft tissues it is roughly proportional to tissue density. When ultrasound encounters a boundary between tissues of different impedances, the mismatch of movements prevents a proportion of the sound energy from being transferred. The rest is reflected and produces the echoes used in diagnostic ultrasound (Fig. 11.2). If the sound meets the boundary at an angle it will be reflected at the same angle, provided the reflecting surface is large compared with the sound wavelength.

Near the edge of the reflector the local sound pressure pushes particles sideways, rounding off the edge of the reflected wave (Fig. 11.3A) at the centre of the reflector pressure balances so the reflected wave is flat. If the reflector is reduced in size, as it approaches half a wavelength the flat portion disappears and the reflection spreads in all directions, spherically (Fig. 11.3B). This form of reflection is known as scattering, since the direction of the reflected sound energy bears no relation to the direction of the incident wave.

Absorption

Ultrasound waves lose energy to the tissue by several mechanisms, viscous, relaxation and thermodynamic losses for instance. Viscous losses are increased in non-homogeneous fluids, whose acoustic impedance varies on a microscopic scale. Relaxation mechanisms arise when at one stage of the sound cycle associated ions become separated and then require a certain specific minimum time to reassociate. Relaxation mechanisms have characteristic variations with frequency which may depend on the chemical state of the tissue. Thermodynamic losses occur because, as the tissue is compressed by the sonic pressure, its temperature rises slightly. Nearby there is another region where the temperature has been reduced by decompression. Any thermal leakage between the two regions is energy lost to the sound wave. In soft tissues at diagnostic frequencies, thermodynamic losses are small compared with viscous and relaxation losses.

Diffraction

The ideal ultrasonic beam for diagnostic purposes would be needle-thin to give the finest detail. Unfortunately, this is not possible because of diffraction. A point source transducer would produce spherical waves similar to a point scatterer. Wider transducer faces produce flatter wave-fronts but

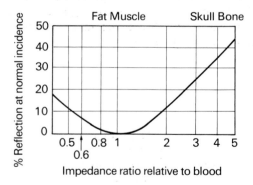

Fig. 11.2 Percentage reflection caused by interfaces of various impedance ratios.

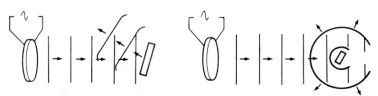

Fig. 11.3 A Reflection. B Scattering.

off-axis waves created at one part of the face may cancel or reinforce those from another. This results in sound being emitted at unwanted angles known as side lobes. It is highly desirable to suppress side lobes and make the angle θ at which the first minima occurs (defining the main lobe) as narrow as possible. For a circular transducer this occurs at an angle

$$\sin^{-1}\theta = \frac{1.22\lambda}{d}$$

where d is its diameter.

Focusing

It is possible to shape the transducer face, fit an acoustic lens, or provide special electronic drive, and thus generate a concave wave, directed to a point. Diffraction effects still limit the effectiveness of this technique, but nevertheless in the region of this focal point the beam is typically half to a third of that from a flat transducer of the same dimensions, improving lateral resolution and raising the echo strength from the desired target (Fig. 11.4).

Ultrasound reception

Just as applying a voltage between the faces of a slice of piezoelectric material produces a press-ure, so pressure on its faces produces a voltage. A slice exposed to the returning ultrasonic echoes produces a corresponding electrical signal. The directional properties of a transducer used as a receiver are usually the same as those used as a transmitter.

The Doppler effect

It is well known that as a police car or fire engine passes, the note of its siren appears to drop. The same effect occurs if sound is reflected off a moving object. If the object is approaching, each sound wave has a shorter distance to travel than the one preceding it. A succession of such waves is received at a higher frequency than the frequency at which it was transmitted. If the reflector moves away from the transducer the delay will increase and the frequency decreases. Mixing the transmitted signal and the echo can produce a new electrical signal at the difference frequency, representing the velocity of the reflector. Doppler systems therefore detect movement rather than distance, and since the difference frequencies are in the audible range they may be fed to a loudspeaker directly for simple instruments.

By suitable filtering to select significant sounds, trigger signals for heart rate meters or flow rate indicators, can be obtained.

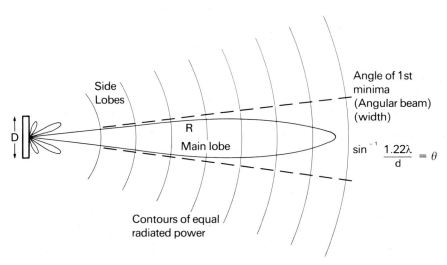

Fig. 11.4 Polar plot of radiated power vector **R** at angle d from a circular transducer of diameter D.

RADIOACTIVITY AND X-RAYS

The term radioactivity refers to occurrences in the nuclei of atoms. The nucleus is the positively charged centre round which the negatively charged electrons of the atom circulate in orbits up to 10 000 times the nuclear diameter. There is continual exchange of energy between particles constituting the nucleus and in some atoms it is possible for sufficient energy to be acquired by a particle to allow it to escape (Fig. 11.5). Protons (carrying one positive charge) or neutrons (uncharged) may leave singly or in a two-plus-two group which is then known as an α particle. Other particles are electrons (called β particles), electrons with positive charges (called positrons) and miscellaneous others such as neutrinos and mesons, which are not of primary importance in medicine yet. Table 11.1 shows some of the radioactive sub-

Table 11.1 Principle parameters of some isotopes associated with medicine

Name	Symbol	Half-life	Radiation energy (MeV)[a] Electromagnetic (γ or X-rays)	Particle (β)
Caesium-137	^{137}Cs	30 years	0.662	0.51[b]
Carbon-14	^{14}C	5760 years		0.155
Cobalt-60	^{60}Co	5.26 years	1.17	0.31[b]
			1.33	0.96
Gold-198	^{198}Au	2.7 d	0.412	
Iodine-125	^{125}I	60 d	0.027	0.61
Iodine-131	^{131}I	8 d	0.36	1.71
Phosphorus-32	^{32}P	14 d		0.167
Sulphur-35	^{35}S	87 d		
Technetium-99m	^{99}Tc^{m}	6 h	0.14	0.018
Tritium (hydrogen-3)	^{3}H	12.3 years		

[a] 1 Mev = 1.6×10^{-19} J.
[b] This form of radiation is not utilised for medical purposes.

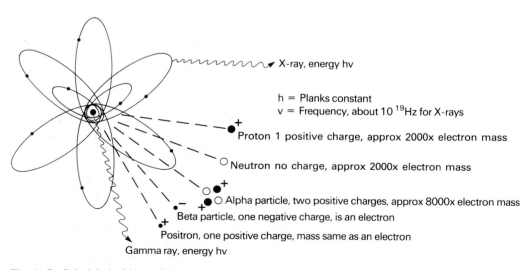

h = Planks constant
v = Frequency, about 10^{19}Hz for X-rays

X-ray, energy hv
Proton 1 positive charge, approx 2000x electron mass
Neutron no charge, approx 2000x electron mass
Alpha particle, two positive charges, approx 8000x electron mass
Beta particle, one negative charge, is an electron
Positron, one positive charge, mass same as an electron
Gamma ray, energy hv

Fig. 11.5 Principle ionising radiations.

stances that do have medical applications and the way in which energy is liberated.

The energy carried away from the nucleus by any particle is limited by wave mechanics to discrete values, and the nucleus may then be left with a surplus energy above its next lowest stable level. The surplus may then be carried away by a burst (quantum) of γ radiation. Since the energy of a γ quantum is proportional to its frequency, any quantity of energy can be carried by an appropriate frequency.

X-rays are also electromagnetic radiation and differ from γ rays only in their origin. They are generated by the circulating electrons of the atom instead of its nucleus.

Ionisation and excitation

Ionisation was the route by which radioactivity was discovered and by which it is usually measured. Excitations may be considered imperfect ionisations, in which sufficient energy is imparted to outer electrons of atoms to put them into orbits of higher energy than usual, but insufficient for them to escape from their parent nucleus.

The biological effects of radiation are due to both phenomena. Both lead to the production of new chemical species inside the cell, some of which lead in turn, to further chains of damaging chemical reaction. DNA disruption is the most critical mode for cell killing but other fatal or disabling reactions, such as impairment of membrane function leading to osmotic changes, release of lysosome contents, mitochondrial damage are also important.

Ionisation is usually considered the dominant effect and as it produces readily detected physical results it is used as a marker or scalar of radiation activity. The ions referred to are those produced by each particle not the particles themselves. An ejected proton, for instance, is travelling in a sea of electrons and exerting an attractive force on them as it passes through the orbital shells of various atoms. If the force is large enough and exerted for long enough an electron may be dragged out of orbit round its parent nucleus (Fig. 11.6a). This produces two new ions, positive and negative. It also slows the proton down slightly as it

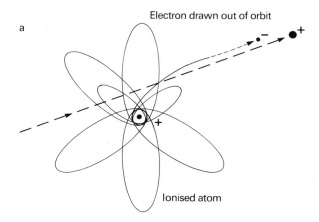

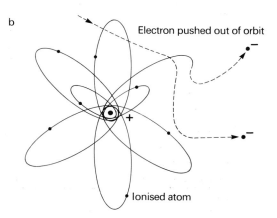

Fig. 11.6 Ion pair production.

gives up energy to the electron, but only slightly because its mass is some 2000 times that of the electron. The proton will continue, ploughing a trail of ion pairs as it goes.

As it gradually loses energy it spends longer in each atom through which it passes and so has greater effect on its electrons, increasing its ionisation efficiency. It eventually captures an electron and becomes a neutral hydrogen atom. Spontaneous radioactivity decay favours the emission of a group of two protons and two neutrons as the heavy positive component (α particle). Having twice the charge and four times the mass of a proton, it is even more efficient at ionisation. A typical α particle moving through air will leave about 25 000 ion pairs per centimetre over most of its 7 cm path length rising to 50 000 in the last centimetre. All nuclear particles have definite air path lengths, although it will be tortuous and so effectively reduced in the case of the lighter and so more easily deflected β and positron particles (Fig. 11.6b).

The electromagnetic X- and γ rays can also transfer energy to electrons in the material through which they pass, in ways that depend on the frequency of the ray. These mechanisms are pair production, Compton scattering and photoelectric absorption, in order of descending ray frequency and energy. The electrons then escape from their parent atoms and cause the ionisation observed, like β particles. The X- or γ ray continues travelling but its frequency is reduced, representing the loss of energy. Unlike the particles, its velocity is unchanged, the probability of interaction with another electron is largely unaltered, and so it dies away exponentially with distance rather than having a well-defined range. It is common to use the thickness of a material that will reduce this ionisation to half its initial value as a measure of the penetrating power of X- or γ rays, corresponding to range in α or β particles. This is known as the half-value layer, HVL.

Quantity of radioactive material

The quantity of radioactive material can be determined chemically, but one usually needs to know how many atoms will disintegrate per second. This is known as activity and is reported in curies (1 Ci is 3.7×10^{10} transformations per second) or in becquerels (1 Bq is 1 transformation per second).

Any such measurement is only true at the moment it is made since the proportion left capable of transforming is continually decreasing. A second parameter, half-life defines the rate at which this is happening as the time required for half the initial quantity to have completed its transformation.

To determine these factors it is only necessary to detect when transformations occur. To determine the effect these disintegrations are having requires measurement of the magnitude of the ionisation caused by the radiation emitted.

Radiation exposure and dose

Measurement of exposure or beam intensity was initially done by collecting and measuring the charged particles produced in 1 g of air interposed in the beam; 1.61×10^{12} ion pairs was defined as 1 roentgen (R). This was later redefined in terms of energy (86.9 erg/g).

When measurement was required in biological situations it was found that the rate of absorption in body tissues varied with the potential used to generate X-rays. A unit to indicate how much energy was actually being absorbed was required and this was the rad. It was defined as the absorbed dose of radiation which imparts 0.01 J/kg of body tissue. When SI units were introduced the 0.01 factor was dropped and the unit 1 J/kg defined as the gray (Gy).

However, the particulate forms of radiation with their various forms of high-density ionisations were being used for their biological effects and it was logical to define a further term to express the relative effectiveness of the way in which the ionisation was delivered. A multiplying factor, defined as Q is used; the quality of Q has the value 1 for X-, γ and β radiation, but 10 for α particles because of the high density of ions along their tracks. For radiation safety purposes it is combined with the rad in the product $Q.rad$ which is defined as the rem (radiation equivalent man). With the introduction of SI units the sievert (Sv), defined as $Q.Gy$, was introduced to replace the rem.

MAGNETIC RESONANCE IMAGING (MRI)

This method does *not* produce ionisation and is called magnetic resonance imaging (MRI) rather than the older Nuclear Magnetic Resonance which had negative associations in patients minds. No beams of light or sound are produced, instead the nuclei of certain atoms in the patient are induced to report their presence and condition by absorbing or sending out radio waves.

The term resonance is borrowed from the study of sound. A guitar string resonates when it continues making a sound after it has been plucked. It is tuned by altering its tension. Just as the string vibrates at a frequency that depends on its nature and the applied tension, so spinning nuclei produce or absorb radio waves at a frequency that depends on their nature and the steady magnetic field they are in. This frequency is known as the Larmor frequency. By analogy this response of nuclei to radio waves, which can be tuned by varying the surrounding magnetic field, is called magnetic resonance.

The converse effect, energy absorption at resonance, can be demonstrated by whistling into a piano while depressing its sustaining pedal. When the whistle ceases, a similar sound is heard coming from the piano. An analogous situation can be set up by supporting a tissue sample in a powerful, steady and very uniform magnetic field to tune the nuclei to the frequency to be absorbed. The whistle is then replaced by a rapidly alternating magnetic field, transverse to the steady main field, referred to as the radio frequency (RF) field. MR spectroscopy generally measures the energy absorbed from the RF field as its frequency is slowly changed. Since different nuclei have different resonant frequencies for the same main magnetic field, their presence and abundance can be determined from the degree of absorption and the frequencies at which they occur, observed during each frequency sweep. This can be plotted to give a series of spectral lines similar to those in optical spectrometry. More importantly, the small magnetic fields each nucleus generates, and the screening effects the electron clouds surrounding molecules exert, modify the main magnetic field. This causes small variations of resonant frequency to be superimposed on these lines, shifting and splitting them. Thus not only can the abundance of the various nuclear species be observed, but also changes in their chemical environment. For example tuning into the phosphorus in muscle enables the availability of ATP during repeated contractions to be followed.

While MR spectroscopy normally measures the energy absorbed from the RF field as it happens, MRI usually depends on observing the signal still being retransmitted by the nuclei some time following a short burst or bursts of the RF field. The signal from individual nuclei is too small to be detected; they have to be synchronised by short bursts of the transverse field, referred to as RF pulses. Hydrogen (a single proton) is the usual nucleus selected for imaging applications, as it is by far the most abundant. In imaging, unlike spectroscopy, the main magnetic field is deliberately made non-uniform to vary the tuning of the protons in different parts of the patient. For instance, suppose the field is made high on one side of the patient and low on the other. Then only one vertical plane in the patient will contain any protons tuned to the same frequency as the RF pulse. If we tune in subsequently with a radio receiver and pick up a signal we will know that it must have come from that plane.

Suppose that during this period the magnetic field is made high at the head end of the patient and low at the feet end. Although the nuclei in the original plane may all still be transmitting, only those in a new plane, orthogonal to the first, will still be tuned to the right frequency to be picked up by the receiver. If there is some signal it must be coming from where these two planes cross, a line through the patient. There are other more subtle ways in which further data can be built into the signal to identify where along the line individual tissue elements are retransmitting. The intensity of the signal is then used to modulate the brightness of a line on a VDU in a position on the screen representing the position of the line in the patient. Increasingly complex pulse sequences have been devised which allow simultaneous reading of the signal from many lines at once and this reduces the time required to scan the patient.

For imaging, some of the spectral detail available in spectroscopy is sacrificed in order to maximise tissue contrast and detail in the image. However, this is partly compensated for by using the dynamic behaviour of the excited protons. Returning to our earlier analogy, if after whistling into the piano the sustaining pedal is released the vibrational energy of the strings is rapidly removed by the felt dampers, and the sound decays quickly. A corresponding effect results from the interaction of nuclei and their surroundings, known as the lattice. The decay of energy is represented by the spin-lattice relaxation time (T_1), which is generally long in liquids and short in structured tissues. Tissues that have similar concentrations of protons may give similar signal strengths soon after excitation by the RF pulse, but if a delay is allowed before measurement large differences in the remaining strength may develop.

Within tissues T_1 may be as short as 0.1 seconds. Fluid-filled cysts have a long T_1, whereas clotted blood and fibrous tissue generally have a short T_1. The longer T_1 of normal blood is generally masked by the fact that it has moved out of the field of view before measurement can be made. Blood vessels usually appear black on the image. The increased T_1 seen in tumours relative to the surrounding tissue is attributed to the increased free water present. Adjustment of measuring delay may increase the contrast between neighbouring tissues of identical proton density but differing internal structure.

Once the RF pulse ceases, some nuclei will resonate slightly faster than average as their local magnetic fields add to the main field and some slower as the local magnetic field subtracts. Then, although there is no energy loss, the increasing lack of synchronisation renders the signal inaccessible to the radio receiver. This is known as spin–spin relaxation, and the time constant describing it is known as T_2. By manipulation of successive RF pulses those nuclei that were fast can be made slow and vice versa. After a delay this results in recovery of synchronisation and the signal reappears. By analogy with sound this is described as a spin-echo. It is extensively used to recover the signal after complicated tissue-selective pulse sequence techniques. By altering the repetition rate of the complete cycle, further mixing of multiple RF pulses, and the timing of the final observation relative to them, the method can be made highly selective to the chemical state of observed tissues with differing T_1, T_2 or T_1/T_2 ratios.

Appendix

THE PRIMARY EXAMINATION OF THE MEMBERSHIP OF THE ROYAL COLLEGE OF OBSTETRICIANS AND GYNAECOLOGISTS
— THE MCQ EXAMINATION

The MCQ examination consists of two papers of 60 multiple choice questions each. It may be taken in London or several other centres in the world, being held twice a year. You can improve your chances by learning and this volume will contain most of the knowledge you will need for the examination but it is recommended that you attend a course to prepare for the examination. The Royal College of Obstetricians and Gynaecologists (27 Sussex Place, Regent's Park, London NW1 4RG) will advise you about the course nearest to you. You should also get from the College a syllabus for the examination which must be studied before sitting for the examination.

You can be helped further by answering questions in the MCQ format. We include a few simple examples but recommend you should try many more of these. Several books of questions in basic science and in obstetrics and gynaecology are on the market. Start with one and do six complete questions a day, only looking at the answers after you have done all you can do in the six questions.

In a multiple-choice question paper, it is probably wise to go through the full paper first, answering those questions which you are sure you know the answers, taking the first 45 minutes or so. By this time you will have answered about half of the questions. Go through the unanswered questions a second time, dealing with those you can logically work out, thus taking another 45 minutes. Do not be disappointed if you are still left with a few questions to which you neither know the facts nor can work out the answers. Do not guess at this stage, for the MRCOG Part I examination has a positive and negative marking system. Hence, although you gain one mark for each correct answer you can also lose a mark for an incorrect one. It is better to leave the mark sheet blank if you do not know or cannot work out an answer so that you will not lose any marks.

MULTIPLE CHOICE QUESTIONS

1. In the metabolism of fats:
   A Triglyceride fats are absorbed into the circulation unchanged
   B Fatty acids are broken down one carbon atom at a time
   C Fatty acids are converted to esters of CoA and oxidised from the carboxyl end
   D The end-product of fatty acid metabolism is lactate
   E Increased dietary fat is always converted directly to depot fat.

2. Plasma glucose is:
   A Directly utilised for energy
   B Phosphorylated before it can be converted into energy
   C Broken down to glycogen
   D Subject to β-oxidation
   E Channelled into the glycolytic pathway.

3. The glycolytic pathway:
   A Involves the synthesis of glycogen
   B Requires oxygen
   C Oxidises sugars to CO_2 and H_2O
   D Is the main energy-producing process of carbohydrate metabolism
   E Can lead to the production of lactate.

4. The hormone insulin is:
   A Secreted by the α cells of the islets of Langerhans
   B Promotes the uptake of glucose by muscle cells
   C Responsible for raising blood glucose concentrations
   D Deficient in diabetes (type 1)
   E Responsible for ketosis.

5. Under aerobic conditions the tricarboxylic acid cycle:
   A Is the major source of CO_2
   B Produces four atoms of hydrogen
   C Oxidises acetyl-CoA
   D Is linked to oxidative phosphorylation
   E Is a source of GTP.

Answers
Cover these up while you try the five questions
opposite.
T = true; F = false.

1. **A**   F
   B   F
   C   T
   D   F
   E   F
2. **A**   T
   B   T
   C   F
   D   F
   E   T

3. **A**   F
   B   F
   C   F
   D   F
   E   T
4. **A**   F
   B   T
   C   F
   D   T
   E   F
5. **A**   T
   B   F
   C   T
   D   T
   E   T